Gynecologic Cytopathology

Gynecologic Cytopathology

Editors

THOMAS A. BONFIGLIO, MD
Professor and Chair
Pathologist-in-Chief
Department of Pathology and Laboratory Medicine
University of Rochester
Rochester, New York

YENER S. EROZAN, MD
Professor, Department of Pathology
Division of Cytopathology
The Johns Hopkins University
Baltimore, Maryland

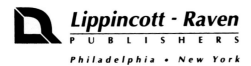

Lippincott - Raven
PUBLISHERS

Philadelphia • New York

Acquisitions Editor: Vickie Thaw
Developmental Editor: Melissa James
Production Editor: Patricia Connelly
Production Manager: Caren Erlichman
Production Coordinator: MaryClare Malady
Design Coordinator: Doug Smock
Indexer: Julia Figures
Compositor: Tapsco
Printer: Mandarin
Printed in Hong Kong

Library of Congress Cataloging-in-Publication Data

Gynecologic cytopathology/editors, Thomas A. Bonfiglio, Yener S. Erozan.
    p. cm.
    Includes bibliographical references and index.
    ISBN 0-397-51501-4
    1. Generative organs, Female—Cytopathology.   2. Generative organs,
Female—Diseases—Cytodiagnosis.   I. Bonfiglio, Thomas A. II. Erozan,
Yener S.
    [DNLM: 1. Genital Diseases, Female—pathology. 2. Cytodiagnosis.
WP 140 G9966 1997]
RG107.G96   1997
618.1′07—dc20
DNLM/DLC
for Library of Congress   96-15640
                                              CIP

9 8 7 6 5 4 3 2 1

To our wives Mary and Brenda

Contributors

Karen M. Atkison, CT (ASCP), M.P.A., *Assistant Professor, Chief Cytotechnologist, Department of Pathology and Laboratory Medicine, University of Rochester Medical Center, 601 Elmwood Avenue, Rochester, NY 14642*

Thomas A. Bonfiglio, M.D., *Professor and Chair, Department of Pathology and Laboratory Medicine, University of Rochester Medical Center, 601 Elmwood Avenue, Rochester, NY 14642*

Parvin Ganjei, M.D., *Professor of Pathology, University of Miami School of Medicine, Department of Cytopathology, Room 2147, 1611 Northwest 12th Avenue, Miami, FL 33136*

Mehrdad Nadji, M.D., *Professor of Pathology, University of Miami School of Medicine, Department of Cytopathology, Room 2147, 1611 Northwest 12th Avenue, Miami, FL 33136*

Mark H. Stoler, M.D., *Associate Professor of Pathology, University of Virginia Medical School, Jefferson Parkway, Old Medical School, Charlottesville, VA 22903*

David C. Wilbur, M.D., *Associate Professor of Pathology and Laboratory Medicine, Department of Pathology and Laboratory Medicine, University of Rochester Medical Center, 601 Elmwood Avenue, Rochester, NY 14642*

Introduction

There are many monographs, specialized books, and texts currently available in the field of diagnostic cytopathology. Even so, we feel there is a need and a place for a new set of publications in the field. Using the traditional cytologic approaches of The University of Rochester and The Johns Hopkins Laboratories, our vision is to publish a series of text-atlases that emphasizes current diagnostic criteria, uses modern terminology, and looks to the future of this rapidly evolving subspecialty of pathology.

Because the emphasis is on useful and practical diagnostic criteria, we devised a format that uses many more illustrations than most standard texts. Although descriptive text is essential, the available vocabulary is limited; more figures are necessary to adequately detail the many possible and variable nuances of cytologic features that are often seen within a single diagnostic category. This design will, we hope, provide the reader with both a better appreciation of the morphologic features that the authors discuss and a useful reference to help solve routine differential diagnostic problems encountered in the typical cytopathology practice.

Thomas A. Bonfiglio, MD
Yener S. Erozan, MD

Preface

This book is intended primarily for practicing pathologists, pathology residents, cytotechnologists, and gynecologists interested in the cytologic method. Cytotechnology students should find it a useful text for their education. It is meant to be a practical yet comprehensive guide to the field of gynecologic cytopathology with an emphasis on illustrating and discussing the spectrum of diagnostic entities encountered in daily practice. Although many of the important articles in the recent and older literature are referred to, there was no attempt to present an all-inclusive review of the literature. Works that the authors felt to be of most importance in establishing cytologic diagnostic criteria or contributing otherwise to our understanding of the cytologic manifestations of gynecologic disease are listed. In addition, other important references related to the field are mentioned.

The success of cytologic screening programs depends not only on an understanding of the cytologic manifestations of premalignant and malignant disease processes and the benign conditions with which they can be confused, but also on a thorough understanding of all aspects of the cytologic method, including sample collection and preparation. Therefore, these topics as well as a discussion of laboratory quality assurance and quality control and proper communication of test results are also addressed in this book. The mainstay of gynecologic cytology is the cervical/vaginal smear and the majority of this work is directed to this type of specimen. Because a through understanding of the process of carcinogenisis in the cervix is essential to the modern practice of gynecologic cytopathology, a thorough review of this topic, including the role of human papillomavirus is included.

Fine-needle aspiration has also become an important aspect of cytopathology practice and is a useful tool for the evaluation of intra-abdominal and pelvic gynecologic neoplasms. Therefore, chapters dedicated to a consideration of this area are included. Because new technologies are rapidly emerging that will have a significant impact on this field, a section is also presented that deals with these exciting advances. Included here is not only an authoritative consideration of new sample preparation instruments but also, for the first time in any standard reference, numerous illustrations of Papanicolaou smears prepared by the new thin-layer technologies are presented and compared with examples of the same cases prepared by standard techniques. Finally, the new computer-based instruments that have recently been approved by the Federal Drug Administration as quality assurance aids for Papanicolaou smear screening and that also offer the potential for at least partial automation of the screening process itself are discussed.

Contents

Gynecologic Cytopathology

Gynecologic Cytopathology. Edited by
Thomas A. Bonfiglio and Yener S. Erozan.
Lippincott–Raven Publishers, Philadelphia, © 1997.

CHAPTER 1

Gynecologic Cytology: Historic Considerations and Current Perspectives

Thomas A. Bonfiglio

HISTORIC CONSIDERATIONS

Cytopathology is a relatively new field, usually considered to have begun with the work of George Nicolas Papanicolaou and a Romanian pathologist named Aurel Babes about 60 years ago. Their findings promoted new interest in the cell and the eventual appreciation of the ability to detect cancer at the level of the individual cell. Observations on the cytology of cancer had been made since the early 19th century. However, these were viewed as nothing more than curiosities or interesting footnotes in the medical literature. Even Papanicolaou's original paper of 1928[1] on the detection of malignant cells in vaginal smears from a patient with cervical cancer aroused little enthusiasm among the establishment. In spite of this paper and a publication by Babes in 1927[2] describing the diagnosis of cervical cancer based on a cervical smear, little was made of this technique until the early 1940s, when a paper and monograph by Papanicolaou and Traut appeared. From that point on, the rest of the story is well known. Pathologists were slow to accept the new technology; it was gynecologists who first adopted it. Making diagnoses by examining cells initially was regarded by most pathologists as impossible, or at best unnecessary, and certainly without a future. However, a few early visionaries among pathologists, including some of the most famous names in the field, saw the potential value of the technique. They pursued it scientifically and clinically, establishing its value through clinical studies and developing its scientific framework through clinical and laboratory experiments. Cytology gained wide acceptance, grew exponentially, and become well established as a discipline.

DIAGNOSTIC TERMINOLOGY

In the beginning, cytology and the cytologic method were not considered diagnostic tools in any sense of the word. There was great debate as to whether the technique could predict the presence of cancer with any degree of accuracy. The biology of cervical cancer was not well understood and the precursor lesions to invasive cancer were not well appreciated. Papanicolaou developed a system that he used in reporting the results of his interpretation of the vaginal cell smears that he examined. This system eventually included five "classes," with class 1 representing a smear with no evidence of cancer and higher classes representing increasing levels of concern for the possible presence of malignancy. Papanicolaou himself apparently seldom used the "class 5" designation. The reports using these class systems did not attain the level of a medical diagnostic consultation, and this contributed in part to the early concern of pathologists about the appropriate place for this test in the laboratory.[3]

The Papanicolaou class system underwent many minor modifications, additions, and enhancements over the years. Unfortunately, many laboratories used the same numbers for different findings. There was no consensus regarding the criteria for including a smear in one class versus another, or regarding the meaning of the classes in relation to the clinical situation or histopathologic findings. In spite of these limitations, the system was used widely until recent times, largely because clinicians and pathologists often claimed to "know" exactly what a certain Papanicolaou classification meant in their

T. A. Bonfiglio: Department of Pathology and Laboratory Medicine, University of Rochester Medical Center, Rochester, New York 14642.

laboratory or practice, and because the system did identify, at least to some extent, those patients who required further investigation.

Although the Papanicolaou system was widely used, particularly in the early years, from the beginning, some pathologists advocated the use of more scientifically accurate terminology that reflected the histologic lesions from which the abnormal cells were derived. Reagan and Patten were early advocates of the now classic dysplasia or carcinoma in situ terminology for reporting Papanicolaou smears. This system was derived from a study of the histology of precursor lesions of cervical squamous cell carcinoma and reflected an attempt to make correlations between the cytologic findings on Papanicolaou smears and those histologic changes.[4-7] This terminology was adopted quickly by most pathologists for reporting biopsy results and by many for relating cytologic findings. Others added this terminology to the Papanicolaou class number on cytology reports, a change that represented an improvement over the simple numeric report.

However, it gradually became clear that the Papanicolaou classification, particularly if used alone, was not acceptable as a modern method of reporting results because of its numerous idiosyncratic modifications, its lack of provision for the diagnosis of noncancerous processes, its inability to reflect current concepts of cervical and vaginal neoplasia, and its lack of equivalent histopathologic terminology.[8]

In the early 1970s, Richart introduced the term *cervical intraepithelial neoplasia* (CIN) to describe the precursor lesions of squamous cell carcinoma of the cervix.[9] This new terminology reflected the widely held concept that cervical cancer developed as a continuum, and that the developing precursors would be classified better as CIN 1, 2, or 3 as they progressed along the continuum. These grades correlated roughly with mild dysplasia (CIN 1), moderate dysplasia (CIN 2), and severe dysplasia or carcinoma in situ (CIN 3). The new terminology did avoid the problems with the older system, which suggested to some that carcinoma in situ was a biologically different disease than severe dysplasia. However, it altered the way in which the process of carcinogenesis in the uterine cervix was viewed. By labeling the entire spectrum of findings as neoplastic, it suggested that every patient with any degree of intraepithelial abnormality had a progressive process and was at high risk for the development of carcinoma. As the role of the human papillomavirus began to be understood in the late 1970s and 1980s, this concept was called into question.

Reporting the results of an examination appropriately to the referring physician is a vital aspect of the practice of cytopathology. The terminology used must convey the message as clearly and precisely as possible within the limitations of the technique. Unfortunately, various methods of reporting have used diverse terminology that sometimes resulted in confusion about the clinical significance of reports.

THE BETHESDA SYSTEM

By the late 1980s, the need for a new, universal terminology system for reporting Papanicolaou smears that once and for all could eliminate the long outdated Papanicolaou classification and could avoid the problems with the other competing terminological systems then utilized became manifest. The ideal was a consistent, reproducible, easily used system that would take into account the current understanding of the biology of cervical carcinogenesis, the role of the human papillomavirus in its development, the limitations inherent in the Papanicolaou smear as a diagnostic method, and the need to communicate clinically relevant information in a clear and concise manner. In December of 1988, the National Cancer Institute convened a workshop to address the issue. The Bethesda system for reporting cervical and vaginal cytologic diagnoses developed out of the deliberations and discussions associated with this conference. After initial experience with its use, the system was modified in 1991 at a second workshop held to evaluate its effect. Finally, a monograph was published in 1994 providing definitions, criteria, and explanatory notes regarding the terminology and specimen adequacy.[10] This brief work, which was the product of the Bethesda system criteria and editorial committees, included illustrations and descriptions and fostered more uniform use of the reporting system.

The Bethesda system terminology is outlined in Table 1-1 and compared with several other classification systems in Table 1-2. The Bethesda system contains both recommended terms for reporting the morphologic observations seen on examination of the Papanicolaou smear and a format for the report. The format for the report includes a statement regarding the adequacy of the specimen, an optional statement specifying the general categorization of the specimen, and the diagnostic statement.

In the Bethesda system, a practical approach is taken to reporting intraepithelial squamous lesions of the cervix that is consistent with current understanding of their biology. For example, squamous lesions are divided into low-grade and high-grade lesions. The low-grade lesions encompass mild dysplasia (CIN I) and lesser intraepithelial abnormalities that show diagnostic evidence of a human papillomavirus effect. The high-grade intraepithelial lesions include moderate dysplasia (CIN II) and severe dysplasia or carcinoma in situ (CIN III). The Bethesda system is a flexible terminology. The use of this system does not preclude the concomitant use of classic diagnostic terminology, and a report may include refer-

TABLE 1-1. *The Bethesda System*

ADEQUACY OF THE SPECIMEN

Satisfactory for evaluation
Satisfactory for evaluation but limited by . . .
   (specify reason)
Unsatisfactory for evaluation . . . (specify reason)

GENERAL CATEGORIZATION (OPTIONAL)

Within normal limits
Benign cellular changes: See descriptive diagnosis
Epithelial cell abnormality: See descriptive diagnosis

DESCRIPTIVE DIAGNOSES

BENIGN CELLULAR CHANGES

Infection
   Trichomonas vaginalis
   Fungal organisms morphologically consistent with
      Canidida species
   Predominance of coccobacilli consistent with shift in
      vaginal flora
   Bacteria morphologically consistent with *Actinomyces*
      species
   Cellular changes associated with herpes simplex virus
   Other*
Reactive Changes
   Reactive cellular changes associated with:
      Inflammation (includes typical repair)
      Atrophy with inflammation ("atrophic vaginitis")
      Radiation
      Intrauterine device
      Other

EPITHELIAL CELL ABNORMALITIES

Squamous Cell
   Atypical squamous cells of undetermined significance
      (qualify[†])
   Low-grade squamous intraepithelial lesion (LSIL)
      encompassing human papillomavirus* and mild
      dysplasia/CIN 1
   High-grade squamous intraepithelial lesion (HSIL)
      encompassing moderate and severe dysplasia, CIS/CIN
      2, and CIN 3
   Squamous cell carcinoma
Glandular Cell
   Endometrial cells, cytologically benign in a
      postmenopausal woman
   Atypical glandular cells of undetermined significance
      (qualify[†])
   Endocervical adenocarcinoma
   Endometrial adenocarcinoma
   Adenocarcinoma, nonspecific

OTHER MALIGNANT NEOPLASM (SPECIFY)

HORMONAL EVALUATION (APPLIES TO VAGINAL
SMEARS ONLY)

Hormonal pattern compatible with age and history
Hormonal pattern incompatible with age and history (specify)
Hormonal evaluation not possible because of . . . (specify)

---

* Cellular changes of human papillomavirus, previously termed koilocytosis, koilocytotic atypia, and condylomatous atypia, are included in the category of LSIL.
[†] Atypical squamous or glandular cells of undetermined significance should be qualified further, if possible, as to whether a reactive or neoplastic process is favored.
CIN, cervical intraepithelial neoplasia; *CIS,* carcinoma in situ.

ences to the grade of dysplasia or CIN and the comparable Bethesda term.

The sections of this book that deal with cervical and vaginal cytology expand on the definitions and criteria provided in the Bethesda system publication edited by Kurman and Solomon. Entities not specifically included in the Bethesda classification also are considered. The Bethesda system terminology generally is used in the discussions along with the traditional terms (dysplasia and carcinoma in situ), with appropriate references made to other terminology when necessary.

A consideration of specimen adequacy and a discussion of the criteria by which it should be judged are presented in Chapter 2. The morphologic criteria for the various diagnoses incorporated in the terminology are discussed in subsequent chapters, which are organized generally along the lines of the Bethesda classification.

ACCURACY OF CERVICAL CYTOLOGY

The cytologic technique as applied to screening for cervical neoplastic processes has improved the human condition significantly, particularly in the area of cancer control and prevention. Cytopathology is a success story in health care and has lived up to its initial promise. However, its success has led to a major problem. The enthusiasm for and extensive promotion of the cytologic method have resulted in unrealistic expectations regarding the accuracy of the technique in detecting uterine cancer and its precursors. The prevalent attitude among the lay public and many health care providers is that the Papanicolaou smear should identify the presence of disease in virtually 100% of the cases, and that failure to do so represents an egregious error and probably professional malpractice. The facts that no test is 100% accurate and that no biologic process is the same in any two individuals often are ignored in these situations.

Great strides have been made toward eliminating many of the correctable factors that diminish the accuracy of this technique. The Papanicolaou smear is much more reliable now than it was during the early years of its use. However, much remains to be done to improve quality in some laboratories. If all laboratories followed existing guidelines and regulations, and if those regulations were strictly enforced, further improvements would occur. This is crucial, and everyone in this field should strive to ensure that all laboratories meet established standards. However, even if the practice of cytopathology is nearly perfected and every woman in the country is screened yearly, the incidence of cervical cancer will not reach zero and false-negative Papanicolaou smears will still occur. Why? The reasons are actually many, but an important factor is that the Papinicolaou smear and those individuals screening them and inter-

TABLE 1-2. *A comparison of the Bethesda System with other Papanicolaou smear reporting terminology*

Bethesda	Classic	CIN	Pap
Within normal limits	Normal	Normal	Class I
Benign cellular changes	Inflammatory, reactive	Inflammatory, reactive	Class II
ASCUS	Atypical cells, squamous type	Atypia	? Class II–III
LSIL	HPV, KA, mild dysplasia	HPV, KA, CIN 1	? Class II–III
HSIL	Moderate, severe dysplasia/CIS	CIN2, CIN 3	? Class III–IV
Invasive carcinoma	Invasive carcinoma	Invasive carcinoma	Class V

CIN, cervical intraepithelial neoplasia; *Pap,* Papanicolaou; *ASCUS,* atypical squamous cells of undetermined significance; *LSIL,* low-grade intraepithelial lesion; *HSIL,* high-grade intraepithelial lesion; *HPV,* human papillomavirus; *KA,* koilocytotic atypia; *CIS,* carcinoma in situ.

preting them are not infallible and never will be. There is an irreducible rate of false-negative results. The exact rate is a matter of debate and depends in part on the way in which a false-negative result is defined, but even in the best laboratories, no less than 4% to 5% and perhaps as many as 10% of patients with epithelial lesions will have falsely negative test results. This has been documented repeatedly in numerous studies. Similar rates have been noted in relation to routine practice situations and in reports of the results of proficiency testing in which those being challenged would be expected to be performing at their best.[11–18]

The cause of false-negative results also has been studied. One well-recognized reason is failure to sample the abnormal area, resulting in the absence of abnormal cells on the slide, even after retrospective review. Another cause may be a problem in the slide preparation process; the abnormal area may have been sampled, but the abnormal cells were not transferred from the sampling device to the slide. This is a relatively newly elucidated method of failure that has been demonstrated in published studies.[19] In a study by Gay and colleagues, sampling failures were the most common cause of false-negative smear results (70%).[11] Other causes include laboratory errors by the cytotechnologist or pathologist, both screening errors (ie, the abnormal cells were not found) and interpretation errors (ie, the abnormal cells were found, but were misinterpreted as normal). In some studies, these causes account for a much larger proportion of the false-negative results than was reported in Gay's study.[20]

Despite its success in decreasing the incidence of cervical cancer over the past 50 years, the Papanicolaou smear is not, and should not be promoted as, an infallible test. Clinicians and patients should be adequately informed regarding the benefits and limitations of this procedure. The benefits of the Papanicolaou smear are well-known, but in the past, we have been reluctant to address its limitations. Interest in addressing the limitations of the technique is growing, however, because of the marked increase in litigation surrounding false-negative results. Some have suggested that all reports should include a disclaimer stating that there is a specified false-negative rate for Papanicolaou smears, even in the best laboratories. However, this may not prevent malpractice suits, and may allow low-quality laboratories to excuse their inadequate performance. Nevertheless, the idea should be considered seriously. It could be considered a matter of truth in advertising, but physicians and patients must be told exactly what the disclaimer means. It is important that patients not assume that the test is inaccurate and unnecessary. Both patients and clinicians would benefit from education regarding the benefits and limitations of the Papanicolaou smear in current practice.[21]

In addition to quality assurance standards, workload limits, and proficiency tests, other methods promise to improve screening for cervical cancer. New technologies are being evaluated to facilitate the process and improve the results[22] (see Chap. 11). Computer assistance with this labor-intensive process has been discussed for years, but the technology only now is becoming available. New preparation techniques are under development and have made more rapid progress. These methodologies have the potential to increase accuracy and decrease cost, improving women's health worldwide. When these technologies come into general use, they will help make accurate cancer screening services more readily available in parts of the world not previously well served.

However, new technology should be evaluated appropriately before it is embraced enthusiastically. Although the instrumentation now available and under development holds considerable promise for improving the efficacy and accuracy of cytology screening, its use needs to be fully evaluated in clinical practice situations.

More accurate methodologies may be available soon. Until that time, every effort must be made to improve the specificity and sensitivity of the Papanicolaou smear, with a clear understanding of its limitations. The interpretation of cervical and vaginal cytologic samples is dependent on a number of prerequisites, all of which must be present to ensure maximum accuracy in the detection and classification of significant abnormalities. Comprehensive sampling of the cervix, including the transformation zone, is necessary, as is appropriate slide preparation, fixation, and staining (see Chap. 2). In addition, a comprehensive laboratory quality assurance program must be in place (see Chap. 12). Finally, each laboratory should educate health care practitioners and the public regarding the advantages and limitations of the Papanicolaou smear in clinical practice.

REFERENCES

1. Papanicolaou GN. New cancer diagnosis. Proceedings Third Race Betterment Conference. Battle Creek: Race Betterment Foundation, 1928:528.
2. Babes A. Diagnostic du cancer du col uterin par les frottis. Presse Med 1927;36:451.
3. Weid GL. History of clinical cytology and outlook for its future. In Wied GL, Keebler CM, Koss LG, Patten SF, Rosenthal DL (eds). Compendium on diagnostic cytology, 7th ed. Chicago: Tutorials of Cytology, 1992:1.
4. Reagan JW, Hamonic MJ. Dysplasia of the uterine cervix. Ann NY Acad Sci 1956;63:1236.
5. Reagan JW, Hamonic MJ. The cellular pathology in carcinoma in situ. A cytohistopathological correlation. Cancer 1956;9:385.
6. Reagan JW, Patten SF. Analytical study of cellular changes in carcinoma in situ, squamous-cell cancer and adenocarcinoma of uterine cervix. Clin Obstet Gynecol 1961;4:1097.
7. Reagan JW, Patten SF. Dysplasia: a basic reaction to injury in the uterine cervix. Ann NY Acad Sci 1962;97:662.
8. National Cancer Institute Workshop Report. The 1988 Bethesda System for reporting cervical/vaginal cytologic diagnoses. JAMA 1989;262:931.
9. Richart RM. Cervical intraepithelial neoplasia. Pathol Annu 1973;7:301.
10. Kurman RJ, Solomon D. The Bethesda System for reporting cervical/vaginal cytologic diagnoses, definitions, criteria, and explanatory notes for terminology and specimen adequacy. New York: Springer-Verlag, 1994.
11. Gay D, Danos LM, Goellner JR. False negative results in cervical cytologic studies. Acta Cytol 1985;29:1043.
12. Van Der Graaf Y, Vooijs GP. False negative rate in cervical cytology. J Clin Pathol 1987;40:438.
13. Van Der Graaf Y, Vooijs GP, Gaillard HLJ, et al. Screening errors in cervical cytologic screening. Acta Cytol 1987;31:434.
14. Koss LG. Diagnostic accuracy in cervicovaginal cytology. Arch Pathol Lab Med 1993;117:1240.
15. Cecchini S, Palli D, Casini A. Cervical epithelial neoplasia III: an estimate of screening errors and optimal screening intervals. Acta Cytol 1985;29:329.
16. Collins DN, Patacsil DP. Proficiency testing in New York: analysis of a 14 year state program. Acta Cytol 1986;30:633.
17. Davey DD, Nielsen ML, Frable WJ, Rosenstock W, Lowell DM, Kramer BB. Improving accuracy in gynecologic cytology: results of the College of American Pathologists Interlaboratory Comparison Program in Cervicovaginal Cytology (PAP). Arch Pathol Lab Med 1993;117:1193.
18. Kreiger P, Naryshkin S. Random rescreening of cytology smears: a practical and effective component of quality assurance programs in both large and small cytology laboratories. (Guest Editorial) Acta Cytol 1994;38:291.
19. Hutchinson ML, Isenstein LM, Goodman A, et al. Homogeneous sampling accounts for the increased diagnostic accuracy using the ThinPrep Processor. Am J Clin Pathol 1994;101:215.
20. Pairwuti S. False negative Papanicolaou smears from women with cancerous and precancerous lesions of the uterine cervix. Acta Cytol 1991;35:40.
21. Koss LG. The Papanicolaou test for cervical cancer detection. A triumph and a tragedy. JAMA 1989;261:737.
22. Wilbur DC, Cibas ES, Merritt S, James LP, Berger BM, Bonfiglio TA. ThinPrep Processor. Clinical trials demonstrate an increased detection rate of abnormal cervical cytologic specimens. Am J Clin Pathol 1994;101:209.

Gynecologic Cytopathology. Edited by
Thomas A. Bonfiglio and Yener S. Erozan.
Lippincott–Raven Publishers, Philadelphia, © 1997.

CHAPTER **2**

Specimen Collection and Determinants of Adequacy

Karen M. Atkison

This text and atlas presents an approach to the study of cytologic material with an emphasis on morphologic classification. This approach does not merely recognize the presence of disease, but permits the recognition of a specific disease process, which then can be transmitted to the physician in the form of standard diagnostic terminology. This approach requires a detailed critical examination of the cytologic material on a slide and the environment within which these cells are found.

To achieve this, certain prerequisites are necessary. The first is a representative cellular sample. The second is adequate cell fixation and optimum staining. The general and specific features that must be considered in arriving at a cytologic diagnosis are reviewed in detail in the discussions of specific diagnostic entities. This section discusses what constitutes an adequate Papanicolaou smear and how this information and the cytologic diagnosis can be helpful for the referring physician in patient management.

EVALUATION OF THE ADEQUACY OF THE SAMPLE

In addition to the cytologic diagnosis, all specimens should be evaluated for adequacy and a statement made on the report as to the result of that evaluation. The Bethesda system for reporting cervical cytologic diagnoses mandates the inclusion of such statements in the body of the report.[1,2] In the original publication describing the system, no criteria or guidelines were provided as to what constituted an adequate specimen. Likewise, no criteria were specified for classifying a sample as satisfactory, unsatisfactory, or limited. Various criteria were being used by different laboratories, but no uniform guidelines had been established. A committee of experts was formed following the 1991 Bethesda conference and was charged with developing criteria for the evaluation of adequacy. The guidelines that were published represented the opinion of these experts and, in general, coincide with the consensus that is well established for the field.[2] The Bethesda system recommends that all cytology final reports minimally qualify the Papanicolaou smear as satisfactory, satisfactory but limited by specified factors, or unsatisfactory.

THE ADEQUATE PAPANICOLAOU SMEAR

The adequate or satisfactory Papanicolaou smear can be defined broadly as follows: the specimen should be properly identified, the glass slide should be received intact, the appropriate clinical and demographic history should be provided, and, microscopically, the smear should exhibit good cellularity with minimal cell overlap, the cells should be well preserved, cellular evidence of the transformation zone should be identified, and no limiting factors such as obscuring blood and exudate should be present.

Most of these adequacy factors are influenced by the individual collecting the specimen, which usually is the responsibility of the clinician. Therefore, the laboratory should assume the responsibility of ensuring that the clinician is informed about the prerequisites for obtaining an adequate smear and provide the recommended methods of specimen identification, collection, fixation, and submission to the laboratory.

K. M. Atkison: Department of Pathology and Laboratory Medicine, University of Rochester Medical Center, Rochester, New York 14642.

SPECIMEN IDENTIFICATION AND INTEGRITY

Proper identification and specimen integrity is as integral a component of specimen adequacy as are cellularity and preservation. To ensure proper identification of a specimen, the patient's name or another identifier, such as a preassigned accession number, should be written on or affixed to the glass slide. The identifier should be unique and should match the information on the accompanying test request form (requisition).

It is the responsibility of the laboratory to develop a written policy detailing what constitutes adequate identification and what course of action should be followed if inadequately identified specimens are received. It is good laboratory practice to document whether a specimen was received improperly labeled and what actions were taken to resolve the problem. These policies should be delineated clearly and communicated to the laboratory's clients.

If specimen integrity is compromised and a broken slide is received that cannot be repaired without cell loss, the sample should be considered inadequate for acceptance. The laboratory should document the event and notify the clinician. Establishing safe methods of transport is essential in the chain of specimen collection.

CLINICAL HISTORY

Information regarding the clinical history of the patient is often essential for the cytotechnologist and pathologist to render an accurate interpretation. At the time of Papanicolaou smear evaluation, the laboratory should have available the patient's age, the time of the patient's last menstrual period, the source of the specimen, and any pertinent history, including previous abnormal cytology, previous gynecologic surgery or treatment, and any other information that may be of potential importance.[3] Some means of providing this information (ie, check boxes) should be included in the laboratory's test request form to facilitate its procurement (Fig. 2-1). Failure to provide the pertinent clinical information requested by the laboratory makes the specimen inadequate and should be reported as satisfactory for evaluation but limited by the specific omission.

SPECIMEN COLLECTION

The accuracy of the Papanicolaou smear depends largely on obtaining a representative cellular sample for examination. To ensure this, it is important that the cervix be visualized adequately and that both the ectocervix and the endocervical canal be sampled thoroughly. Because most of the abnormalities of interest occur in the area of the transformation zone, it is particularly important that cells from this region be obtained for examination.

Several methods using a variety of devices are available for obtaining cervical samples (Fig. 2-2). The Ayre spatula or modified Ayre spatula typically is used to obtain a sample from the ectocervix. The modified Ayre spatula with an elongated tip was developed to provide a better sample of the canal, but it now is recognized that other instruments are superior to the spatula alone in reliably obtaining a sample that contains material from the transformation zone. Although cotton swabs or a pipette for aspiration of the canal were used to sample the transformation zone in the past, the Endocervical brush and Cervex brush have proven to be better instruments for this purpose.[4-14] Using the presence of endocervical and metaplastic cells as a marker of adequacy, several studies have demonstrated the superiority of the combined use of the Cytobrush and spatula for sampling compared with the spatula alone or the spatula and cotton swab. The Cervex brush used alone also has been reported to provide a reliably adequate sample.

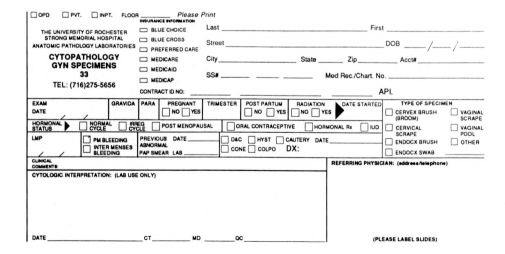

FIG. 2-1. Sample test requisition illustrating the use of check boxes and designated spaces to facilitate the procurement of pertinent clinical information from the referring clinician.

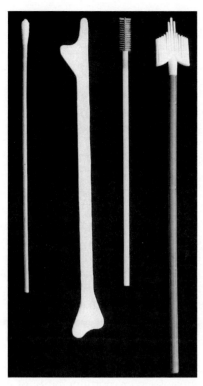

FIG. 2-2. Papanicolaou smear sampling devices. From left to right: endocervical swab, Ayre spatula with extended tip, endocervical brush, and Cervex brush.

The adequacy of the sample does not depend solely or even primarily on the device used, but also on the technique of the individual taking the specimen. No matter which device is used, it is important that the entire circumference of the cervix be sampled and that the smear be prepared properly. The manufacturer's instructions or specific instructions established by the laboratory can be used to illustrate the appropriate use of the device for obtaining material from the ectocervix and endocervix, and for transferring the material to the glass slide. The sensitivity of the technique is diminished if the smear is not spread on the slide evenly and if the cells are not preserved adequately by rapid and complete fixation.

FIXATION

Proper preservation of cell detail is crucial to accurate interpretation. To ensure adequate fixation, rapid immersion of the smear in 95% ethanol is the method of choice. However, regulations regarding the acquisition and transportation of 95% ethanol and the sheer bulkiness of the method often make it impractical. Other wet fixation methods are available using substitute fixatives such as 100% methanol, 80% isopropanol, or denatured ethyl alcohol.[15]

When wet fixation is not a viable option, the most commonly used alternative method is spray fixation.

With commonly available commercial fixatives, this technique can produce a satisfactory smear, but care must be taken to prevent artifactual distortion of the cells. Used inappropriately, the aerosol may "freeze" the cells, or the force of the aerosol may disperse cellular material. The nonaerosol or pump method is recommended over the aerosol spray fixatives. It should be noted that spray fixatives may contain protective agents such as Carbowax.[15] If these wax-like agents are not removed prior to staining, they can inhibit appropriate penetration of the Papanicolaou stain, altering optimum staining reaction. To enhance the cellular preservation of cytologic material that is spray-fixed, the slides should be soaked in 95% alcohol (or substitute) for 30 minutes to 1 hour prior to hydration and staining with hematoxylin. This additional soaking time in alcohol will aid in the removal of the protective coat.

If conventional wet and spray fixation methods do not meet the needs of the laboratory, wet fixation of Papanicolaou smears in 95% ethanol or substitute for 30 minutes can be used. The glass slides then can be removed and allowed to air dry. To reconstitute the cellular material, the glass slides should be soaked for at least 1 hour in a 50:50 solution of glycerin and distilled water prior to staining using the standard Papanicolaou method.

Newly proposed methods of preparation involving a monolayer technique do not require smear preparation by the clinician. The cell sample is placed directly in a liquid preservative and the monolayer is prepared on a slide by special equipment in the laboratory. This virtually eliminates the possibility of drying artifact or poor cell preservation. This technique is still under evaluation, but initial clinical studies are promising. Details of these methodologies are presented in Chapter 11.

STAINING

Smears should be stained with a standard Papanicolaou stain, a polychromatic stain that consists of hematoxylin, eosin, and orange G. Many variations of the stain are commercially available, and the choice is based on personal preference for color differentiation. The range of staining reactions encompasses blue and pink to green and red or orange. Staining intensity (light to dark) can be regulated by varying the staining time.

CRITERIA FOR ASSESSING ADEQUACY

To report cytologic findings more accurately, each laboratory should establish criteria for Papanicolaou smear adequacy and quantitative guidelines defining the categories of "satisfactory," "satisfactory but limited by specified factors," and "unsatisfactory." These guidelines aid cytotechnologists in uniformly applying consistent criteria when making judgments regarding specimen adequacy at the microscopic level.

The Bethesda Committee has published the following definitions and recommended criteria for adequacy[2]:

Satisfactory for evaluation: Well-preserved and visualized squamous epithelial cells covering more than 10% of the slide surface, with a minimum of two clusters of at least five cells of well-preserved endocervical or squamous metaplastic cells.

Satisfactory for evaluation but limited by:obscuring blood, inflammation, thick areas, poor fixation, or air drying that preclude the interpretation of approximately 50% to 75% of the epithelial cells, or by the absence of an endocervical component.

Unsatisfactory for evaluation: Well-preserved and visualized squamous epithelial cells covering less than 10% of the slide surface, or limited by such factors as obscuring blood, inflammation, thick areas, poor fixation, or air drying artifact that preclude the interpretation of approximately 75% or more of the epithelial cells.

The Bethesda system provides guidelines for interpreting specimen adequacy, which can be modified based on each laboratory's preference. Using these definitions and recommendations, this author's laboratory has specified the criteria for classifying a smear as satisfactory, satisfactory but limited, or unsatisfactory.

A satisfactory specimen is quantitatively defined as a cellular specimen (at least 50% of the glass slide covered by epithelial cells) with cellular evidence of an endocervical component (three to five cells and/or groups of columnar and/or metaplastic cells). The smear should exhibit good cellular preservation and no other limiting factors should be identified (Fig. 2-3). A satisfactory

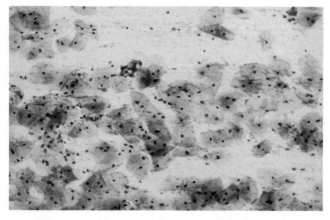

FIG. 2-3. Low-power magnification. This is an adequate Papanicolaou smear interpreted as satisfactory for evaluation and within normal limits. Notice the good cellular preservation, evidence of transformation zone sampling, even cell spread, high cellularity, and absence of limiting factors such as obscuring blood or exudate, or air-drying artifact.

smear that exhibits no cytologic abnormality would be interpreted and reported using the Bethesda system terminology as follows: Specimen adequate for interpretation. Within normal limits. No recommendation.

LESS THAN SATISFACTORY AND UNSATISFACTORY SPECIMENS

Many factors can limit the interpretation of a smear. Laboratories may use different terminology for similar factors (ie, poor preservation versus air-drying artifact) and not all laboratories report the same number or types of limiting factors. Each laboratory should establish the factors to be considered. For example, at the University of Rochester, air-drying artifact, no endocervical component, obscuring blood or exudate, scant or limited sample, and cytolysis are factors that are evaluated and reported on in regard to determining specimen adequacy.

Once these factors have been established, the laboratory should provide written quantitative guidelines for laboratory personnel to apply when determining specimen adequacy. Studies have shown that the interobserver and intraobserver reproducibility of categorizing smears as satisfactory or unsatisfactory are excellent and good, respectively. However, there is relatively low concordance between observers categorizing smears as satisfactory but limited by category, largely because of the lack of established criteria.[16] Quantitative guidelines provide a framework for cytotechnologists in making these subjective judgments.

In evaluating an inadequate sample, this author's laboratory uses the ranges 50% to 80% and 80% to 100% to define smears as satisfactory but limited by and unsatisfactory, respectively. For example, a suboptimal smear could be reported as follows: specimen adequate for interpretation, but limited by air-drying artifact altering 50% to 80% of the cellular material; or specimen adequate for interpretation, but limited by scant cellularity (50% to 80% of the glass slide area shows no cellular elements). An unsatisfactory smear would be reported as follows: specimen unsatisfactory for evaluation due to air-drying artifact altering 80% to 100% of the cellular material; or specimen unsatisfactory for evaluation due to scant cellularity (80% to 100% of the glass slide area shows no cellular material). Caution should be exercised in differentiating obscuring exudate and blood from the same elements in the background that do not obscure cellular detail. In addition, a smear that contains identifiable abnormal cells should not be reported as unsatisfactory. Any cellular abnormality should be reported, regardless of whether the smear is otherwise unsatisfactory because of inherent limitations in its quality. The illustrations in Figures 2-4 through 2-9 compare the three categories of adequacy in relation to cellularity and exudate.

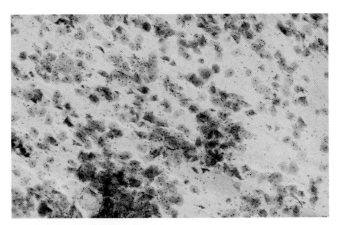

FIG. 2-4. Low-power magnification. This figure and the next two figures (Figs. 2-5, 2-6) represent an overall pattern of cellularity. Adequate cellularity (minimally 50% of the glass slide is covered with epithelial cells).

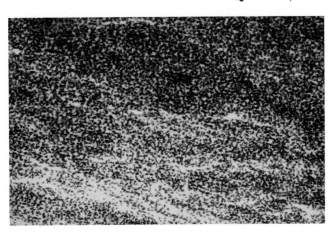

FIG. 2-7. Low-power magnification. This figure and the next two figures (Figs 2-8, 2-9) represent the overall cellular pattern of inflammatory exudate as it relates to adequacy. Specimen is unsatisfactory for evaluation due to inflammatory exudate obscuring 80% to 100% of the cellular material. Note cellular material is not visible. However, if an abnormality is detected it must be reported, even though the smear is technically unsatisfactory for evalutation.

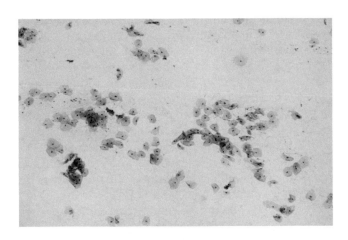

FIG. 2-5. Low-power magnification. Specimen satisfactory for evaluation but limited by scant cellularity (50% to 80% of the glass slide area shows no cellular elements).

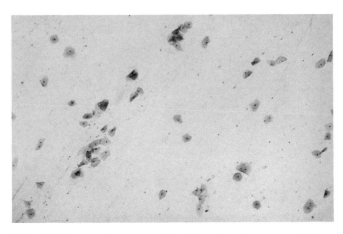

FIG. 2-6. Low-power magnification. Specimen unsatisfactory for evaluation due to scant cellularity (80% to 100% of the glass slide area shows no cellular elements).

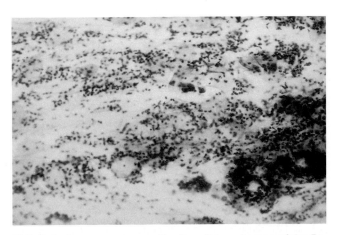

FIG. 2-8. Low-power magnification. Several areas of the Papanicolaou smear exhibited this pattern of partial obscuring with inflammatory exudate. The total area obscured encompasses approximately 50% to 80% of the cellular material. This pap smear is satisfactory for evaluation but limited by inflammatory exudate.

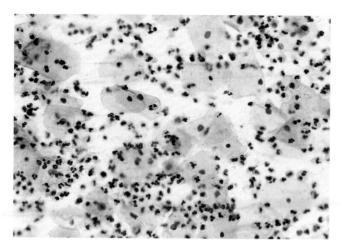

FIG. 2-9. Low-power magnification. This figure shows inflammatory cells in the background that do not obscure cellular detail. The Papanicolaou smear is satisfactory for evaluation.

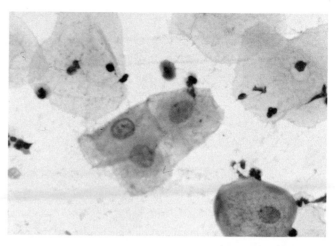

FIG. 2-11. High-power magnification. Note 'muddy'' and polychromatic staining reaction secondary to air drying.

Limiting factors hinder the ability of the cytologist to make an accurate assessment of the cellular changes present on the glass slide. Air-drying artifact results in cellular and nuclear enlargement, making changes in the nuclear-to-cytoplasmic ratio difficult to assess. Drying artifact alters the staining reaction, resulting in poorly or lightly stained eosinophilic or amphophilic cells. The most debilitating effect of air-drying artifact is the loss of nuclear and chromatin detail (Figs. 2-10 through 2-13). Taken together, the effects of air-drying may result in high false-positive rates, especially in the category of atypical squamous cells of undetermined significance, or

in ambiguous reporting when the abnormality cannot be graded. Immediate fixation should be stressed to the clinician to prevent air-drying artifact.

Obscuring exudate may mask or completely cover abnormal cells, making their detection difficult on routine screening. Hatem and Wilbur reviewed Papanicolaou smears of apparently rapidly progressive lesions that previously had been interpreted as negative, and showed most of the false-negative reports to be in the background of obscuring exudate.[17] Often, the abnormal cells were small, mimicking immature squamous metaplasia. They were imbedded in the exudate, making visualization difficult. Care should be taken in evaluating smears with obscuring exudate.

Blood may obscure or dilute the cellular specimen

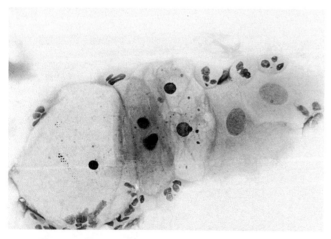

FIG. 2-10. High-power magnification. This figure and the next three figures (Figs 2-11–2-13) illustrate the cytologic effects of air-drying artifact. Note nuclear enlargement with lack of nuclear chromatin detail in the two cells exhibiting air-drying artifact. These cells may mimic atypical squamous cells of undetermined significance resulting in a false-positive interpretation.

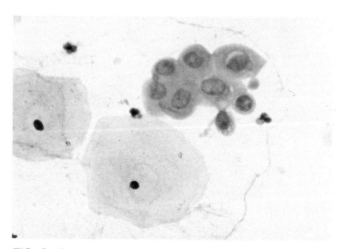

FIG. 2-12. High-power magnification. Air-drying artifact exhibited in this cluster of cells makes determination of origin and biologic potential of these cells difficult. The cells most likely represent benign sqaumous metaplasia or columnar endocervical cells.

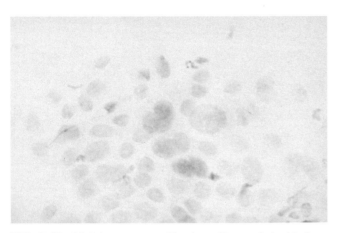

FIG. 2-13. High-power magnification. Sheet of air-dried endocervical cells illustrating the lack of nuclear chromatin detail and poor staining reaction secondary to air-drying artifact. Proper fixation will eliminate air-drying artifact.

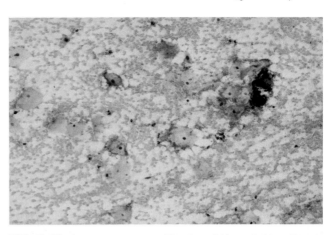

FIG. 2-15. Low-power magnification. Although blood is obscuring cellular detail, only 50% to 80% of the cellular material was obscured. This case should be interpreted as satisfactory for evaluation but limited by blood obscuring the cellular material.

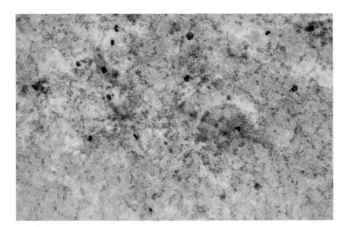

FIG. 2-14. Low-power magnification. This figure and the next two (Figs. 2-15, 2-16) compare the cellular patterns of obscuring blood. Note visualization of the epithelial cells is obscured by blood. The overall pattern on this smear exhibited blood obscuring 80% to 100% of the cellular material. This smear should be interpreted as unsatisfactory for evaluation.

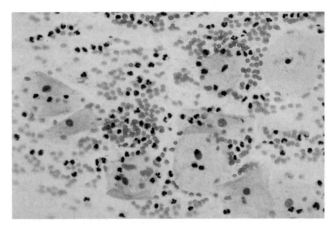

FIG. 2-16. High-power magnification. Note the blood and exudate in the background. These elements are not obscuring cellular detail. This case would be interpreted as satisfactory for evaluation.

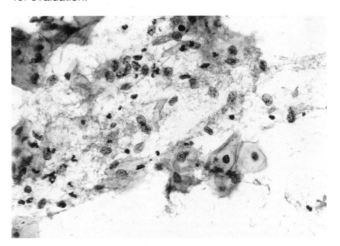

FIG. 2-17. Low-power magnification. This figure and the next two (Figs. 2-18, 2-19) represent the limiting effects of cytolysis. Cytolysis results in the fragmentation of cytoplasm with resultant stripped nuclei in the background. This fragmentation may be so pronounced that sufficient viable, intact cells for evaluation may not be present.

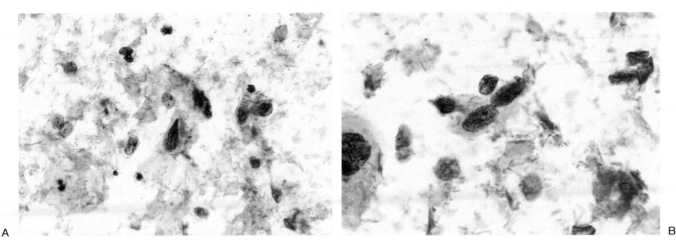

A   B

FIG. 2-18. (A,B) These figures show a high-grade squamous intraepithelial lesion on a patient exhibiting extensive cytolysis. Assessment of true nuclear enlargement and nuclear to cytoplasmic ratio is difficult due to the cytoplasmic fragmentation. Detection and grading of the lesion may be hindered by the effects of cytolysis.

(Figs. 2-14 through 2-16). Extensive cytolysis also can be a limiting factor. Fragmentation of the cytoplasm and the resultant stripped nuclei may make assessment of an abnormality difficult (Figs. 2-17 through 2-18*B*). Thick cell areas, the result of inappropriate cell spread by the clinician, makes visualization of all cell layers impossible (Fig. 2-19).

Brown artifact, or corn flaking, is caused by air trapped under the coverslip and results in a golden brown, refractile artifact that obscures both individual cells and cell clumps. The brown artifact obscures all cellular detail (Fig. 2-20). Corn flaking occurs during the coverslipping

process and can be monitored and controlled by the laboratory.

THE CLINICAL IMPACT OF REPORTING ON ADEQUACY

Although it is somewhat subjective, the inclusion of a statement in the report describing the adequacy of the specimen and the nature of any factors which limit the quality of a smear is important. This provides the clinician with a clearer understanding of the cytologic presen-

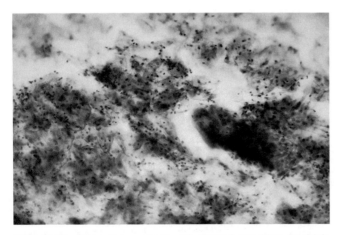

FIG. 2-19. Note the uneven cell spread resulting in thick groups in which not all levels are able to be visualized with conventional light microscopy. This artifact is the result of improper cell transfer and spread by the referring clinician. Communication with the referring physician can eliminate this artifact.

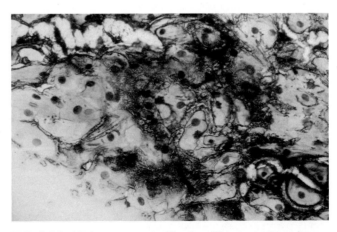

FIG. 2-20. High-power magnification. The amorphous brown material present in this slide is the result of trapped air under the coverslip. This artifact occurs during the coverslipping process, when the clearing agent is allowed to air dry before the mounting media is applied. "Brown artifact" or "corn flaking," as it is commonly referred to, can extensively obscure cellular detail.

tation as it relates to the effectiveness of the collection technique, the preservation of the cellular material, and the correlation with the clinical situation. In some circumstances, a diagnosis of "inadequate" may prompt the clinician to repeat the Papanicolaou smear in a shorter interval than she or he normally would for a "negative" diagnosis. However, the final decision regarding the adequacy of an individual smear for a particular patient is ultimately the responsibility of the clinician, as the individual who can best correlate the details of the report with his or her knowledge of the patient.

THE ENDOCERVICAL COMPONENT AS A DETERMINANT OF ADEQUACY

Most intraepithelial lesions arise in the transformation zone, an area of variable size and extent wherein the process of squamous metaplasia occurs. This area is located on the face of the cervix in young women and gradually becomes more proximal with age, so that in older women, it often is found within the endocervical canal. It has been argued logically that this area of the cervix must be sampled for the Papanicolaou smear to have the highest probability of revealing developing lesions. Cytologic evidence of transformation zone sampling has been defined as the presence of columnar (endocervical) and/ or squamous metaplastic cells.[2] Based on this reasoning, the presence of an endocervical component has come to represent one of the key markers of specimen adequacy.

The significance of an endocervical component as an indicator of specimen adequacy was discussed by Gondos and colleagues in 1972. They cited earlier studies from 1965 comparing false-negative rates associated with the detection of squamous carcinoma in situ using the collection methods of vaginal pool aspiration (45%) versus endocervical os aspiration (4%). These investigators concluded that the presence of endocervical cells was associated with a lower false-negative rate for cervical neoplasia and that endocervical canal sampling should be part of the routine Papanicolaou test. They also suggested that cytology reports on cyclic women should indicate the presence or absence of endocervical cells.[18]

Several subsequent studies have established a relation between the identification of an endocervical component and the rate of detection of squamous intraepithelial lesions.[8,13,19-24] Using three different cervical sampling techniques (a cotton swab with an Ayre spatula, a Cytobrush with a spatula, and a Cervex Brush), Henry and associates reported that high-grade squamous intraepithelial lesions were detected two times more frequently on specimens that exhibited an endocervical component than on those that did not.[21]

Case control, longitudinal, and cross-sectional studies similarly have demonstrated that the rate of detection of squamous intraepithelial lesions is increased in specimens that contain an endocervical component.[8,13,19-24] However, an increased rate of reporting an endocervical component is not related directly to an increased incidence of reportable squamous intraepithelial lesions. These studies also pointed out that the presence of squamous metaplastic cells had a greater association with the detection of squamous intraepithelial lesions than did the presence of endocervical columnar cells.[22]

The use of an endocervical component (ie, columnar and/or squamous metaplastic cells) as a measure of adequacy is valid but not absolute. Cytologic evidence of an endocervical component ensures that the cervix, and not the vagina, has been sampled.[22] If the patient has clinical evidence of cervical neoplasia and cytology reveals squamous metaplasia, studies indicate that the sensitivity of the test for the detection of cervical neoplasia should be increased. In addition, with the increasing incidence of endocervical neoplasia, direct sampling of the endocervical canal should increase the sensitivity of the test in detecting endocervical adenocarcinoma and its precursor lesion, adenocarcinoma in situ. However, smears may provide evidence of a lesion, even though they do not contain evidence of an endocervical component. In addition, short-term studies demonstrate no significant increase in the frequency of the subsequent detection of lesions in patients whose initial smears showed no evidence of an endocervical component compared with those whose smears did show such evidence.[24,25]

Care should be taken not to use the presence of an endocervical component as the sole indication of specimen adequacy. The presence of an endocervical component does not indicate that all the targeted region has been sampled. For example, endocervical cells may be derived from more distal portions of the endocervical canal and may not represent true sampling of the transformation zone. The sampling device itself may not sample the full circumference of the cervix, and may miss a lesion entirely, even though an endocervical component is present on the slide.

THE RELATION OF THE NUMBER OF SLIDES PREPARED PER CASE TO ADEQUACY RATES AND SENSITIVITY

Historically, in addition to the best sampling devices and optimal types of samples, debate has surrounded the ideal number of slides to prepare from each patient. It has been conventional practice to prepare one slide per sampled site, regardless of the type of sampling device used. For example, when three sites (ie, vagina, endocervix, and ectocervix) are sampled, the cellular material is transferred onto three separate glass slides. This technique is supported by the theory that diagnostic accuracy improves as the volume of tissue sampled increases.

However, concerns regarding the adequacy, sensitivity, and cost-effectiveness of Papanicolaou smear screening led to several studies evaluating the relation of these factors to the number of slides prepared.[26-34]

The One-Slide Versus the Two-Slide Method

One of the earliest studies evaluating the effect of using one slide rather than multiple slides was reported by Wied and Bahr in 1959. Using the Ayre spatula, vaginal aspirator, and endocervical swab, they investigated the technique of placing three samples on one slide. The slide was prelabeled to designate each anatomic area sampled: "V" for vagina, "C" for cervix, and "E" for endocervix (VCE). The technique required sequential sampling of the vagina, cervix, and endocervix, keeping the material on the sampling devices. Then, in reverse order, each specimen was transferred to the glass slide in the designated area corresponding to the sampled site of origin.[33]

The results showed that diagnostic accuracy and false-negative rates were comparable to those of the conventional three-slide method. In addition, although the total surface area available for the cell spread was reduced from 606 mm^2 to 450 mm^2, the area required to make an optimal cytologic interpretation was only 150 mm^2. The advantages of the one-slide method included the use of fewer glass slides, coverslips, and staining materials; the need for less filing space; and reduced screening times resulting in a cost savings. Further studies performed by Willbanks and associates in 1968, using two sampling devices (cervical aspirator and cervical scraper) and one slide, corroborated the original findings in regard to accuracy and cost savings.[34]

Some studies, such as the one reported by Tabbara and colleagues in 1992, have produced contradictory results. These authors reported a 28% false-negative rate associated with one-slide preparations when the endocervix and ectocervix were sampled compared with a 12% to 15% false-negative rate associated with two-slide preparations. They attributed the increased false-negative rate to artifactual problems associated with the technique of smearing itself. Factors such as uneven cell spread of material resulting in areas that were too thick to evaluate, and areas of excessive mucus trapping epithelial cells hindering visualization were problems they identified.[32] Nevertheless, based on the data in the literature and cost-effectiveness concerns, most laboratories recommend the preparation of a single slide per case in routine circumstances.

The Role of Sampling Devices in the One-Slide Versus the Two-Slide Method

The incentive to use a single slide per case without compromising adequacy played a major role in directing research and development strategies for manufacturers of Papanicolaou smear sampling devices. Although the combined use of a cervical scraper and endocervical brush is touted as the best method of collection, it is difficult to use one slide for two sampling devices without inducing unacceptable air-drying artifact during slide preparation. In response to this problem, several new devices that sample both the endocervix and ectocervix have been developed. The Cervex Brush, Acellon Combi, CytoPick, and Tech Touch are examples of such devices.

Regardless of the device used and the number of slides prepared, it is essential that the transformation zone be sampled, the cells be transferred appropriately, and the specimen be well fixed for an accurate cytologic assessment to be made.

Do Duplicate Papanicolaou Smears Improve Accuracy?

The false-negative rate associated with the Papanicolaou smear has been reported to be as high as 40%.[35] One common cause of false-negative cytology results is sampling error. Sampling error is considered to have occurred when a lesion is present on the cervix, but the Papanicolaou smear contains no abnormal cells. This may occur in one of two circumstances. The specimen taken may not contain any abnormal cells because the lesion was not sampled, or the lesion may have been sampled but the abnormal cells were not transferred to the glass slide.

Based on the premise that increased sampling of a site might reduce the number of false-negative results secondary to these events, several studies were initiated. Using a pointed-tip spatula, Sedlis and associates took duplicate smears in succession with the same device. Of 262 abnormal cases identified, 50% and 30% were interpreted as squamous intraepithelial lesions and carcinoma in situ, respectively, on only one slide. There was no significant difference in false-negative rates between the first and second slides.[31] In a similar study, Meisels performed repeated Papanicolaou smears at 3-month intervals on patients with previous squamous intraepithelial lesions and documented agreement in less than 50% of the cases.[29]

Luthy and colleagues evaluated the effectiveness of using a cervical scraper and vaginal pool aspirator on the first slide and a cervical scraper alone on the second slide. Of 3524 patients enrolled in the study, 93 were found to have abnormal cytology. The rates of positive results were 76% and 80% for the first and second samples, respectively. These researchers determined that the use of a second smear increased the rate of detection of squamous intraepithelial lesions by 26.3%. However, projected onto the study population of 3524 patients, the second smear detected only 28 additional abnormal cases, for a 0.8% increase in the detection of cervical intraepithelial neoplasia. Overall, this does not represent a significant increase in sensitivity when compared with the additional cost of required resources.[27] Using the Ayre spatula and endocervical aspiration, Davis and associates reported only a 7% lower rate of false-negative results using the consecutive or duplicate sampling method.[26]

Although an additional smear may improve sensitivity, the cost may not outweigh the benefits. However, these findings substantiate the high false-negative rate associated with Papanicolaou smear sampling and support the recommendation that consistent annual Papanicolaou testing be done to minimize the result of sampling errors.

THE RELATION OF THE TYPE OF SAMPLING DEVICE TO SPECIMEN ADEQUACY

The association between the type of sampling device used and one measure of Papanicolaou smear adequacy, the presence of an endocervical component, has been the subject of considerable discussion in the literature. Several reports compare the endocervical component yield for techniques using different devices.[4–14] In general, the combination of an endocervical brush and a cervical scraper has yielded endocervical component rates of 88% to 99% in the general population. The Cervex Brush has yielded endocervical component rates of 73% to 96%, compared with 62% to 92% for the combination of a cotton swab and a cervical scraper. This wide range of values has been attributed to variability in the skill levels of the sample takers and the clinical situations of the patients.

The University of Rochester experience with sampling devices includes data on the combined use of a cervical scraper and a cotton swab, a cervical scraper and an endocervical brush, and the Cervex Brush. The endocervical component yield in 3000 patients (1000 for each device) was 90% with the scraper and cotton swab combination, 88.7% with the cervical scraper and endocervical brush combination, and 92.7% with the Cervex Brush. In a high-risk family planning population of 9478 patients, an overall 96.6% endocervical component yield was realized. The predominant sampling device used was the Cervex Brush. However, the combination of a cervical scraper and an endocervical brush was used occasionally.[14]

In pregnant and postmenopausal patients, the transformation zone may be difficult to sample. The sampling device used to obtain this material with minimal jeopardy or discomfort for the patient is an important factor. Our laboratory compared the endocervical component yield in pregnant patients using three devices (1000 patients per study, of which approximately 8% per study were pregnant). The endocervical component yield was 66.2% using the cotton swab and scraper, 53.2% using the endocervical brush and scraper, and 70.5% using the Cervex Brush. For postmenopausal patients, the endocervical component yield was 50% with the cotton swab, 60.7% with the endocervical brush, and 88.6% with the Cervex Brush (1000 patients per study, of which approximately 2% per study were postmenopausal).

Several authors have evaluated the relation between the sample taker, sampling device, endocervical component yield, and other microscopic factors of adequacy, such as cellularity and preservation. Neinstein and Church concluded that endocervical component yield using the combination of a cervical scraper and an endocervical brush or the Cervex Brush was related directly to the level of training, experience, and skill of the sample taker. Adequacy rates were 85% for attending physicians, 94% for nurse-practitioners, and 65% for trainees.[10]

Boon and associates compared five sampling methods using five sample takers with 5 to 10 years of extensive clinical experience. These practitioners were familiar with only one of the five methods evaluated, but received training in the other four methods. The results showed a wide variability in the endocervical component yield per sample taker per device. Using the spatula only, the method the group was familiar with, 7.86% to 11.0% of samples had no endocervical component. Using the endocervical brush and spatula, 0.20% to 1.29% of samples had no endocervical component, and using the cotton swab, 4.08% to 13.89% had no endocervical component.[4]

The specific design of a sampling device alone cannot account for the clinical variability between patients and sample takers. Specific training and familiarity with the use of any sampling device is necessary to ensure the best results. Ferris and colleagues demonstrated that a minimal variation in technique, such as the number of rotations used with the Cervex Brush, can have an effect on adequacy and the rate of detection of squamous intraepithelial lesions. Varying the number of rotations from 1 to 5 complete turns affects the amount of obscuring blood, the cellularity, the endocervical component yield, and the rate of detection of squamous intraepithelial lesions.[7]

When a device designed to sample only the endocervical canal (eg, the endocervical brush) is used, a cervical scraper must be included in the technique. The endocervical brush alone does not adequately sample the ectocervix. Studies have shown that reduced numbers of squamous cells are found on pure endocervical brush samples. In addition, fewer low-grade squamous intraepithelial lesions are detected when the endocervical brush is used without the cervical scraper.[6,20,36,37]

The ideal Papanicolaou smear sampling device would be inexpensive, easy for the clinician to use, and relatively comfortable for the patient, and would obtain adequate material from the endocervix and ectocervix.

IN SEARCH OF THE ADEQUATE PAPANICOLAOU SMEAR

Since the introduction of the Papanicolaou test as a routine screening tool for cervical neoplasia, the rate of death from cervical cancer has decreased dramatically. Significant effort has been made to enhance the sensitivity and specificity of this screening test by improving collection methods and laboratory procedures, and establishing better reporting systems to provide more useful information to clinicians. Communication is the key to maintaining a quality test. Continued evaluation of the process involved in Papanicolaou smear testing from the point of collection to the final report will contribute to the overall quality of the test. It is the responsibility of the laboratory to assess the factors that affect specimen adequacy and to recommend changes that will improve the ability of the Papanicolaou test to aid in the detection of cervical neoplasia.

REFERENCES

1. Solomon D. The Bethesda system for reporting cervical/vaginal cytologic diagnoses: an overview. Int J Gynecol Pathol 1991;10:323.
2. Kurman R, Solomon D. The Bethesda system for reporting cervical/vaginal cytologic diagnoses, pp 4-8. New York: Springer-Verlag, 1994.
3. Wied G, Keebler C, Rosenthal D, Schenck U, Somrak T, Vooijs P. Compendium on quality assurance, proficiency testing and workload limitations in clinical cytology. Tutorials of Cytology, pp 90-94. Chicago, 1995.
4. Boon M, de Graaff Guilloud J, Rietveld W. Analysis of five sampling methods for preparation of cervical smears. Acta Cytol 1989;33:843.
5. Chakrabarti S, Guijon F, Paraskevas M. Brush vs. spatula for cervical smears: histologic correlation with concurrent biopsies. Acta Ctyol 1994;38:315.
6. Buntinx F, Boon M, Beck S,et al. Comparison of Cytobrush sampling, spatula sampling and combined Cytobrush-spatula sampling of the uterine cervix. Acta Cytol 1991;35:64.
7. Ferris D, Berrey M, Ellis K, et al. The optimal technique for obtaining a Papanicolaou smear with the Cervex-Brush. J Fam Pract 1992;34:276.
8. Kristensen G, Holund B, Grinsted P. Efficacy of Cytobrush versus the cotton swab in the collection of endocervical cells. Acta Cytol 1989;33:849.
9. McCord M, Stoval T, Meric JL, et al. Cervical cytology: a randomized comparison of four sampling methods. Am J Obstet Gynecol 1992;166:1772.
10. Neinstein L, Church J. Comparison of Cytobrush with Cervex-Brush for endocervical cytologic sampling. J Adolesc Health 1992;13:520.
11. Rammou-Kinia R, Anagnostopoulou I, Gomousa M. Comparison of spatula and nonspatula methods for cervical sampling. Acta Cytol 1991;35:69.
12. Hoffman M, Gordy L, Cavanagh D. The use of Cytobrush for cervical sampling after cryotherapy. Acta Cytol 1990;3:79.
13. Szareski A, Curran G, Edwards R, et al. Comparison of four cytologic sampling techniques in a large family planning center. Acta Cytol 1993;37:457.
14. Atkison K, Mulford D, Wilkinson P, Wilbur D. A comparison of endocervical component yield pre- and post-introduction of the Cervex Brush Pap smear sampling device in a rural and metropolitan population. Acta Cytol 1995;39:983.
15. Keebler C, Somrak T. The manual of cytotechnology, pp 412-417. Chicago: American Society of Clinical Pathologists, 1993.
16. Spires S, Banks E, Weeks J, Banks H, Davey D. Specimen adequacy according to the Bethesda system: interobserver and intraobserver reproducibility. Acta Cytol 1993;37:778
17. Hatem F, Wilbur D. High grade squamous cervical lesions following negative Papanicolaou smears: false-negative cervical cytology or rapid progression. Diagn Cytopathol 1995;12:135.
18. Gondos B, Marshall D, Ostergard D. Endocervical cells in cervical smears. Am J Obstet Gynecol 1972;15:833.
19. Campion M. The adequate cervical smear: a modern dilemma. J Fam Pract 1992;34:273.
20. Elias A, Linthorst G, Bekker B, Vooijs P. The significance of endocervical cells in the diagnosis of cervical epithelial changes. Acta Cytol 1983;27:225.
21. Henry M, Germain M, Heaton R, Erickson D, O'Connor D. Evaluation of the effect of endocervical component on the adequacy of cervical specimens. Acta Cytol 1993;37:770.
22. Mitchel H, Medley G. Influence of endocervical status on the cytologic prediction of cervical intraepithelial neoplasia. Acta Cytol 1992;36:875.
23. Woodman C, Williams D, Yates M, Tomlinson K, Ward W, Luesley D. Indicators of effective cytological samping of the uterine cervix. Lancet 1989;2:8653.
24. Sidawy M, Tabbara S, Silverberg S. Should we report cervical smears lacking endocervical component as unsatisfactory? Diagn Cytopathol 1992;8:567.
25. Kivlahan C, Ingram E. Papanicolaou smears without endocervical cells: are they inadequate? Acta Cytol 1986;30:258.
26. Davis J, Hindman W, Paplanus S, Trego D, Wiens J, Suciu T. Value of duplicate smears in cervical cytology. Acta Cytol 1981;25:533.
27. Luthy D, Briggs R, Buyco A, Eschenbach A. Cervical cytology: increased sensitivity with a second cervical smear. Am J Obstet Gynecol 1978;51:713.
28. Meisels A. Superiority of the V-C-E smear. Acta Cytol 1969;13:1.
29. Meisels A. Are two smears better than one? Acta Cytol 1990;34:459.
30. Saitas V, Hawthorne C, Cater J, Bibbo M. Single-slide versus double-slide Papanicolaou smear: a comparative study. Acta Cytol 1993;37:779.
31. Sedlis A, Walters H, Balin, H, et al. Evaluation of two simultaneously obtained cervical cytological smears. Acta Cytol 1974;18:291.
32. Tabbara S, Horbach N, Sidawy M. The adequacy of the one-slide cervical smear in the detection of squamous intraepithelial lesions. Am J Clin Pathol 1994;101:647.
33. Wied G, Bahr G. Vaginal, cervical and endocervical cytologic smears on a single slide. Obstet Gynecol 1959;14:362.
34. Willbanks G, Ikomi E, Prado R, Richart R. An evaluation of a one-slide cervical cytologic method for the detection of cervical intraepithelial neoplasia. Acta Cytol 1968;12:157.
35. Baker R. Improving the adequacy of Pap smears. Am Fam Physician 1989;39:109.
36. Vooijs PG. Endocervical brush device. Lancet 1989;2:784.
37. Longfield J, Grimshaw R, Monaghan J. Simultaneous sampling of the endocervix and ectocervix using the Profile brush. Acta Cytol 1993;37:472.

Gynecologic Cytopathology. Edited by
Thomas A. Bonfiglio and Yener S. Erozan.
Lippincott–Raven Publishers, Philadelphia, © 1997.

CHAPTER 3

Normal Uterine Histology and Cytology

Thomas A. Bonfiglio

NORMAL HISTOLOGY OF THE UTERINE CERVIX

The vagina and the outer portion of the uterine cervix are lined by a squamous mucosa. The squamous epithelium is stratified and is composed of a basal layer of immature cells, a parabasal layer, an intermediate cell layer, and a superficial layer. In the normal state, neither a granular cell layer nor a cornified layer is present (Fig. 3-1).

The endocervical canal and a variable portion of the ectocervix in the young female is lined by a glandular type of epithelium consisting of a single layer of tall, columnar, mucin-producing cells with basally located nuclei that are round to oval with vesicular chromatin (Fig. 3-2). Ciliated columnar cells are also present (Fig. 3-3). Below the columnar cells, a layer of small primitive-appearing cells called *reserve cells* is often identified. This columnar epithelial–lined mucosa invaginates into the endocervical stoma, forming the "endocervical glands." This pattern of epithelium extends upward throughout the endocervical canal to the region of the internal cervical os and lower uterine segment. In this region, the columnar lining is transformed into one composed of non–mucin-secreting columnar epithelium of endometrioid type. Also in the upper portions of the endocervical canal, it is common to see an epithelial lining that is histologically similar to that of tubal epithelium, including the presence of intercalated cells and terminal bars and cilia (Fig. 3-4). This is referred to as *tubal metaplasia,* but it is unclear whether the almost ubiquitous presence of this type of epithelium represents a metaplastic event or a common variation of normal. The recognition of this type epithelium is important because it often appears in cytologic samples, particularly with the extensive endocervical sampling that is now common with the newer sampling devices.

The point of junction between the squamous epithelium of the ectocervix and the endocervical columnar epithelium is referred to as the *squamocolumnar junction* (Fig. 3-5). It is in this area that the process of squamous metaplasia occurs that gradually transforms the preexisting area of glandular epithelium into a squamous epithelium. This process moves the squamocolumnar junction up the endocervical canal, creating a zone of metaplasia and proliferating epithelium referred to as the *transformation zone.* This physiologic process occurs in all females beginning at about the time of menarche and continuing to some extent throughout the reproductive years. Its etiology is uncertain, but it appears to be related to menarchal changes in bacterial flora and a lowering of vaginal pH. Adequate cellular samples that include material from the transformation zone in cyclic women, therefore, would be expected to contain immature metaplastic cells as a normal finding.

The first morphological manifestation of the squamous metaplastic process is the appearance of a layer or layers of the very immature cells termed *reserve cells* immediately below the columnar endocervical–type epithelium in a portion of the transformation zone (Fig. 3-6). These cells subsequently develop evidence of squamous differentiation in the form of more cytoplasm and the development of well-defined cell borders. The overlying columnar epithelium may persist, and at this point, the appearance is referred to as *subcolumnar squamous metaplasia* (Fig. 3-7). This stage is followed by loss of the columnar epithelium, which results in the pattern that is recognized as common squamous metaplasia (Figs. 3-8, 3-9). Eventually, this epithelium matures and becomes indistinguishable from the native squamous epithelium on the face of the cervix save for the presence of underlying endocervical-type glands.

T. A. Bonfiglio: Department of Pathology and Laboratory Medicine, University of Rochester Medical Center, Rochester, New York 14642.

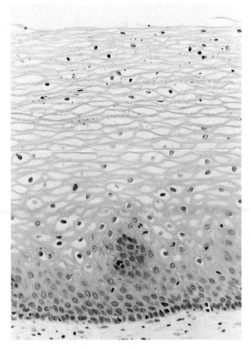

FIG. 3-1. Normal squamous epithelium of ectocervix.

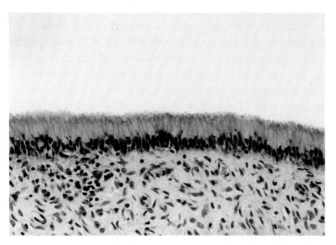

FIG. 3-2. Normal columnar mucinous epithelium of cervix.

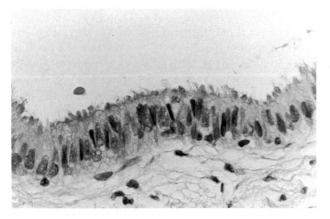

FIG. 3-3. Ciliated columnar epithelium of cervix.

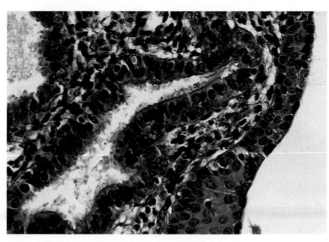

FIG. 3-4. Tubal metaplasia. Ciliated columnar cells with interspersed intercalated cells.

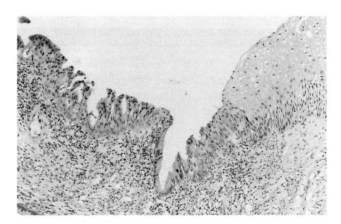

FIG. 3-5. Low-power view of cervical transformation zone. Immature squamous metaplasia is present in the area between the squamous epithelium on the right and the columnar epithelium on the left.

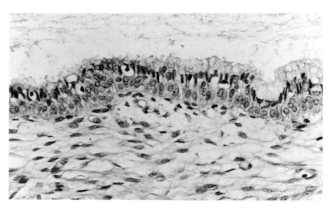

FIG. 3-6. Early reserve cell hyperplasia. A single layer of very immature appearing cells is present below the columnar epithelium.

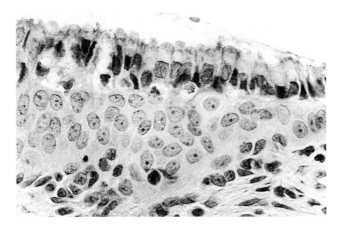

FIG. 3-7. Subcolumnar squamous metaplasia. There are multiple cell layers in the subcolumnar location. Some cells show definite evidence of squamous differentiation with the appearance of more cytoplasm and well-defined borders.

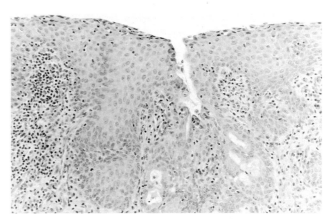

FIG. 3-9. Immature squamous metaplasia. The maturation of metaplastic process on the surface is more advanced in this area but the epithelium still has an immature appearance with immature cells with a high nuclear-cytoplasmic ratio in the superficial layers.

Although this is a normal process the involved area, the transformation zone, is of great importance because it is in this relatively small region of the cervix that the process of carcinogenesis occurs in the great majority of instances. Figure 3-10 depicts in graphic form the physiologic changes that occur in this area as compared to the events that are believed to occur in the process of carcinogenesis. Current theory holds that the immature epithelium of the transformation zone is that which appears to be most sensitive to the carcinogenic events that are associated with the development of cervical squamous carcinoma and its precursors. It is apparently this epithelium that is most susceptible to the oncogenic effects of the human papillomavirus, and it is in this region that we see the precursor lesions develop (see Chap. 5). The

histology and corresponding cytology of the changes mediated by this virus and its cofactors make up the substance of diagnostic cytopathology of the uterine cervix covered in the subsequent chapters of this text. In order to gain a clear understanding of the features of abnormal cytology, a thorough familiarity with the spectrum of appearances of normal histology and cytology of the cervix is necessary.

NORMAL CYTOLOGY OF THE CERVIX AND VAGINA

The normal cells found on a Papanicolaou smear reflect the tissue from which they are derived. Basically, three types of normal squamous cells are present: the superficial squamous cells, derived from the most superficial portions of the epithelium; the intermediate squamous cells, derived from slightly deeper portions of the epithelium; and the squamous metaplastic cells, immature squamous cells derived from areas of immature squamous metaplasia in the transformation zone. The superficial squamous cells are polygonal, with thin eosinophilic or cyanophilic cytoplasm and small pyknotic nuclei. The intermediate cells are similar in appearance to the superficial cells except that their nuclei are more vesicular in their appearance and are larger, averaging approximately 35 μm^2 in area (Figs. 3-11 and 3-12). The immature metaplastic squamous cells are smaller than both the superficial and intermediate cells, and are round to oval with denser cytoplasm and a much higher nuclear-to-cytoplasmic ratio. The nuclei of these cells are round, vesicular, and average 50 μm^2 in area. Their overall appearance, however, varies with their degree of maturity. The most immature forms are quite small and resemble reserve cells or even cells derived from some

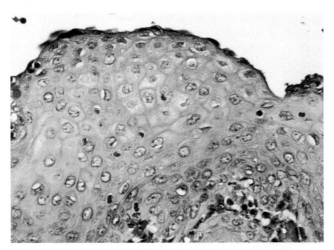

FIG. 3-8. Immature squamous metaplasia. The columnar epithelium has been replaced by an immature squamous epithelium.

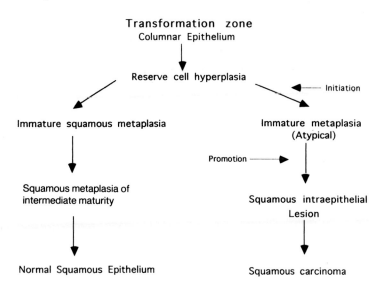

Transformation zone
Columnar Epithelium

Reserve cell hyperplasia

<-------- Initiation

Immature squamous metaplasia

Immature metaplasia
(Atypical)

Promotion -------->

Squamous metaplasia of
intermediate maturity

Squamous intraepithelial
Lesion

FIG. 3-10. Diagramatic comparison of physiologic squamous metaplasia (left) as compared with the neoplastic process as it theoretically develops in the transformation zone.

Normal Squamous Epithelium

Squamous carcinoma

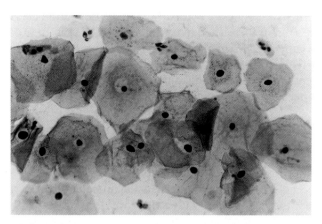

FIG. 3-11. Normal superficial squamous cells. Note the pyknotic nuclei.

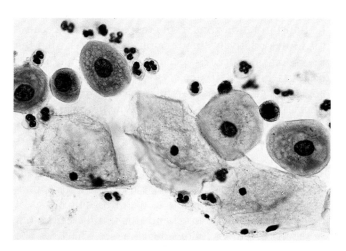

FIG. 3-13. Squamous metaplastic cells and superficial cells. The metaplastic cells have a round to oval configuration and denser cytoplasm.

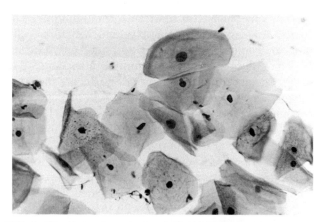

FIG. 3-12. Normal squamous cells. Note the larger, more vesicular nuclei of the cells in the upper center.

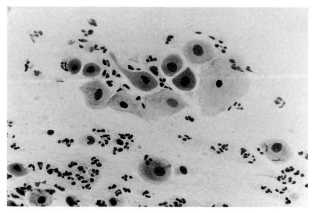

FIG. 3-14. Immature squamous metaplastic cells intermingled with intermediate cells.

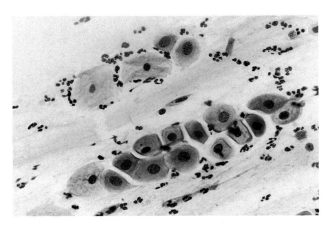

FIG. 3-15. A cluster of immature squamous metaplastic cells.

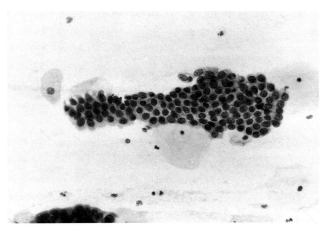

FIG. 3-17. Normal endocervcal cells seen "en face". Note "honeycomb" appearance.

forms of high-grade squamous intraepithelial lesions. This is an important differential diagnostic problem discussed in the chapter on squamous intraepithelial lesions. As the cells mature, they acquire more cytoplasm and, therefore, lower nuclear-to-cytoplasmic ratios, gradually approaching the appearance of mature squamous cells (Figs. 3-13 through 3-15).

Reserve cells, which were relatively uncommon in cervical cytologic samples prior to the use of the endocervical brush sampling devices, are now more commonly identified, particularly in the endocervical samples.

These cells, which are quite undifferentiated in their cytologic appearance, must be distinguished from similar immature-appearing cells of high-grade intraepithelial lesions. Reserve cells tend to appear in tight aggregates, often with more mature-appearing columnar cells attached to a portion of the cellular group. They have scant cytoplasm, round nuclei with smooth nuclear envelopes, and small, distinct nucleoli (Fig. 3-16).

The endocervical cells present in Papanicolaou smears as tall, columnar, mucin-secreting cells with basally located nuclei. Some endocervical cells may be ciliated. Endocervical epithelial cells may be identified as single cells or they may occur as strips or sheets of cells. When viewed on end instead of from the side, the cells look smaller and cuboidal. When seen in a group from this perspective, they have a honeycomb-like appearance. The cytoplasm is finely granular or vacuolated and stains either eosinophilic or cyanophilic. The nuclei are round to oval with finely granular, evenly distributed chromatin. Nucleoli, although present, are generally inconspicuous (Figs. 3-17 through 3-21).

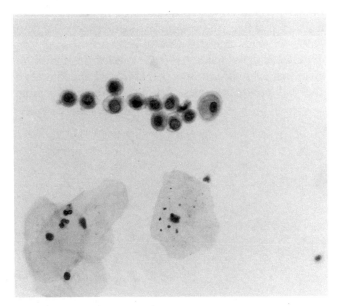

FIG. 3-16. Probable reserve cells. These very small immature-appearing cells are probably derived from reserve cell hyperplasia or very immature subcolumnar metaplasia. Note the very high nuclear cytoplasmic ratio, the smooth nuclear outlines, and absence of hyperchromasia. Superficial squamous cells and a single, slightly more mature metaplastic cell provide size comparisons.

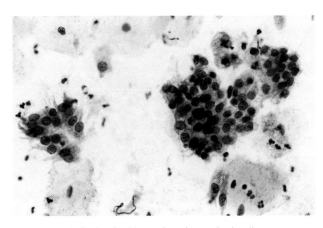

FIG. 3-18. Normal endocervical cells.

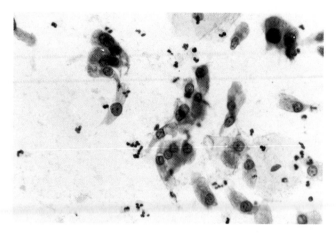

FIG. 3-19. Normal endocervical cells appearing singly and in small aggregates with a side-by-side arrangement.

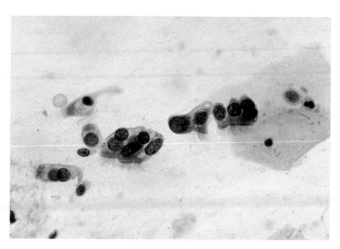

FIG. 3-21. Cilated endocervical cells.

Cells derived from tubal metaplasia have a columnar configuration, with nuclei that are larger and more hyperchromatic than the nuclei of other endocervical cells. They are arranged in sheets or side-by-side configurations and, in the well-preserved state, demonstrate terminal bars and cilia. Single cells with larger nuclei are often evident interspersed between the columnar cells. These apparently represent the intercalated cells seen histologically (Figs. 3-22 and 3-23). Tubal metaplasia can cause differential diagnostic problems in cytologic samples. (See Chapter 7)

Endocrine Effects on Squamous Epithelium

The cellular patterns encountered in normal smears vary with the hormonal state of the patient. Intermediate squamous cells predominate in smears taken during the late luteal and early follicular phases of the cycle. Super-ficial cells predominate around the time of ovulation at the height of estrogen effect. In the postmenopausal patient and in the immediate postpartum period, an atrophic pattern is often seen. Here, the dominant cell is the parabasal cell, which is characterized by relatively small size and oval to round configuration, similar to the immature metaplastic cell.

Exfoliative cytology was used as a means to evaluate hormonal status for many years. Direct determination of hormonal levels, however, has largely supplanted cytologic studies for these evaluations in recent years. Nevertheless, the cytologist is still sometimes asked to estimate hormonal activity based on cytologic observations. Although the squamous epithelium of the cervix is hormonally reactive, the common occurrence of inflammatory changes and the normal presence of squamous metaplastic cells make cervical samples unsuitable for hormonal evaluation. Smears taken from the lateral vaginal wall are the samples of choice for these determina-

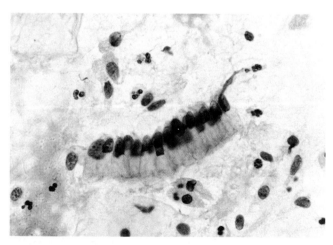

FIG. 3-20. Normal mucin-containing endocervcal cells in a typical picket-fence-like arrangement.

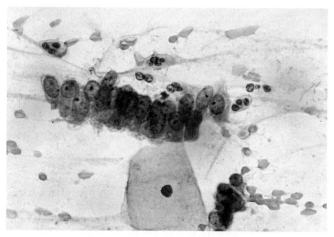

FIG. 3-22. Cells derived from tubal metaplasia. Note cilia and enlarged, somewhat hyperchromatic nuclei.

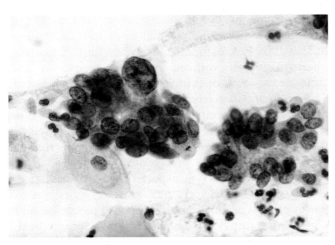

FIG. 3-23. Tubal metaplasia. Notice the large nucleus of one of the cells in this group along with the pseudostratified appearance and mild hypeerchromasia. These features, which are common manifestations of tubal metaplasia, give this aggregate a somewhat atypical appearance.

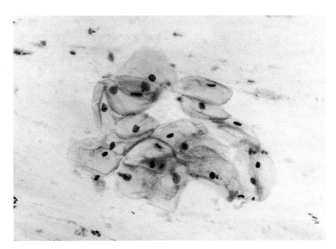

FIG. 3-25. "Folded" intermediate squamous cells. These are typical of a smear taken during the esecond half of the menstrual cycle.

tions, representing a more reliable indication of hormonal status.

Cytologic findings in respect to hormonal assessments have been typically reported in the form of indices. A number of such indices have been utilized. The most commonly preferred index is the "maturation index," which is calculated from a count of parabasal, intermediate, and superficial cells present as a ratio. This index reports the relationship between the parabasal cells (PB), intermediate cells (I), and superficial cells (S), written as PB:I:S. A predominance of superficial cells indicates estrogenic effect, whereas a predominance of parabasal cells indicates the absence of estrogenic effect. It should be noted, however, that in any valid index, only one or two of the places should contain numbers, because no hormonally stimulated situation exists in which all three

cell types occur at the same time. The presence of all three cell types indicates the likelihood of an infectious process or contamination of the sample with material from the cervix. Possible hormonal patterns consist of parabasal cells alone, parabasal and intermediate cells, intermediate cells alone, intermediate and superficial cells, or superficial cells alone. It should be noted, however, that these hormonal evaluations are of value only when compared to other similarly reported evaluations from the same patient. A single evaluation can only indicate the presence or absence of estrogen stimulation. Even with multiple studies, the value of the indices is limited because there is no direct correlation between hormonal levels and the epithelial response.[1]

The "normal" cytologic hormonal patterns vary with the hormonal status of the patient. During infancy, the pattern is an atrophic one, except for the first few days of

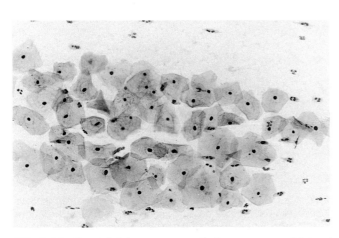

FIG. 3-24. Superficial squamous cells from a smear obtained from a patient on day 14 of her menstrual cycle.

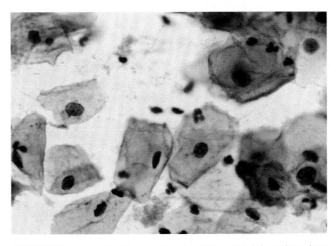

FIG. 3-26. Intermediate squamous cells containing abundant glycogen, from a smear taken during pregnancy.

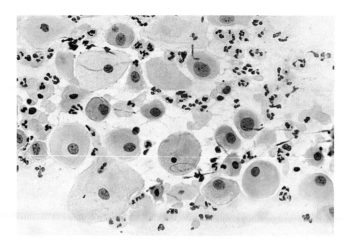

FIG. 3-27. Atrophic cellular pattern in a smear taken from a postmenopausal patient. A similar pattern is seen in the immediate postpartum period.

life, when it is influenced by maternal hormones. A few years prior to the beginning of menstruation, this is replaced by an intermediate pattern, which subsequently changes to a typical cyclic pattern with the onset of adult ovarian function. Throughout the reproductive years, the normal pattern varies with the phase of the menstrual cycle. During the proliferative phase, there is a gradual increase in the proportion of superficial cells in the smear, reaching a maximum at the time of ovulation (Fig. 3-24). The percentage of superficial cells present at ovulation varies considerably from individual to individual. An individual patient, however, consistently shows the same maturation index at ovulation each month. After ovulation, cellular folding begins to occur and the relative number of superficial cells begins to decrease within the next week. An intermediate pattern consisting of crowded, folded intermediate cells exists until menstruation begins.

During pregnancy, an intermediate pattern (MI 0/100/0) is seen because of the high levels of progesterone, but may take several months to develop fully. Numerous intermediate cells with an angulated appearance and abundant amount of cytoplasmic glycogen are present. These cells are often referred to as *navicular cells* because of their supposed configurational resemblance to a boat (Figs. 3-25 and 3-26). In addition, the smear obtained from a pregnant patient is also often marked by marked cytolysis related to the presence of lactobacilli. In the postpartum state, the typical pattern is one of atrophy up to 6 weeks after delivery. This pattern can persist for longer periods of time in the presence of lactation and is not reversed until estrogen production is resumed with the return of normal ovarian function and ovulation.[1,2]

In the postmenopausal patient, the patterns observed may vary. Atrophy may occur quickly, that is, within several months (Figs. 3-27 through 3-29). In other patients, an intermediate pattern may persist indefinitely. The pattern is related to the amount of residual estrogen production. Exogenously administered hormones may alter these patterns. The exact effect of these hormones depends on the status of the epithelium prior to administration, the nature of the hormone, and the dose.

In the Bethesda system terminology for reporting cervical and vaginal smears, the hormonal patterns are reported (only on vaginal smears) simply as being compatible with age and history or not being compatible with age and history. In the latter case, the type of incompatibility should be specified (ie, evidence of marked estrogen effect in a postmenopausal patient with no history of estrogen replacement therapy). If the specimen is unsuitable for hormonal evaluation, the reason (eg, inflammation) should be specified.

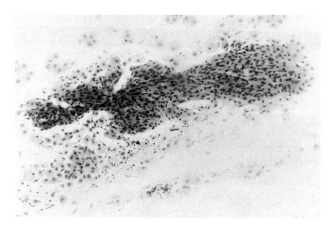

FIG. 3-28. Atrophic smear characterized by numerous parabasal type cells both singly and in large sheet-like aggregates.

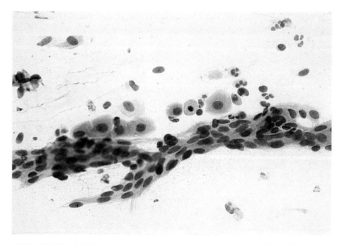

FIG. 3-29. Higher power view of aggregate of atrophic cells. These cells shold not be confused with syncytial like aggregates seen in high-grade intraepithelial lesions. The regularity of the nuclei and the bland chromatin are typical of atrophy.

NORMAL HISTOLOGY
OF THE ENDOMETRIUM

The histology of the normal endometrium varies with the hormonal status of the patient and the time of the cycle in the cyclic woman. Prior to menarche, the endometrial mucosa is relatively thin and consists of simple tubular glands within a moderately cellular background composed of stromal cells. With the onset of ovarian activity and ovulation, the endometrium undergoes cyclic changes in association with hormonal activity. Under the influence of estrogen during the follicular phase of the normal menstrual cycle, the endometrial glandular epithelium and stroma undergo proliferation (Fig. 3-30). The glands become elongated and tortuous, and the endometrial mucosa becomes thickened. With the onset of ovulation, the endometrium comes under the influence of progesterone produced by the corpus luteum. This induces the endometrium to become secretory and the proliferative activity within the glandular epithelium ceases. The first morphologic indication of ovulation and the onset of secretory activity is the appearance on the first day after ovulation of subnuclear vacuoles within the columnar cells lining the endometrial glands (Fig. 3-31). The vacuoles, which are uniformly present by the third postovulatory day, become supranuclear and extrude their contents by the process of decapitation secretion into the gland lumina. At this point, on about the fifth day after ovulation, the gland lumina are seen to contain secretory material. The stroma becomes edematous and then develops a pseudodecidual reaction marked by an increase in the number of stromal cells and the amount of cytoplasm they contain as the endometrium becomes prepared for possible implantation. If fertilization does not occur, the endometrial stroma becomes infiltrated by granulocytes and breakdown of the stroma and glandular structures occurs as the progesterone level produced

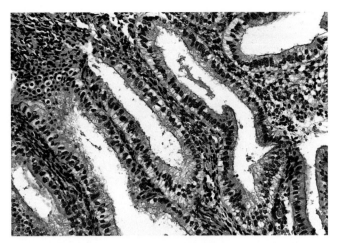

FIG. 3-31. Early secretory endometrium characterized by longer more complex glands and numerous subnuclear secretory vacuoles within the lining cells.

by the corpus luteum drops. With the onset of the breakdown of the endometrial tissue that is no longer under hormonal support, menstrual bleeding begins, marking day 1 of the next menstrual cycle (Fig. 3-32).

After the cessation of ovarian function and the onset of menopause, the endometrium ceases its pattern of cyclic changes and becomes inactive. Eventually, in the absence of hormonal stimulation, atrophy occurs. In the postmenopausal state, no endometrial cells are shed and, therefore, endometrial cells are not normally found in cervical vaginal cytologic samples.

NORMAL CYTOLOGY
OF THE ENDOMETRIUM

Endometrial cells are normally shed from the endometrium in the first half of the menstrual cycle and,

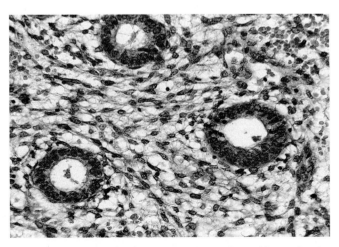

FIG. 3-30. Early proliferative endometrium. Note simple, small tubular glands.

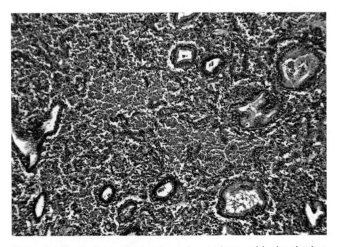

FIG. 3-32. Early menstrual endometrium with beginning breakdown of the stroma.

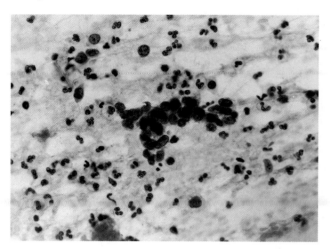

FIG. 3-33. Normal endometrial cells in a smear taken on day 4 of cycle.

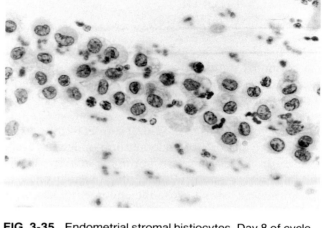

FIG. 3-35. Endometrial stromal histiocytes. Day 8 of cycle.

therefore, can be expected to be identified in the normal female in smears made from day 1 through about day 12. They normally are not present after day 14 of the normal cycle or in the postmenopausal state.

Normal endometrial epithelial cells can be identified as groups of cells in small clusters and, less commonly, as single cells. The cells have small, round nuclei that range from 30 to 35 μm^2 in area. The cytoplasm is scant, basophilic, and sometimes vacuolated (Figs. 3-33 and 3-34). The cluster arrangements are three-dimensional and vary from being composed of a few cells to larger groups made up of numerous cells. Stromal cells vary in appearance from round to oval cells resembling small histiocytes that are thought to be derived from the more superficial portions of the endometrial stroma to small spindle-shaped cells with scant cytoplasm that are derived from the deeper portions of the endometrial stroma (Figs. 3-35 and 3-36). During the first few days of the

cycle, numerous fragments of degenerating endometrial tissue are present as part of the menstrual material. In the period from day 4 through day 8, the Papanicolaou smear is marked by the presence of numerous endometrial "histiocytes" and ball-like clusters of endometrial stroma surrounded by endometrial epithelial cells (Figs. 3-37 and 3-38). This pattern is well recognized and the period encompassed by its appearance has been termed *exodus*.

INCIDENTAL FINDINGS ON NORMAL SMEARS

In addition to the normal cells derived from the vagina, cervix, or endometrium, it is not unusual to note a variety of other cellular or noncellular elements in normal smears. Spermatozoa, for example, are readily identified (Fig. 3-39). Very rarely, cells that may be derived from the seminal vesicles of the male may be encoun-

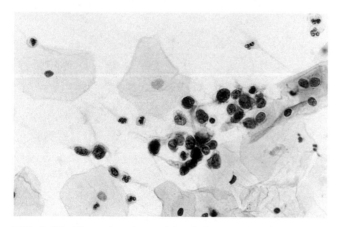

FIG. 3-34. Normal endometrial cells in a smear taken on day 4 of cycle.

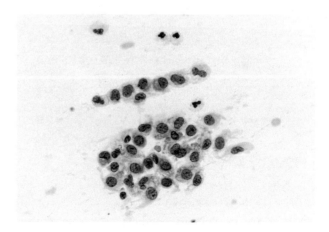

FIG. 3-36. Deep endometrial stromal cells.

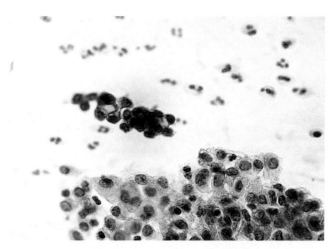

FIG. 3-37. Normal endometrial cells and superficial stromal cells. Day 6.

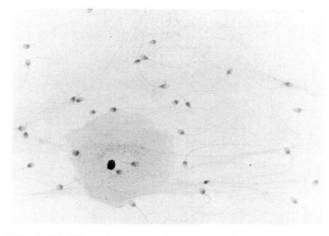

FIG. 3-39. Normal sperm with a superficial squamous cell from a cervical smear.

tered. These cells, which apparently may be present in seminal fluid, have an atypical appearance. Their origin may be suggested by the presence of the brown pigment in the cytoplasm that is characteristic of these cells, as seen in histologic sections of these structures.[3] Occasionally, normal-appearing transitional cells may occur in Papanicolaou smears (Fig. 3-40). Except in the unusual circumstance of a vaginal-vesical fistula, these types of cells are usually the result of the inadvertent or intentional sampling of the area of the urethral os. It should also be noted that transitional metaplasia of the cervical epithelium can occur and, therefore, transitional-type epithelial cells may actually originate from the cervix.

Other structures found represent artifacts or contaminants of one kind or another. The so-called "blue blobs," as depicted in Figure 3-41, are found in association with atrophy and atrophic vaginitis. Their exact nature is de-

bated. Although originally thought by most observers to represent inspissated mucus, it is now believed by others that these structures represent degenerated parabasal cells. In any event, the presence of these bodies is of no significance. Their identification is of importance only insofar as they are not confused with other more significant findings.

Psammoma-like bodies may be seen in cervical smears. Although such structures have been traditionally associated with papillary neoplasms, particularly papillary serous neoplasms of the ovary, their presence does not necessarily indicate a neoplastic process. They may also be seen as part of a reactive process such as papillary mesothelial hyperplasia or in association with cells that appear to be otherwise entirely normal (Fig. 3-42).

Alternaria may appear on Papanicolaou smears as an airborne contaminant that may find its way onto a slide

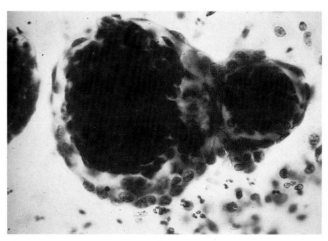

FIG. 3-38. Normal endometrial epithelial cells and stroma (dark cells in center of cluster, as seen as part of the "exodus" pattern. Day 6.

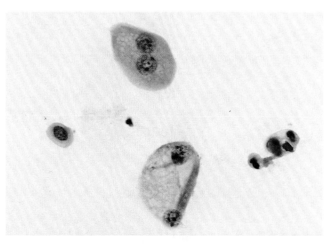

FIG. 3-40. Normal transitional epithelial cells, a rare finding in routine Papanicolaou smears.

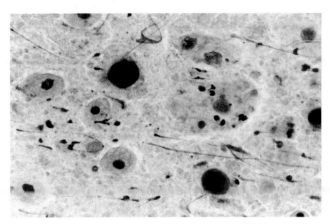

FIG. 3-41. "Blue blobs" in an atrophic smear. These structures are felt to most likely represent degenerative parabasal cells.

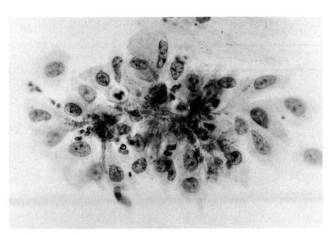

FIG. 3-44. Hematoidin crystals ("cockle burrs") surrounded by histiocytes.

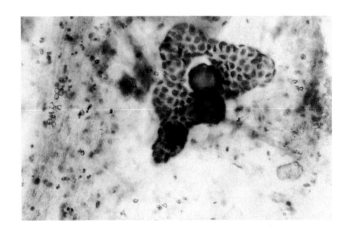

FIG. 3-42. Psammoma bodies associated with cytologically benign epithelial cells. An uncommon finding which in itself is not diagnostic of a neoplastic process.

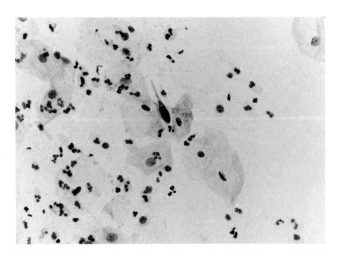

FIG. 3-43. *Alternaria.* A fungal organism that is a contaminant in Papanicolaou smears.

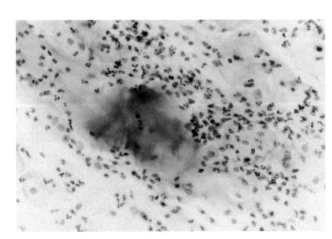

FIG. 3-45. Lubricating jelly. This amorphous-appearing material typically has a light blue tinge when present on smears.

during preparation or processing procedures. Its characteristic form is depicted in Figure 3-43. Hematoidin crystals with a characteristic appearance likened to "cockle burrs" are sometimes identified (Fig. 3-44) and, occasionally, lubricating jelly in the form of amorphous bluish staining material on the slide may be found as a contaminant[4] (Fig. 3-45).

Starch granules, vegetable fibers, and insect parts have also been reported as smear contaminants.

REFERENCES

1. Wied GL, Bibbo M, Keebler CM. Evaluation of the endocrinologic condition of the femal genital tract by exfoliative cytology. In Wied GL, Keebler CM, Koss LG, et al (eds). Compendium on diagnostic cytology, 7th ed. Chicago: Tutorials of Cytology, 1992:44.
2. Meisels A. Hormonal cytology. In Wied GL, Keebler CM, Koss LG, et al (eds). Compendium on diagnostic cytology, 7th ed. Chicago: Tutorials of Cytology, 1992:52.
3. Meisels A, Ayotte D. Cells from the seminal vesicles: contaminants of the V.C.E. smear. Acta Cytol 1976;20:211.
4. Capaldo G, LeGolvan DP, Dramczyk JE. Hematoidin crystals in cervicovaginal smears. Acta Cytol 1983;27:237.

ADDITIONAL READING

Bibbo M. Comprehensive cytopathology. Philadelphia: WB Saunders, 1991:85.
Keebler CM, Somrak TM (eds). The manual of cytotechnology. Chicago: ASCP Press, 1993.
Koss LG. Diagnostic cytology and its histologic basis. Philadelphia: JB Lippincott, 1992:251.
Meisels A, Morin C. Cytopathology of the uterine cervix. Chcago: ASCP Press, 1991:15.
Patten SF. Cytology of normal epithelia and benign proliferative reactions of the uterine cervix. Chicago: Tutorials of Cytology, 1973.
Patten SF. Diagnostic cytology of the uterine cervix. New York: S Karger, 1978:30.

Gynecologic Cytopathology. Edited by
Thomas A. Bonfiglio and Yener S. Erozan.
Lippincott–Raven Publishers, Philadelphia, © 1997.

CHAPTER 4

Benign Cellular Changes

Thomas A. Bonfiglio

The vaginal and cervical epithelia are subject to a variety of stimuli that result in morphologic alterations in their component cells. Infectious or physical agents, chemotherapy, radiation, and trauma all can cause damage to epithelium and result in reactive changes that are manifest cytologically. These benign changes are evident in cellular samples taken from the involved areas and must be distinguished from the often morphologically similar cellular changes that are due to preneoplastic or neoplastic processes. In the Bethesda classification system, these benign cellular changes are divided into those associated with specific infectious agents and other reactive cellular changes.

CYTOLOGIC CHANGES ASSOCIATED WITH INFECTION

The vagina and the uterine cervix both harbor microbial organisms, including bacteria, viruses, and fungi. Some of these are pathogenic and cause infection and inflammation in most women. Other organisms result in neither inflammation nor symptoms and are considered normal flora. Even these organisms, however, may cause symptomatic inflammation in some circumstances. Lactobacilli, *Staphylococcus epidermidis,* and *Streptococcus viridans,* for example, are frequently present and do not result in symptomatic lesions. *Gardnerella,* on the other hand, may be found in many asymptomatic women, but also is a common finding in bacterial vaginosis, a condition characterized by a nonirritating, malodorous vaginal discharge. In this condition, the vagina is colonized by a polymicrobial mixture of *Gardnerella,* other aerobes, and anaerobes.

In addition to the identification of organisms and specific cytologic changes that are related to certain types of

T. A. Bonfiglio: Department of Pathology and Laboratory Medicine, University of Rochester Medical Center, Rochester, New York 14642.

infections on cytologic smears, there are also a number of less specific cytologic findings that are associated with vaginal or cervical inflammation. Small numbers of neutrophils may be found in normal smears, but very large numbers of these cells characterize acute infection. Indeed, these inflammatory cells may be so numerous in acute infections that other cellular elements are obscured. In long-standing chronic cervicitis, a dense lymphoid infiltrate with the formation of germinal centers may be present. This condition, termed *chronic follicular (lymphocytic) cervicitis,* is characterized in cytologic samples by the presence of numerous lymphocytes and tinctorial body macrophages[1] (Figs. 4-1 and 4-2).

As a nonspecific response to inflammation, mild nuclear enlargement, in the range of 1.5 to 2 times normal, may be seen in squamous cells. Endocervical cells may show even greater nuclear enlargement (Fig. 4-3). The nuclear envelope of both types of cells remains smooth and only mild hyperchromasia, if any, is present. Binucleation may be evident in some squamous cells in inflammatory smears (Fig. 4-4). Cellular degeneration may also occur and is manifested in a number of ways on smears. Cytoplasmic degenerative changes may result in the presence of small, ill-defined perinuclear halos that must be distinguished from the halos that are characteristic of human papillomavirus infection (Figs. 4-5 and 4-6). Nuclei also show degenerative changes in the form of pyknosis, karyorrhexis, or simply loss of nuclear detail (Fig. 4-7). Inflammatory changes of this type may occur in either squamous or glandular epithelial cells.

INFECTIOUS PROCESSES CAUSED BY COMMON, SPECIFIC ORGANISMS

Lactobacillus (Döderlein's Bacilli)

As mentioned earlier, *Lactobacillus* species are considered to be part of the normal vaginal flora and are not included as a specific category in the Bethesda system.

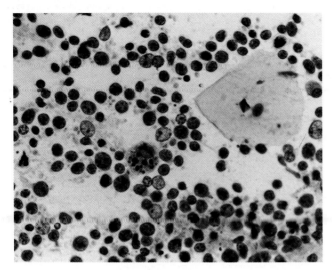

FIG. 4-1. Chronic follicular cervicitis. There are numerous lymphocytes and tinctorial body macrophages.

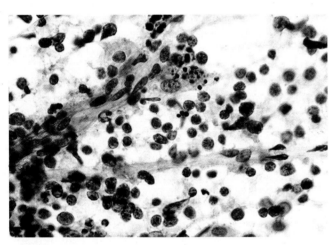

FIG. 4-2. Chronic follicular cervicitis. Note capillary structure on left.

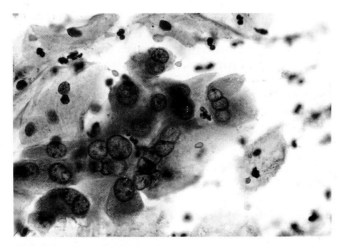

FIG. 4-3. Endocervical cells demonstrating reactive nuclear changes.

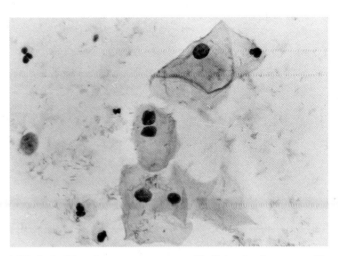

FIG. 4-4. Binucleate squamous epithelial cells. A nonspecific change associated with inflammation.

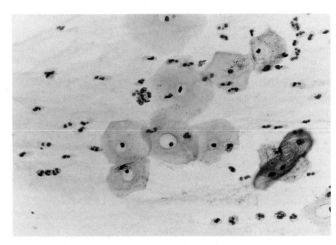

FIG. 4-5. Squamous cells demonstrating small perinuclear halos and normal nuclei. This type of halo is a nonspecific change and is not indicative of human papillomavirus effect.

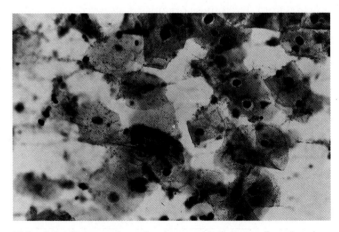

FIG. 4-6. Squamous cells demonstrating small perinuclear halos as a result of inflammation.

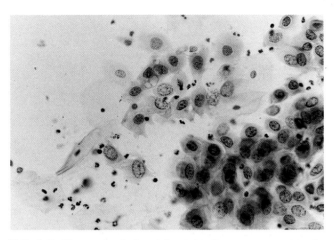

FIG. 4-7. Karyorrhexis involving immature squamous metaplastic cells. This degenerative nuclear change as well as simple loss of nuclear detail is sometimes seen as a manifestation of inflammation.

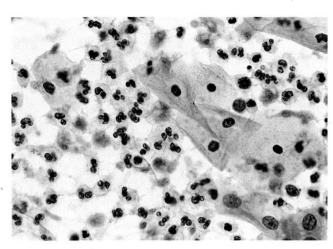

FIG. 4-10. Trichomoniasis. Note organisms, numerous neutrophils, and small perinuclear halos in squamous cells.

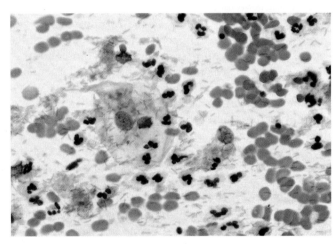

FIG. 4-8. Lactobacilli and secondary cytolysis.

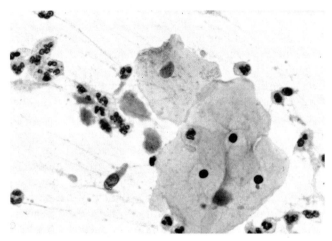

FIG. 4-11. Trichomoniasis. Two relatively large organisms are noted in the center of the slide. The ill-defined eccentric nuclei are an important diagnostic feature.

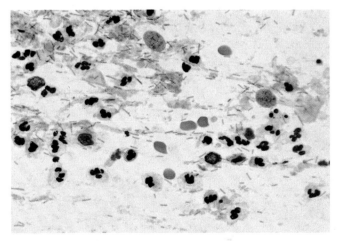

FIG. 4-9. Bare nuclei and cytoplasmic debri secondary to lactobacilli.

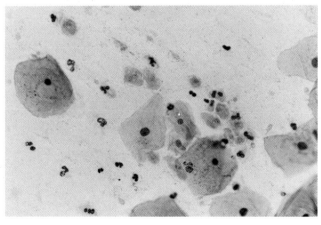

FIG. 4-12. Trichomoniasis. Numerous organisms are noted in this field.

Although numerous strains of this organism have been identified, *Lactobacillus acidophilus* is the one most commonly found in the vagina. However, the organism is found in only a relatively small percentage of patients. These rod-shaped bacteria are associated with an acidic vaginal pH and typically cause cytolysis of the glycogen-rich intermediate cells that are present. Superficial cells, however, are resistant to cytolysis by lactobacilli. Cytologic specimens in which this process is evident have a crowded cellular appearance with a relatively clean background, except for the numerous organisms present. There is usually no significant accompanying inflammation[2] (Figs. 4-8 and 4-9).

Trichomonas vaginalis

Perhaps the most common example of cytologic changes induced by an inflammatory process are those seen in association with trichomoniasis. The organisms, in the well-preserved state, appear as oval to round structures measuring from 10 to 25 μm in diameter. The cytoplasm stains a pale gray-blue with Papanicolaou stain. The nucleus is eccentric, and is usually ill-defined and degenerated-appearing (Figs. 4-10 through 4-13). However, identification of the nuclear structure is important for accurate diagnosis of infection because mucus, degenerated metaplastic cells, or neutrophils or cytoplasmic fragments occurring in association with cytolysis may mimic the appearance of the organism (Figs. 4-14 and 4-15). The presence of red cytoplasmic granules also helps in identifying organisms. Flagella, which are characteristic and provide the motility typical of the parasite in wet preparations, are seldom seen in fixed cervical smear samples.[3,4] The inflammation induced by this protozoan results in mild to moderate enlargement of squamous cell nuclei, usually in the range of 1.5 to 2 times

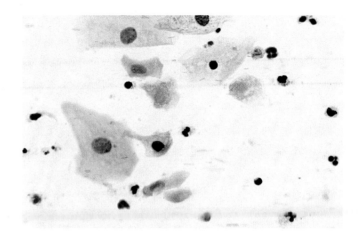

FIG. 4-14. Degenerating cells mimicking the appearance of *Trichomonas*.

normal. In addition, small, ill-defined perinuclear halos may become evident within the cytoplasm (see Fig. 4-13). The relatively minor degree of nuclear enlargement and the absence of hyperchromasia usually permits easy differentiation of these changes from those of intraepithelial lesions. The presence of the etiologic agent explains the changes seen and usually negates the necessity for other than routine cytologic follow-up. In some cases wherein the nuclear alterations are more severe, the distinction from an early intraepithelial lesion may be more difficult and classification as atypical squamous cells of undetermined significance may be appropriate. In these instances, repeat cytologic examination after treatment of the infection may be indicated. Inflammation-related cellular changes rapidly revert to normal with resolution of the inflammatory process. Despite early interest in the possibility, there is no evidence that trichomoniasis is related to the etiology of cervical neoplasia.[5,6]

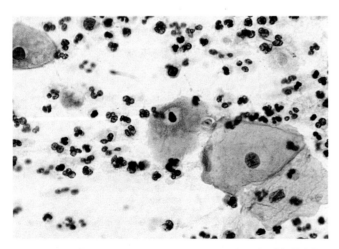

FIG. 4-13. Small perinuclear halos associated with *Trichomonas* infection.

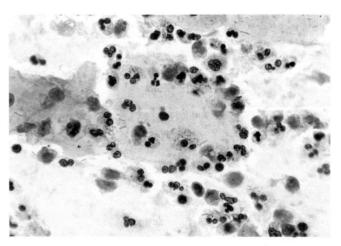

FIG. 4-15. Degenerating cells associated with inflammation resembling trichomoniasis.

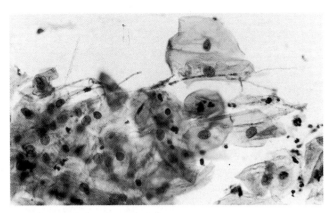

FIG. 4-16. *Candida.* Both pseudohyphae and spore forms are evident.

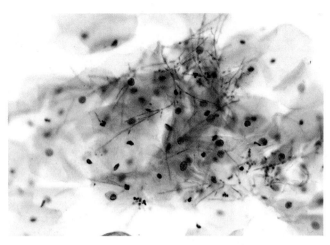

FIG. 4-18. *Candida.* Low-power view showing numerous organisms and clumped epithelial cells.

Candida albicans

Candida albicans is the most common fungal organism to infect the lower female genital tract. The fungus is identified in some patients who are asymptomatic, but in most cases, infection is associated with pruritus and a white vaginal discharge. The organisms appear as pseudohyphae forms and as round to oval budding yeasts. Typically, there is an associated heavy neutrophilic infiltrate. The epithelial cells may show a moderate degree of nuclear enlargement and other nonspecific changes, such as indistinct perinuclear halos and nuclear degeneration (Figs. 4-16 through 4-18). *Torulopsis glabrata* and other fungal types may also be encountered in cervicovaginal smears and are often difficult to distinguish from *Candida* on Papanicolaou-stained preparations. *Torulopsis glabrata* may produce a vaginitis similar to candidiasis, whereas other fungi are often present only as contaminants.[7]

Bacterial Vaginosis

Formerly referred to as nonspecific vaginitis, bacterial vaginosis is a condition characterized by a malodorous vaginal discharge. A polymicrobial bacterial etiology is proposed based on the frequent detection of a mixed bacterial population on vaginal smears. The organism, *Gardnerella vaginalis* (formerly called *Haemophilus vaginalis*) has been isolated from up to 90% of patients with this syndrome and is felt to be etiologically related to the process in the majority of cases.[8] The prevailing concept, however, is that bacterial vaginosis is a synergistic infection involving a variety of bacterial organisms. Reflecting this concept, this condition in the Bethesda classification system is reported as "Predominance of coccobacilli consistent with shift in vaginal flora."

In addition to the mixed bacterial flora and relative absence of lactobacilli, the characteristic cytologic finding is the presence of "clue cells," mature squamous epithelial cells that are covered by coccobacilli, typically extending beyond the cell margins[9] (Figs. 4-19 and 4-20).

Herpes Simplex Genitalis

Herpesvirus infection is a disease that is manifest clinically by the occurrence of painful vesicles involving the skin and mucous membranes at various body sites. Two distinct viral types exist, herpes simplex virus type 1 (HSV-1) and herpes simplex virus type 2 (HSV-2). The former usually involves the perioral area and results in the typical cold sore or fever blister, whereas the latter, which is transmitted through genital secretions, involves the genital or perianal areas. Clinically, HSV-2 infection results in painful, blistering eruptions of the genital skin or mucous membranes. The infection is almost always symptomatic in the acute phase in men, but may be relatively asymptomatic in women.

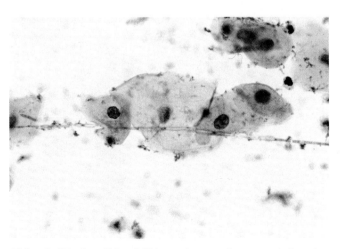

FIG. 4-17. *Candida.* Mild nuclear enlargement is also evident.

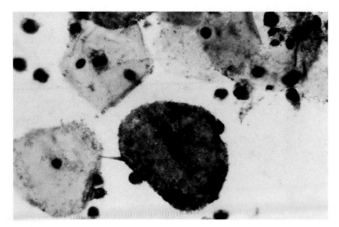

FIG. 4-19. Bacterial vaginosis. A typical "clue cell" is pictured with coccobacilli covering the cytoplasm.

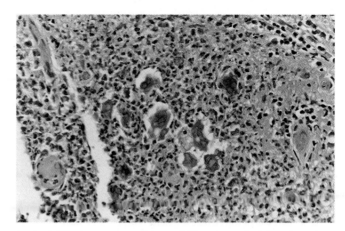

FIG. 4-21. Low-power view of biopsy material from a herpetic lesion. Note numerous mutinucleated cells with typical features of herpesvirus effect and marked inflammation.

Infection results in well-recognized and diagnostic cytologic alterations consisting of intranuclear, eosinophilic inclusions; multinucleation; nuclear molding; chromatin margination; and a "ground-glass" appearance of the chromatin in infected cells (Figs. 4-21 through 4-24). Other nonspecific cytologic changes commonly associated with herpetic infections include karyomegaly of squamous cells and reparative or regenerative changes. The changes specified are most commonly caused by HSV-2 in the genital tract, but similar changes can occur with HSV-1 infection.[10,11] Although it was formerly believed that herpesvirus may play an etiologic role in the development of carcinoma of the cervix, the evidence to support this theory has never been adequate.[12] As discussed in Chapter 5, current molecular techniques have provided very strong evidence that it is another virus, the human papillomavirus, that is the etiologic agent.

Actinomyces

Actinomyces organisms do not occur as part of the normal flora of the genital tract. Their presence is usually the result of an ascending infection, often found in association with a foreign body, such as an intrauterine device, vaginal pessary, or vaginal tampon, that has been left in place for a prolonged period. Although the organisms frequently represent a commensal infection, they are capable of tissue invasion and are known to be associated with serious pelvic infections in some patients. For a detailed review, see the excellent paper by Gupta.[13]

Actinomyces appear in cervical or vaginal smears as clumps of dark, basophilic, filamentous organisms. The centers of the clumps are dense and opaque, with the filamentous nature of the individual structures visible at the margins (Figs. 4-25 through 4-28). These may be as-

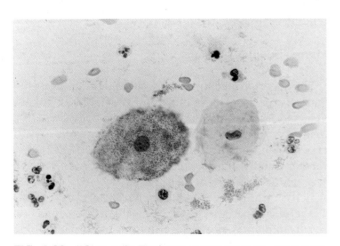

FIG. 4-20. "Clue cell" The coccobacilli typically extend beyond the cell margins.

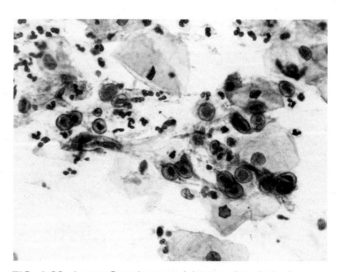

FIG. 4-22. Large Cowdry type A intranuclear inclusions are evident in these cells. These are typical of herpes infection.

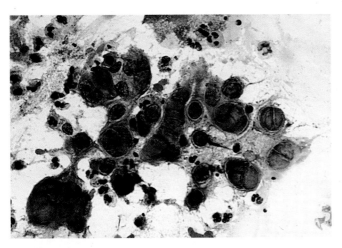

FIG. 4-23. Numerous mutinucleated giant cells typical of herpesvirus cytopathic effect. Note the nuclear moulding, ground glass appearance and chromatin margination.

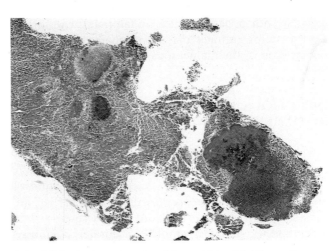

FIG. 4-26. *Actinomyces* involving endometrial tissue in a curettage sample. Although in most cases *actinomyces* cause only a superficial comensal infection, in some instances, tissue invasion occurs and serious pelvic infection results.

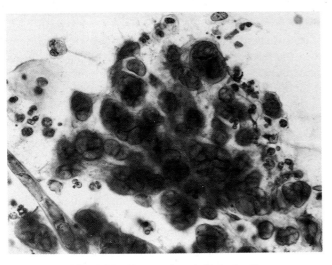

FIG. 4-24. Herpesvirus-infected cells.

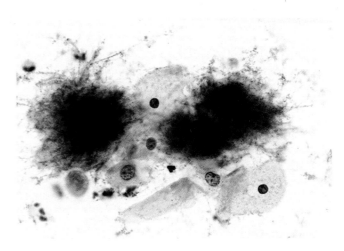

FIG. 4-27. *Actinomyces*-like organisms in a smear from a patient wearing an intrauterine device.

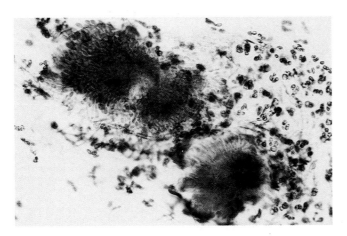

FIG. 4-25. *Actinomyces*-like organisms in a cervical smear associated with marked inflammation.

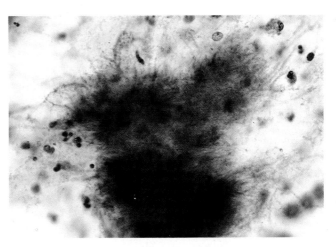

FIG. 4-28. *Actinomyces*-like organisms. Note the fine filaments radiating from the periphery of the clumps.

sociated with a dense, acute, inflammatory infiltrate. Typical sulfur granules may occasionally be seen, and calcification of the filamentous structures is sometimes noted.

INFECTIOUS PROCESSES CAUSED BY OTHER ORGANISMS

A wide variety of other organisms that are not included in a specific category of the Bethesda system may also be identified in cervical or vaginal smears. Some of these, such as the *Lactobacillus* mentioned earlier, are considered part of the normal flora. Others, such as *Chlamydia* species (see later), cannot be accurately diagnosed in routine cervical or vaginal cytologic specimens and, therefore, do not appear as a diagnostic category. Other pathogenic organisms, however, do have specific diagnostic characteristics, and it is often appropriate to mention their presence on the cytopathology report.

Leptotrichia buccalis

Formerly called *Leptothrix vaginalis*, *Leptotrichia buccalis* are usually found on cervical smears in the form of thin, filamentous, hair-like, gray-staining structures. Alone, they seldom result in significant inflammation, but they are commonly found with trichomonads, and in this situation, are associated with inflammation. *Leptotrichia* should be distinguished from the previously described *Actinomyces*, another filamentous organism that occurs in cervical or vaginal smears (Figs. 4-29 and 4-30).

Cytomegalovirus

Cytomegalovirus is a common DNA virus belonging to the herpesvirus group. More than 50% of the adult

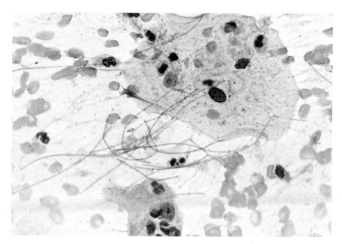

FIG. 4-30. *Leptotrichia* in association with *Trichomonas*. These two organisms often coexist.

female population can be demonstrated to have antibodies to this agent. Its identification in cytologic specimens from the female genital tract is unusual. The infections are usually asymptomatic, but diagnostic inclusions can be identified in cervical smear specimens from both immunocompetent and immunocompromised hosts. The detection rate in cytologic samples appears to have increased in recent years. This may be related to the more widespread use of brush devices to sample the endocervical canal. Indeed, the infected cells appear to be of endocervical glandular origin, and cytomegalovirus is recognized to be tropic for glandular rather than squamous epithelium.

Cytologically, although the changes may be confused with those of herpesvirus, the morphologic features are usually quite distinct. The classic finding is a single, very large, round to oval, red to purple, intranuclear inclusion surrounded by a thin halo (Figs. 4-31 through 4-33*B*). In

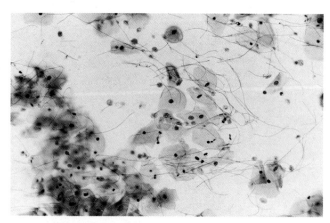

FIG. 4-29. *Leptotrichia.* The long, thin filamentous structures are characteristic.

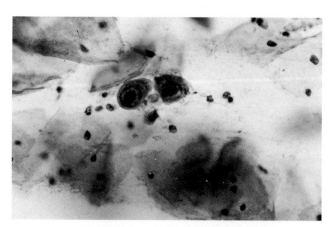

FIG. 4-31. Cytomegalovirus cervicitis. The intranuclear inclusion is much larger than those associated with herpesvirus.

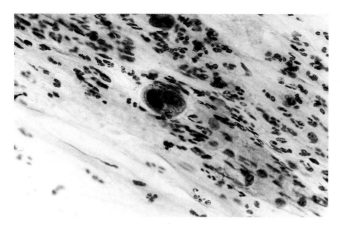

FIG. 4-32. Cytomegalovirus intranuclear inclusion.

some cases, small, basophilic-staining cytoplasmic inclusions may also be present.

Other Viral Infections

Other viruses may infect the cervical tissues. The most common is the human papillomavirus, which, because of its key role in the carcinogenic process in the cervix, is discussed in detail in Chapter 5. Viruses much less commonly identified in cervical cytologic material include the human polyomavirus and adenovirus.[14]

Chlamydia trachomatis Infections

Chlamydia species have been implicated in a number of human infections, including trachoma inclusion conjunctivitis, lymphogranuloma venereum, and other sexually transmitted inflammatory reactions that involve the genital tract. The morphologic changes associated with chlamydial infections of the cervix have been studied by Gupta and colleagues,[15] but the diagnostic value of these morphologic findings is limited. These authors divided the cytologic alterations associated with chlamydial infections into three stages. In general, affected cells are either metaplastic squamous or endocervical glandular cells and are frequently multinucleate. In stage I, the earliest recognizable alterations are described as consisting of a diffuse, acidophilic or cyanophilous "coccoid granularity" within a "porous" cytoplasm. In the second stage, this diffuse coccoid granularity is joined by single or multiple cytoplasmic inclusion bodies measuring 1 to 2 μm in diameter. In the final stage, multiple, often molded, cyanophilic inclusion bodies surrounded by a clear zone are described, intermixed with the diffuse, acidophilic coccoid particles in the cytoplasm. In all stages of chlamydial infection, nuclear enlargement also occurs (Figs. 4-34*A* through 4-34*B*).

Other investigators also have studied the cytologic changes associated with *Chlamydia* and have attempted to correlate cytologic findings with the results of cultures and immunocytochemical antibody studies.[16–18] In general, there has been relatively poor correlation between cytologic diagnoses and confirmatory studies by tissue culture and antibody techniques. In view of this, the cytologic diagnosis of *Chlamydia* infection in gynecologic cytology specimens cannot be considered to be an accurate methodology. Recent advances in other diagnostic methodologies, including cultures, immunostaining techniques, and methods based on enzyme-linked immunosorbent assays, have established these as the diagnostic methods of choice.

An interesting observation noted in relation to the studies of chlamydial infections is that the cytologic finding that appears to have the best correlation with infection with this agent is the presence of chronic follicular cervicitis (see Figs. 4-1 and 4-2). There are reports that

A
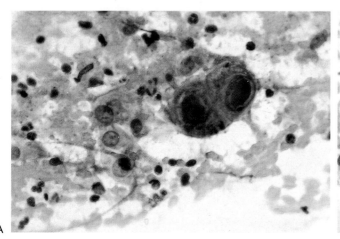

B
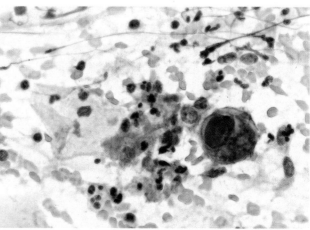

FIG. 4-33. (A,B). Cytomegalovirus virus cervicitis. Note the reddish-purple color of the typical large intranuclear inclusions. The basophilic cytoplasmic structures are also characteristic.

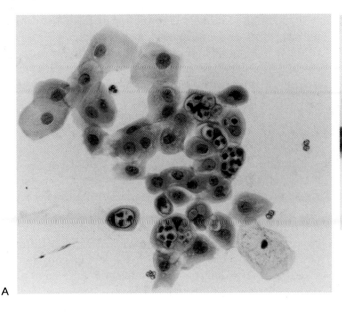

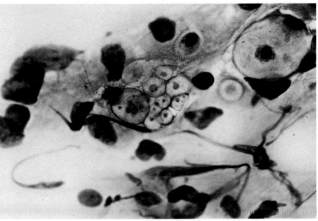

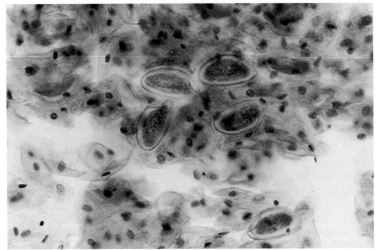

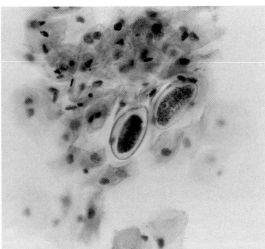

FIG. 4-34. (A,B) Cytoplasmic inclusions of the type originally thought to be indicative of *Chlamydia.* This type of alteration, however, has not been shown to be a reliable diagnostic indicator of a Chlamydia infection.

FIG. 4-35. (A,B) *Enterobius vermicularis* ova in a cervical smear.

as many as half of the patients with this finding may have a *Chlamydia* infection.[19,20]

Unusual Organisms

Several varieties of protozoan and parasitic organisms may rarely be seen in cervical or vaginal smears. *Entamoeba histolytica* are identified fairly frequently in this type of specimen in parts of the world where intestinal tract infection is common. Similarly, infection with *Balantidium coli* has been reported in the vagina. Schistosomiasis and the ova of several worms, particularly pinworms *(Enterobius vermicularis)* (Figs. 4-35 *A,B*), may also be identified in Papanicolaou smear samples.[2,21]

REACTIVE CELLULAR CHANGES

The category of reactive cellular changes encompasses those benign changes that are associated with inflammation, radiation therapy, the presence of an intrauterine device, and other, less specific causes.

Cytopathology of Epithelial Repair and Regeneration

Specific and characteristic modifications of epithelial cells occur in association with epithelial injury that results in the necessity to regenerate or repair the injured epithelium. It is important that those who evaluate cytologic material be familiar with these manifestations of epithelial repair and regeneration as they occur in cytologic samples. The cytologic changes of typical repair are included in this category. The more atypical reactions of this type are included in the categories of atypical squamous or glandular cells of undetermined significance.

Typical reparative reactions involve both squamous

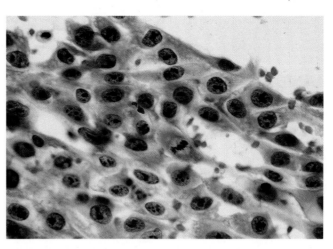

FIG. 4-37. Loose sheet of cells derived from a reparative epithelial reaction. Note mitotic figure, a common finding.

and columnar epithelium and are characterized morphologically by the presence of sheets or syncytium-like arrangements of cells with nuclear enlargement and prominent nucleoli (Figs. 4-36 through 4-39). The nucleoli may be multiple and may vary in both size and configuration. Chromatin remains finely granular and evenly distributed, and nuclear outlines are smooth. Mitoses are identified and may be frequent, but the mitotic figures are morphologically normal. Single cells with similar features are rare.[22]

Cytopathologic Changes Related to Therapy

The morphologic characteristics of both normal and abnormal epithelial cells of the cervix are altered by various therapeutic procedures. Cryosurgery, electrocautery, and biopsy all cause short-term cellular alterations

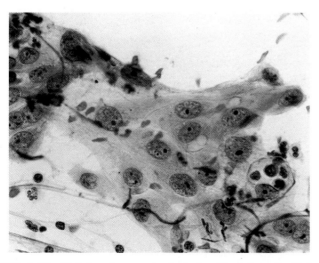

FIG. 4-36. Cellular changes typical of epithelial repair. Note the large nuclei, prominent nucleoli and bland chromatin.

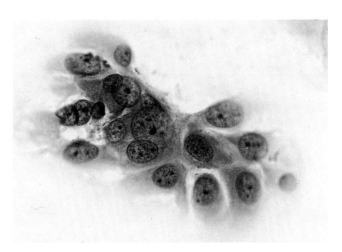

FIG. 4-38. Reparative changes involving cells that appear to be of endocervical origin.

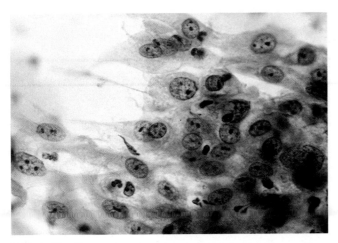

FIG. 4-39. Reparative changes. Note the multiple nucleoli in some of the cells.

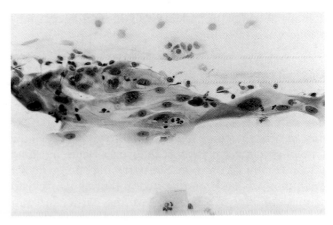

FIG. 4-41. Reparative reaction in radiated patient.

that are identifiable in cervical samples. Usually, these changes are similar to those described in the section on reparative reactions. Cryosurgery and electrocautery may also produce degenerative and reactive changes, including nuclear enlargement and hyperchromasia, which could be confused with cells originating from an intraepithelial neoplastic process. Because of this, it is often advisable not to perform cytologic studies within the first 2 months after cautery or cryosurgery.[23,24]

Radiation therapy, which is commonly utilized for the treatment of cervical carcinoma, has profound effects on epithelial cells. These changes have been described in detail in the literature.[25,26] In the acute phase, the cellular manifestations of radiation in normal cells include a marked increase in size, cytoplasmic vacuolation, and a polychromatic staining reaction. Nuclei are enlarged and typically demonstrate degenerative changes, including

loss of nuclear detail and vacuolation. Bizarre nuclear and cytoplasmic forms may be encountered (Figs. 4-40 through 4-42). Similar changes occur within the malignant cell population and tend to emphasize many of the cytologic features of malignancy. The acute radiation effect usually dissipates a few weeks after the completion of treatment, but may persist for several months in some instances. Tumor cells, however, should disappear within 4 to 8 weeks after the completion of therapy. The persistence of tumor cells without evidence of a radiation effect beyond this time suggests residual carcinoma.

Although in the majority of cases, the effects of radiation disappear from the cellular sample after a period of time, in some patients, changes persist. These include nuclear enlargement, mild hyperchromasia, and a polychromatic staining reaction of the cytoplasm. These changes need to be distinguished from recurrent or new intraepithelial lesions (ie, postirradiation dysplasia).[27] These lesions are morphologically identical to classic squamous intraepithelial lesions. It is important to note, however, as Patten has pointed out, that patients in

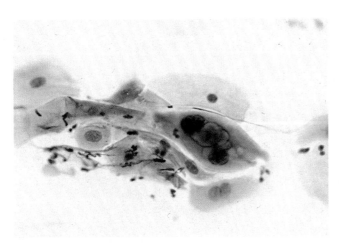

FIG. 4-40. Acute radiation effect. Nuclear enlargement, mutinucleation, cytoplasmic vacuolation, and amphophilia are evident.

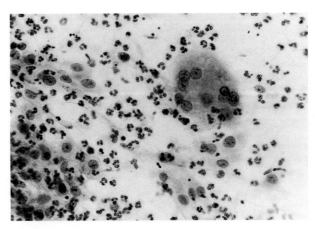

FIG. 4-42. Acute inflammatory cells and mutinucleated histiocytes in a patient undergoing pelvic radiation.

whom postirradiation dysplasia develops within 3 years of the completion of radiation therapy may have a poorer prognosis than those in whom it develops later. Some patients with early recurrence of squamous intraepithelial lesions are found to have recurrent or residual carcinoma.

Cellular Changes Associated With the Intrauterine Device

Soon after the introduction of the intrauterine device as a contraceptive method, a number of cytologic changes began to be identified that were associated with its use.[28] As the use of this device has declined, the incidence of these findings in cytologic samples has also declined. Nevertheless, it is important to recognize the morphologic manifestations of the "intrauterine device effect" in order to avoid confusion with more serious cytologic changes. The presence of an intrauterine device may be associated with irregular shedding of cells from the endometrial cavity. It is not uncommon, therefore, to find endometrial cells outside of the period when they are normally encountered (ie, the first half of the menstrual cycle). Although these cells may look entirely normal, in some instances, they are enlarged. This may lead to their confusion with cells derived from a hyperplastic or neoplastic endometrial process.

The presence of an intrauterine device may also be associated with atypical changes in immature metaplastic cells derived from the endocervical canal. These changes may be related to the irritating effect of the portion of the device that lies in the canal. The affected cells have enlarged nuclei, an increased nuclear-to-cytoplasmic ratio, and, often, vacuolated cytoplasm. The changes may again mimic those seen with endometrial hyperplastic or neoplastic processes (Figs. 4-43 through 4-45). In other

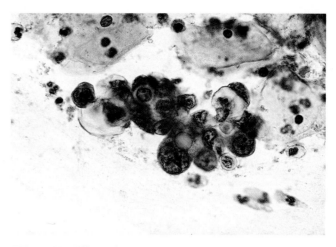

FIG. 4-44. Effect of intrauterine device (IUD). There is more nuclear abnormality noted in these cells than is usually seen with IUD-related changes, however, this is within the range of what may be seen.

instances, nuclear enlargement occurs alone. Single cells with this type of change may be confused with those from high-grade intraepithelial squamous lesions (Fig. 4-46). The lack of nuclear irregularity, the scant number of abnormal cells, and the absence of other changes associated with high-grade squamous intraepithelial neoplasia, such as syncytial aggregates, helps distinguish these cells from those derived from intraepithelial lesions.

Atrophic Vaginitis

Atrophy of the squamous epithelium of the cervix and vagina is associated with a general enlargement of the nuclei of basal and parabasal types of cells without evidence of hyperchromasia or any significant alterations in

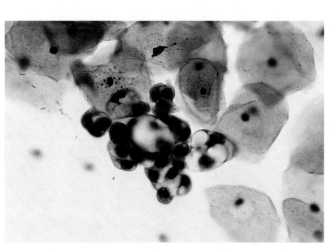

FIG. 4-43. Effect of intrauterine device. There is nuclear enlargement and cytoplasmic vacuolation. These changes may simulate those of endometrial adenocarinoma.

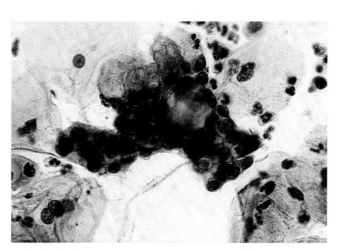

FIG. 4-45. Atypical endocervical cells in a smear from a patient with an intrauterine device. Note the hyperchromasia and mild nuclear enlargement.

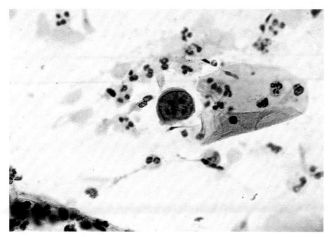

FIG. 4-46. Effect of intrauterine device (IUD). Single cells such as this may also be seen secondary to an IUD. These cells may be confused with those derived from a high-grade intraepithelial lesion.

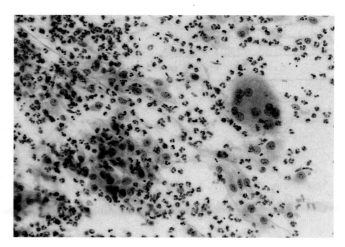

FIG. 4-48. Atrophic vaginitis.

Hyperkeratosis and Parakeratosis

the configuration of the nuclear envelope. These cells may appear in smears as single cells or as sheets of cells with ill-defined cell borders, which may resemble syncytium-like arrangements. However, the lack of any significant nuclear changes, other than the generalized enlargement of the nuclei, usually allows ready differentiation of these cells from those derived from a squamous intraepithelial process.

When atrophy is associated with inflammation, a prominent inflammatory infiltrate is typically present. This may be associated with autolysis and cell degeneration, which results in numerous bare nuclei or the presence of pyknotic basal and parabasal cells with eosinophilic or orangeophilic cytoplasm resembling parakeratosis (Figs. 4-47 and 4-48).

The terms *hyperkeratosis* and *parakeratosis* are not officially included in the Bethesda system terminology, but are widely used to describe epithelial changes that are considered to be benign proliferative changes.[29] The problem is that these terms, particularly *parakeratosis,* have been used inconsistently in the past for a variety of cellular changes, including some that are more appropriately included in the category of atypical squamous cells of undetermined significance.

The normal squamous epithelium of the cervical mucosa does not contain a granular cell layer or a keratin layer. Under some circumstances, however, particularly in response to chronic irritation, the epithelium undergoes hypermaturation and a granular cell layer with overlying keratinization develops. This occurrence is referred to as *hyperkeratosis.* A common situation associated with this process is uterine prolapse, but any irritating stimulus, be it traumatic or inflammatory, may result in the development of hyperkeratosis (Fig. 4-49).

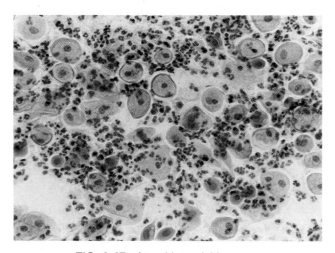

FIG. 4-47. Atrophic vaginitis.

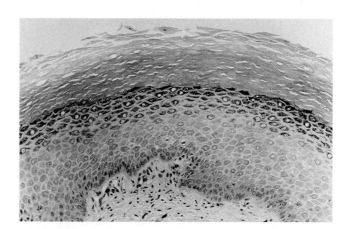

FIG. 4-49. Hyperkeratosis of cervix in a biopsy specimen.

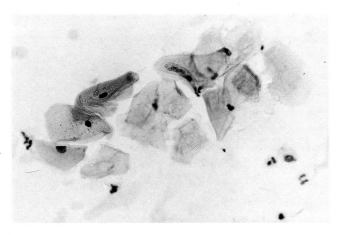

FIG. 4-50. Anucleate squames in clusters consistent with hyperkeratosis.

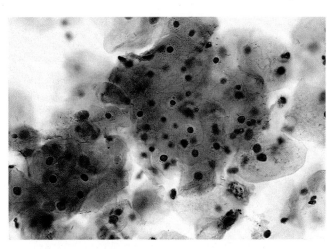

FIG. 4-52. Parakeratotic cells in a cervical smear.

Hyperkeratosis is diagnosed in cytologic samples by the identification of variable numbers of anucleate squames that stain eosinophilic or orangeophilic with the Papanicolaou stain (Figs. 4-50 and 4-51). The finding of hyperkeratosis alone does not appear to be associated with the presence or future development of a more significant epithelial lesion. Although some significant intraepithelial processes and certain cases of invasive squamous carcinoma are marked by keratinization, these conditions almost always are identifiable on cytology by the concurrent presence of other significant cytologic abnormalities.

Parakeratosis is a process that is similar to and may coexist with hyperkeratosis. It is characterized by multiple layers of miniature keratinized cells with small pyknotic remnants of cell nuclei identifiable within their cytoplasm. The process occurs in squamous epithelium

that is undergoing rapid turnover and, in its typical form, is considered to be a benign cellular change (Fig. 4-52). In some cases, however, a similar process overlies an abnormal epithelium. For example, atypical parakeratosis, which has also been referred to as "dyskeratosis," may be a feature associated with human papillomavirus–related epithelial changes. These cells are characterized by pleomorphic miniature forms, occurring singly or in clusters, with caudate and spindle shapes and irregular, often elongated, miniature hyperchromatic nuclei. Most typically, when this process is present as part of an intraepithelial lesion, other cytologic abnormalities are present. Sometimes, however, the presence of these pleomorphic parakeratotic forms on a Papanicolaou smear is the only evidence that a significant lesion may be present (Fig. 4-53). Atypical parakeratosis should be reported as atypical squamous cells of undetermined significance or as a

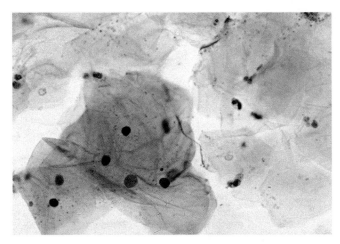

FIG. 4-51. Cellular evidence of hyperkeratosis.

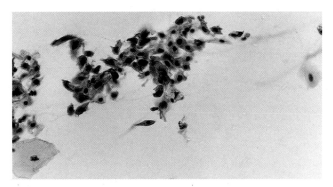

FIG. 4-53. "Pleomorphic" parakeratosis (dyskeratosis). This type of change is generally associated with human papilloma virus and should be reported as atypical squamous cells of undetermined significance or as an intraepithelial lesion, depending on the degree of nuclear abnormality.

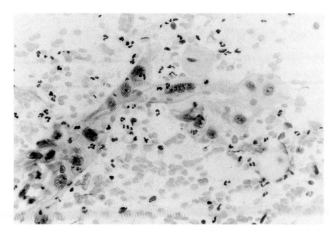

FIG. 4-54. Medium-power view of cells derived from a decidual reaction.

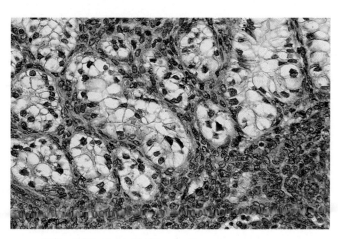

FIG. 4-56. Arias-Stella reaction in tissue section.

squamous intraepithelial lesion, depending on the degree of nuclear changes present and the severity of associated abnormalities.

CELLULAR CHANGES RELATED TO PREGNANCY

The cytologic findings during pregnancy are in general identical to those in the nonpregnant state, in regard to both normal cells and cytologic manifestations of disease states. Cellular changes that may occur during pregnancy and are rather specific include those associated with decidua, the Arias-Stella reaction, and trophoblastic tissue. These are important because of the possibility that they may be confused with potentially significant abnormalities.

The decidual reaction typically involves the endometrium of pregnancy. Cells of this origin are seldom found on Papanicolaou smears. In some patients, however, endocervical tissue may be involved. In this circumstance, cells derived from this reaction may be expected to be found in routine smears. These cells are typically polygonal, with abundant cytoplasm and large nuclei. They may resemble squamous cells derived from a low-grade intraepithelial lesion, except that the nuclei are bland, generally not hyperchromatic, and often contain one or more prominent nucleoli. This last characteristic is often the most important differential diagnostic feature because prominent nucleoli are not seen in cells derived from an intraepithelial process (Figs. 4-54 and 4-55). The distinction from squamous epithelial repair may be more difficult, but does not present a problem of significant clinical importance.[30]

The Arias-Stella reaction, characterized by the presence of atypical, large columnar cells with hyperchromatic, sometimes irregular nuclei, is a common finding involving endometrial glands during early pregnancy

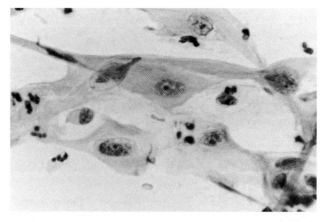

FIG. 4-55. High-power view of decidua cells, demonstrating enlarged nuclei and nucleoli. The cells resemble those derived from a low-grade intraeithelial reaction, but the latter lack prominent nucleoli.

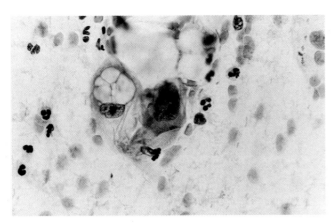

FIG. 4-57. Atypical cells of glandular type in a smear taken during early pregnancy, probably originating in an Arias-Stella—like reaction. There was no evidence of a significant lesion.

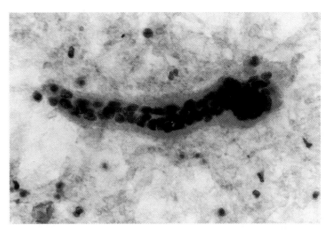

FIG. 4-59. Syncytial trophoblast in a cervical smear from a pregnant patient.

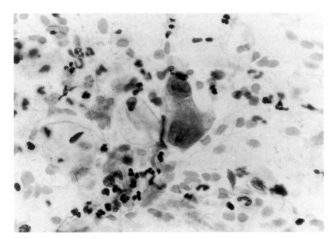

FIG. 4-58. Similar atypical glandular cells from the same patient as Fig 4-57.

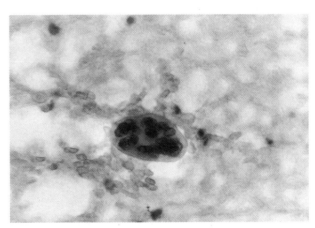

FIG. 4-60. Syncytial trophoblast.

(Fig. 4-56). This type of reaction also sometimes involves the endocervical epithelium. In this situation, the appearance of the cells on the Papanicolaou smear may present a picture that can easily be confused with adenocarcinoma (Figs. 4-57 and 4-58). Therefore, the possibility of an Arias-Stella reaction should be considered in any case in which the cytologic diagnosis of adenocarcinoma is entertained during pregnancy.[31,32]

Trophoblastic cells may also rarely be found on a Papanicolaou smear taken during pregnancy (Figs. 4-59 and 4-60). The presence of these cells is an incidental finding that has no prognostic significance.[32]

REFERENCES

1. Roberts TH, Ng APB. Chronic lymphocytic cervicitis: cytologic and histopathologic manifestations. Acta Cytol 1975;19:235.
2. Bibbo M, Wied GL. Inflammatory reactions and microbiology of the female genital tract. In Wied GL, Keebler CM, Koss LG, et al (eds). Compendium on diagnostic cytology, 7th ed. Chicago: Tutorials of Cytology, 1992:63.
3. Jirovic O, Petru M. Trichomonas vaginalis and trichomoniasis. Adv Parasitol 1968;6:117.
4. Honigberg BM, Gupta PK, Spence MR, et al. Pathogenicity of Trichomonas vaginalis: cytopathologic and histopathologic changes of the cervical epithelium. Obstet Gynecol 1984;64:179.
5. Koss LG, Wolinska WH. Trichomonas vaginalis cervicitis and its relationship to cervix cancer. Cancer 1959;12:1171.
6. Patten SF, Hughes CP, Reagan JW. An experimental study of the relationship between Trichomonas vaginalis and dysplasia in the uterine cervix. Acta Cytol 1963;7:187.
7. Siapco BJ, Kaplan BJ, Bernstein GS, et al. Cytodiagnosis of Candida organisms in cervical smears. Acta Cytol 1986;30:477.
8. Gardner HL, Dykes CD. Hemophilus vaginalis vaginitis. Ann NY Acad Sci 1959;83:280.
9. Gupta PK, Hustis DG, Bonfiglio TA, et al. Cytology of the female genital tract. In Astarita RW (ed). Practical cytopathology. New York: Churchill Livingstone, 1990:28.
10. Yen SSC, Reagan JW, Rosenthal MS. Herpes simplex infection in the female genital tract. Obstet Gynecol 1965;26:91.
11. Ng ABP, Reagan JW, Lindner E. The cellular manifestations of primary and recurrent herpes genitalis. Acta Cytol 1970;14:124.
12. Amstey MS, Patten SF, Turk M. Herpes cervicitis and cervical neoplasia: a clinical review. Cancer 1972;32:1321.
13. Gupta PK. Intrauterine contraceptive device: vaginal cytology, pathologic changes and their clinical implications. Review and lead article. Acta Cytol 1982;26:571.
14. Laverty CR, Russel P, Black J, et al. Adenovirus infection of the cervix. Acta Cytol 1977;21:114.
15. Gupta PK, Lee EF, Erozan YS, et al. Cytologic investigations in Chlamydia infection. Acta Cytol 1979;23:315.
16. Lindner L, Geerling S, Nettum JA, et al. The cytologic features of chlamydial cervicitis. Acta Cytol 1985;29:676.
17. Kiviat NB, Paavonen JA, Brockway J, et al. Cytologic manifestations of cervical and vaginal infections. I. Epithelial and inflammatory cellular changes. JAMA 1985;253:989.
18. Kiviat NG, Peterson M, Kinney-Thomas E, et al. Cytologic manifestations of cervical and vaginal infections. II. Confirmation of Chlamydia trachomatis infection by direct immunofluorescence using monoclonal antibodies. JAMA 1985;253:997.
19. Hare MJ, Toone E, Taylor-Robinson D, et al. Follicular cervicitis: colposcopic appearances and association with Chlamydia trachomatis. Br J Obstet Gynaecol 1981;88:174.
20. Winkler B, Crum CP. Chlamydia trachomatis infection of the female genital tract. Pathogenic and clinicopathologic correlations. Pathol Annu 1987;22:193.
21. San Cristobol A, DeMundi A. Enterobius vermicularis larvae in vaginal smears. Acta Cytol 1976;20:190.
22. Geirsson G, Woodworth F, Patten S, et al. Epithelial repair and regeneration in the uterine cervix. I. An analysis of the cells. Acta Cytol 1977;21:371.
23. Gondos B, Smith LR, Townsend DE. Cytologic changes in cervical epithelium following cryosurgery. Acta Cytol 1970;14:386.
24. Hasegawa T, Tsutsui F, Kurihara S. Cytomorphologic study on the atypical cells following cryosurgery for the treatment of chronic cervicitis. Acta Cytol 1975;19:533.
25. von Haam E. Radiation cell changes. In Wied GL, Keebler CM, Koss LG, et al (eds). Compendium on diagnostic cytology, 6th ed. Chicago: Tutorials of Cytology, 1988:239.
26. Graham RM. The cytologic diagnosis of cancer. Philadelphia: WB Saunders, 1972:155.
27. Patten SF. Postradiation dysplasia of the uterine cervix: cytopathology and clinical significance. In Wied GL, Keebler CM, Koss LG, et al (eds). Compendium on diagnostic cytology, 7th ed. Chicago: Tutorials of Cytology, 1992:191.
28. Fonari ML. Cellular changes in the glandular epithelium of patients using IUCD: a source of cytologic error. Acta Cytol 1974;18:341.
29. Patten SF. Benign proliferative reactions of the uterine cervix. In Wied GL, Keebler CM, Koss LG, et al (eds). Compendium on diagnostic cytology, 7th ed. Chicago: Tutorials of Cytology, 1992:77.
30. Schneider V, Barnes L. Ectopic cervical decidual reaction: frequency and cytologic presentation. Acta Cytol 1981;25:616.
31. Schneider V. Arias-Stella reaction of the endocervix: frequency and topographic location. Acta Cytol 1981;25:224.
32. Schneider V. Cytology in pregnancy. In Wied GL, Keebler CM, Koss LG, et al (eds). Compendium on diagnostic cytology, 7th ed. Chicago: Tutorials of Cytology, 1992:58.

ADDITIONAL READING

Bibbo M, Keebler CM, Wied GL. The cytologic diagnosis of tissue repair in the female genital tract. Acta Cytol 1971;15:133.
Gupta PK. Microbiology, inflammation and viral infections. In Bibbo M. Comprehensive cytopathology. Philadelphia: WB Saunders, 1991:115.
Koss LG. Diagnostic cytology and its histologic basis. Philadelphia: JB Lippincott, 1992:314.

Gynecologic Cytopathology. Edited by
Thomas A. Bonfiglio and Yener S. Erozan.
Lippincott–Raven Publishers, Philadelphia, © 1997.

CHAPTER 5

The Biology of Human Papillomaviruses and Their Role in Cervical Carcinogenesis

Mark H. Stoler

An appreciation of human papillomavirus (HPV) biology is central to an understanding of cervical carcinogenesis and is currently influencing both the pathologic classification of cervical neoplasia as well as the clinical management of these lesions. The expansion of our knowledge regarding the pathology, epidemiology, and molecular biology of these viruses has defined them as the major and best understood class of true human tumor viruses. The interaction of the papillomavirus genome with its host cell produces the majority of cytologic abnormalities at which cervical cancer screening is directed. It is the purpose of this chapter to review briefly our understanding of HPV biology, with special reference to the mechanisms by which the HPV produces abnormal cytology. This provides a foundation for the subsequent detailed presentation of our criteria-based approach to cytologic diagnosis and classification.

HISTORICAL PERSPECTIVE

Based on their characteristic gross morphology, skin warts have been recognized since antiquity. In the first decade of the 1900s, Ciuffo established the viral etiology of human warts (papillomas) by using cell-free extracts from wart tissue as an inoculum for man-to-man transmission experiments. In 1933, Shope described the first papillomavirus in cottontail rabbits. When the virus was isolated from naturally occurring papillomas of wild rabbits and inoculated into domestic rabbits, papillomas were produced that progressed to carcinomas in a significant subset of cases.[1-3] Carcinoma development could be promoted by the application of coal tar to the

papillomas. Thus, the Shope cottontail rabbit papillomavirus system stimulated our early concepts of cancer initiation and promotion, and produced one of the first examples of a DNA tumor virus, as well as a mammalian cancer virus. With the advent of electron microscopy, the morphology of the papillomaviruses became evident. It also became clear that different kinds of warts were more productive of virions than others. For example, plantar warts often had abundant viral particles, whereas genital warts had few.[4-7] Because papillomaviruses were resistant to tissue culture and could not be transmitted to laboratory animals, their characterization was arduous. Limited biochemical characterization and immunology was carried out on viral proteins derived from direct extracts of warts. Based on these studies, it was believed that there was a single type of HPV, a view that was held through the 1960s.[8] In the 1970s, the tools of modern molecular biology permitted the molecular characterization of the papillomavirus family. Clones of the HPV genomes could be used to probe different pathologic processes to establish the relationship of those lesions with HPVs, and analysis of the genomes isolated from these lesions revealed the plurality of HPV types based on differences in their DNA content.[9,10]

Today, it is recognized that papillomaviruses infect essentially all vertebrate species and induce primarily, albeit not exclusively, squamous epithelial neoplasia. In humans, more than 70 molecular types have been cloned, some two dozen of which are trophic for the anogenital tract.[11] Anogenital HPV infections are the most common sexually transmitted diseases.[12] When they involve the cervix, a major by-product of these infections is the development of cervical neoplasia. Major interest in the pathology of this very small area of the female anatomy is justified because of the morbidity and mortality caused by cervical epithelial cancers and their pre-

M. H. Stoler: University of Virginia School of Medicine, Charlottesville, Virginia 22908.

cursors. Worldwide, cervical cancer is the most common cancer of women. During 1995, there were approximately 15,000 cases of cervical cancer and about 5000 associated deaths in the United States.[13] Despite a dramatic decrease in incidence, from 32.6 per 10^5 in the 1940s to 8.3 per 10^5 in the 1980s, directly attributable to the efficacy of cytologic screening, squamous cancer of the uterine cervix remains the most common cancer of the female genital tract and the fourth most common cause of female cancer death worldwide.[14] Coincident with the decrease in invasive cancer in countries where screening has been productive, there has been a dramatic increase in the frequency and attendant costs of detecting and treating the precursors of cervical cancer. The incidence of cervical intraepithelial neoplasia (CIN) 3 is roughly four times that of invasive squamous cancer. It is currently estimated that 2.5 million women are diagnosed with low-grade squamous intraepithelial lesions (LSILs) each year. By some estimates, the attendant costs for the management of these lesions could approach $6 billion.[15] In recent years, it has become increasingly clear that all this clinical activity is directly attributable to the interaction of HPVs with the cervical mucosa.

STRUCTURE AND CLASSIFICATION OF HUMAN PAPILLOMAVIRUSES

A more detailed review of this subject is available elsewhere.[16,17]

Historically, the papillomaviruses have been classified as members of the papovavirus family. This family was named by combining the first two letters of each of the major genera: *pa*pillomavirus, *po*lyomavirus, and simian *va*cuolating virus, respectively. All members of the family are small, double-stranded DNA viruses that replicate in the nucleus and have icosahedral capsules that form nonenveloped virions. However, it has become apparent that the papillomaviruses are biologically distinct from simian vacuolating virus 40 and polyomavirus, and should be classified in separate families, or at least subfamilies. The capsids of papillomaviruses measure 55 nm rather than 40 nm in diameter, reflecting the fact that the approximately 8000–base pair papillomavirus genome is 60% larger than the polyomavirus genome. Moreover, the polyomavirus genome does not crosshybridize with papillomaviruses under low-stringency conditions, and the molecular organization of viral transcription is very different in HPV and polyomavirus. Papillomaviruses transcribe all their genes off one strand of the double-stranded genome. In contrast, simian vacuolating virus 40 and polyomavirus use bidirectional transcription strategies involving both strands.

The circular, 7900–base pair, double-stranded DNA genome of HPV is divided into early and late regions, encoding seven or eight early and two late genetic open reading frames (ORFs), which, through gene splicing, code for all viral gene products (Fig. 5-1 and Table 5-1). In addition, there is a noncoding region of approximately 1000 base pairs, often referred to as the *upstream regulatory region* or *long control region,* which contains the sequences regulating the expression of the ORFs. More than 20 messenger RNAs are expressed, many in a differentiation- and cell type–specific manner, and a detailed discussion of the regulation of transcription is beyond our scope. (For an up-to-date review of viral gene transcription and regulation, refer to the publication by Howley.[18]) Briefly, and in order of occurrence distal to

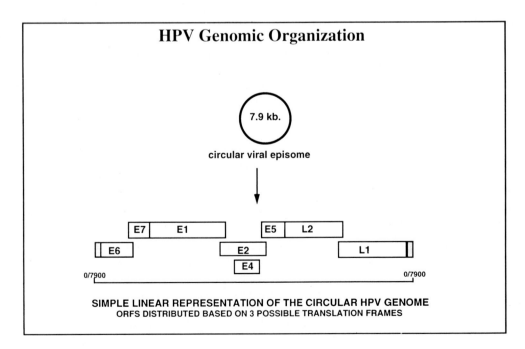

HPV Genomic Organization

7.9 kb.

circular viral episome

| E7 | E1 |
| E6 |

| E5 | L2 |

| E2 |
| E4 |

| L1 |

0/7900

0/7900

SIMPLE LINEAR REPRESENTATION OF THE CIRCULAR HPV GENOME
ORFS DISTRIBUTED BASED ON 3 POSSIBLE TRANSLATION FRAMES

FIG. 5-1. Simple linear representation of the circular human papillomavirus (HPV) genome. The open reading frames (ORFs) are distributed based on three possible translation frames.

TABLE 5-1. *Human papillomavirus open reading frames*

Open reading frame	Major functions
E6	Cell transformation, p53 binding, and degradation
E7	Cell transformation, retinoblastoma protein binding, and cellular transcription activation
E1	Viral DNA replication and plasmid maintenance
E2	Regulation of viral transcription
E4	Cytokeratin binding, ? other functions
E5	Cell transformation through growth factor receptor interactions
L2	Minor capsid protein
L1	Major capsid protein

the upstream regulatory region: E6 and E7 encode proteins that are capable of inducing cell proliferation and transformation, but are also involved in regulating viral gene expression or replication and recruiting the host enzymatic machinery for these purposes. These are the only ORFs that are conserved and expressed in *all* HPV-associated pathologies, and I explore their host interactions in more detail later in this chapter. The proteins encoded by E1 are involved in genome maintenance and replication. E2 encodes the major transregulatory proteins that interact with the upstream regulatory region, having both positive and negative effects on transcription. The E4 ORF is the most abundantly transcribed message in a wart and is most highly expressed in differentiated cells. Some forms of E4 encode a protein that binds to and disrupts the cytoplasmic keratin network, producing what we recognize as a koilocyte in cells that are appropriately differentiated. E5 seems to be involved in cell transformation. E5 encodes a small protein that seems to bind to a variety of host membrane proteins, including growth factor receptors. It also contains 3′ regulatory and polyadenylation sequences for all the E-region genes. Because expression of E5 is often lost during viral integration, its role in human carcinogenesis is controversial. L2 and L1 encode the minor and major viral capsid proteins, respectively. The expression of these proteins and their messages is also tightly regulated in a cell differentiation–dependent manner (Fig. 5-2).

All papillomaviruses have a similar structure and genetic organization. As noted earlier, there are more than 70 HPV types. Given the absence of serologic reagents or viral culture systems, these viruses are classified not by serotype, but by genotype. Within a species, a different genotype was initially defined by a greater than 50% homology difference using a specific liquid hybridization assay and stringent reassociation kinetics. This assay overestimated sequence differences and has been supplanted by the analysis of nucleotide sequence differences of the E6, E7, and L1 ORFs. A new HPV type should have less than 90% sequence homology in these regions to any of the known HPV types. From these definitions and computerized analysis of these sequences, it is clear that the papillomaviruses have had a long evolution, probably coevolving with humans and vertebrates in general[19-21] (Fig. 5-3). Different viral types are not the products of simple point mutations. Remarkably, the grouping of papillomaviruses that is derived from sequence analysis closely predicts the recognized clinical groupings.[22] Broadly speaking, there are cutaneous and mucosotropic groups. In the cutaneous group, there are HPVs common to the general population, such as HPV 1 (the agent of plantar warts) and HPVs 2 and 4 (which cause common warts), and there is a large group of 20 or more HPV types that are associated with the rare disease epidermodysplasia verruciformis. Interestingly, most of the epidermodysplasia verruciformis warts that progress to cancer are associated with HPVs 5 and 8 (ie, there is a "high-risk" subgroup analogous to the subgroups recognized in the mucosotropic HPVs). In the mucosotropic group, the viruses may be broadly classified into those with a low risk of lesion progression to cancer and those with a moderate to high risk. Viruses classified as low risk are defined by the fact that they are almost never found in invasive cancers. In contrast, high-risk viruses are those that are most often found in invasive cancers. It should be noted that infection with a high-risk virus does not imply the inevitable development of cancer. It should also be pointed out that the molecular epidemiology of most of the moderate- or intermediate-risk viruses is incompletely developed because of a relative lack of probes and the comparatively recent description of members of this group. The four mucosotropic viruses, HPVs 6, 11, 16, and 18, form the prototypes for the high- and low-risk groups and, together, account for approximately two thirds of HPV-associated anogenital neoplasms[23,24] (Table 5-2). Types 6 and 11 primarily cause benign exophytic genital warts, or condylomata acuminata. These are the viruses present in more than 90% of condylomata, with about two thirds caused by HPV 6 and one third by HPV 11. They are also associated with LSILs and are only rarely associated with high-grade squamous intraepithelial lesions (HSILs) or invasive squamous cancers. Related viruses that produce a similar spectrum in the cervix are HPVs 26, 42 through 44, 53 through 55, 62, and 66. In contrast, HPV 16 is the most prevalent virus to infect the uterine cervix and is closely associated with the entire range of intraepithelial and invasive squamous neoplasia as well as, less commonly, cervical glandular neoplasia. The moderate- to high-risk types most closely related to HPV 16 include types 31, 33, 35, 52, 58, and 67. HPV 18 is the other cancer-associated prototype that is also most commonly associated with nonsquamous cervical neoplasms. The viruses most related to type 18 include types 39, 45, 59, and 68. Other types, such as 51 and 56, seem

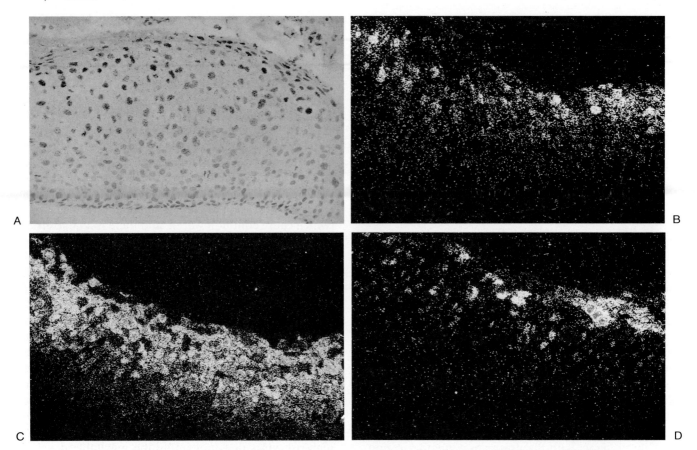

FIG. 5-2. Patterns of human papillomavirus (HPV) gene expression in low-grade squamous intraepithelial lesions (LSILs). In situ autoradiograms with tritium-labeled riboprobes, hematoxylin counterstain, magnification on film plane 50×. **(A)** Bright-field image of LSIL probed for HPV 11 DNA. Note the amplification of the nuclear DNA signal with squamous maturation **(B)** Adjacent section probed for HPV 11 E6E7 RNA under dark-field optics. Most of the E6 and E7 message is expressed in differentiated, ie, nondividing cells. **(C)** E4E5 expression in an adjacent section. These genes are the most highly expressed genes in LSILs and again are expressed in a very differentiation-dependent manner. **(D)** L1 expression under dark-field optics. L1, which encodes for the HPV major capsid protein, is expressed in a subset of the most differentiated cells. With high-resolution in situ hybridization, one can follow the maturation of the message from nucleus to cytoplasm as the cells differentiate.

to have some association with cervical cancer, but are genetically also related to the cutaneous group. Morphologically similar lesions at different mucosal sites by and large are caused by the same mucosal viruses. Thus, laryngeal and conjunctival papillomas, which are pathologically and biologically equivalent to condylomata, are most often caused by HPVs 11 and 6. In contrast, bowenoid dysplasia of the vulva, penis, anus, and oral cavity is most often associated with HPV 16. As will become clear, all HPV types, even the high-risk viruses, must induce the pathologic equivalent of a wart, condyloma, or LSIL, because this is the pathology that supports viral replication and virion production.

During the past two decades, three major lines of evidence have converged to strengthen markedly the association of HPVs with squamous carcinomas of the ano-genital tract, particularly the uterine cervix. Koilocytotic atypia, the *morphologic* hallmark of HPV cytopathic effect, is recognized as the earliest manifestation of CIN. Squamous cell carcinoma of the cervix and its precursors have the *epidemiologic* characteristics of a venereal disease. The *molecular biology* of HPVs provides a rational link explaining both the epidemiology and much of the morphology of cervical neoplasia.

MORPHOLOGY OF HUMAN PAPILLOMAVIRUSES

In a sense, much of the remainder of this text describes the cytologic and histologic manifestations of papillomavirus expression in cervical epithelial cells. Thus, the

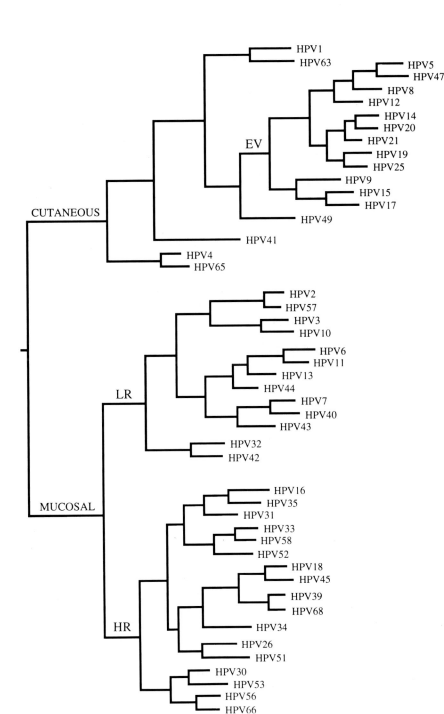

FIG. 5-3. Phylogenetic tree constructed from the alignment of 384 nucleotides in the human papillomavirus (HPV) E6 genes using maximum parsimony analysis. The branch labeled **cutaneous** contains HPV types, which group together and are found to infect keratinized epithelium. The branch labeled **mucosal** contains the mucosotropic group, and is divided into those associated with a low risk for cancer (LR) versus those with a high risk (HR). EV: epidermodysplasia verruciformis group. (Figure courtesy of Dr. R.D. Burk and adapted from Van Ranst MA, Tachezy R, Delius H, et al. Taxonomy of the human papillomaviruses. Papillomavirus Report 1993;3:61.)

cytology of the uterine cervix is very much the cytology of papillomavirus-associated neoplasia. In 1956, Koss and Durfee coined the term *koilocytotic atypia* to describe the cells derived from flat "warty lesions" of the cervix because of their histologic resemblance to skin warts.[25] Cells demonstrating koilocytotic atypia are defined as intermediate squamous cells with a cave-like vacuole surrounding an atypical (ie, 2 to 4 times enlarged) hyperchromatic nucleus, often with nuclear membrane irregularity and no nucleoli (Fig. 5-4).

Nuclear atypia is essential to the diagnosis. Cells with large vacuoles and no atypia are not diagnostic. Koilocytotic atypia is often referred to as being pathognomonic for HPV infection or as an *HPV cytopathic effect* because it is the cytologic abnormality most often described as being associated with the virus. In fact, it is the cell in which virions are most often detected, and is highly correlated with productive HPV infection. However, the cytologic or histologic absence of koilocytotic atypia does not in any way imply the absence of HPV, or more spe-

TABLE 5-2. *Common clinical lesions associated with different human papillomavirus types*

Clinical lesion	Human papillomavirus types
Common warts (verruca vulgaris)	2, 4
Plantar warts	1
Flat warts	3, 10, 28, 41
Epidermodysplasia verruciformis	5, 8, 9, 12, 14, 15, 17, 19, 20–25, 36–38, 47, and 49
Butcher's warts	7
Condyloma acuminatum (genital warts)	6, 11
Laryngeal papillomatosis	11, 6
Low-grade squamous intraepithelial lesion or equivalent	Essentially all mucosotropic types (more than 24)
High-grade squamous intraepithelial lesion	Same as invasive squamous cancer
Invasive cervical cancers	**16, 18, 31,** 33, 35, 39, **45,** 51, 52, 56, 58, 59, 66, 67, and 68
Invasive squamous cancer of other anogenital sites	Mainly 16
Bowenoid high-grade dysplasia	Mainly 16

cifically, the absence of pathogenic HPV gene expression. Indeed, as will be shown, essentially all the neoplastic cytologic abnormalities of the cervix are associated with HPV. Koilocytotic atypia, which under the Bethesda classification is considered an LSIL, is the most common definite abnormality in cytologically screened populations today, being present in 1% to 4% of Papanicolaou smears.[26,27] In retrospect, similar cells were illustrated in all the early cytology atlases, and perhaps were described best by J. Earnest Ayre as the "halo cells" of his nearocarcinoma or precancer cell complex.[28,29] In 1976, Meisels and Fortin in Canada and Purola and Savia in Scandinavia both recognized the existence of flat and inverted condylomata of the uterine cervix and reported that these lesions not only can be found in the spectrum of CIN, but also are associated with the HPV.[30–33]

These landmark papers and numerous subsequent morphologic studies have contributed greatly to our understanding of the role of these viruses in carcinogenesis.

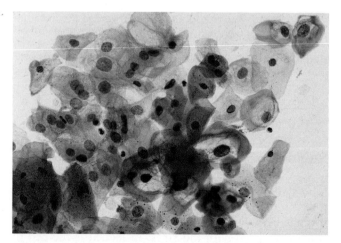

FIG. 5-4. Koilocytotic atypia meeting the criteria described in the text. Note also the cells in the background without nuclear halos, but having nuclear abnormalities sufficent to diagnose either mild dysplasia (low-grade squamous intraepithelial lesion) or atypical squamous cells of undetermined significance. Papanicolaou stain, magnified, on film plane 80×.

Supporting morphologic data come from studies of the distribution of HPV capsid protein or HPV virions in intraepithelial neoplasia. Using a broadly reactive group-specific antisera against the L1 protein, papillomavirus capsid antigen, the expression of which is a highly differentiation-dependent phenomenon, is present in 50% to 60% of condylomata or LSILs, decreasing in frequency as the cytohistologic grade increases.[34–38] Similarly, if one uses transmission electron microscopy to search cell nuclei for virions, there is an inverse correlation between cytologic lesion grade and detection of the virus.[37–39]

EPIDEMIOLOGY OF HUMAN PAPILLOMAVIRUSES

(For a consolidated review, see the excellent World Health Organization (WHO)/International Agency for Research on Cancer (IARC) monograph.[40])

In 1842, Rigoni-Stern reported an analysis of the death records of Verona, Italy and noted that cancer of the uterus (undoubtedly primarily cancer of the cervix) was much more common among married women and widows than among unmarried women and nuns.[41,42] Since then, numerous epidemiologic studies have linked cervical cancer to sexual behavior, suggesting a venereal etiology.[12,14,43–53] The finding that promiscuity on the part of a woman or her partner confers increased risk for cervical cancer supports the concept of a sexually transmitted agent.[54] The strongest epidemiologic risk factor is the number of sexual partners. Young age at first intercourse and early age of parity, both in part markers of promiscuity, also seem to confer risk, although beginning sexual activity during adolescence may also confer risk on the basis of an altered hormonal environment.[55,56] In most epidemiologic studies, cigarette smoking also remains a risk factor after sexual factors are controlled for. Rates of cervical cancer also vary among different ethnic communities, which may again partially reflect ethnic group differences in sexual behavior. For example, the rates of cervical cancer in New York City were found to be 12 to 25 times higher in Hispanic and black women as compared with white Jewish women.[57–59] Similarly, there are major differences between the rates of cervical cancer in geographically or ethnically similar but culturally different populations (eg, Denmark versus Greenland and Colombia versus Spain).[60–62] Although these differences may indeed be related to differences in sexual behavior, recent data may suggest a genetic predisposition as well.[63–65] Morphoepidemiologic studies demonstrate that the precursors of cervical cancer precede invasive cancer, with LSILs being most prevalent in patients who are in their early 20s, HSILs in patients who are in their late 20s to early 30s, and invasive cancers in patients who are in their 40s. In more recent cohorts, there is a trend toward an earlier age for each of these stages.

But which of the many sexually transmitted agents is responsible? In the 1970s, based on seroepidemiologic studies, herpes simplex virus type 2 was considered the strongest candidate.[66] After all, it is a ubiquitous sexually transmitted agent, and some studies have demonstrated a much greater prevalence in patients compared with control subjects.[43] However, in many studies, the serologic methods used were quite variable.[67] In 1984, Vonka's much-cited seroepidemiologic analysis failed to demonstrate a significant difference between the rate of herpes simplex virus type 2 in patients with cervical dysplasia or cancer and that in control subjects.[68] By this time, the case for HPV as *the* cervical cancer agent was rapidly gaining strength.[69–72]

As of 1995, suffice it to say that the epidemiology of genital HPV infection accounts for the epidemiology of cervical neoplasia.[45,46,48] This statement is based on modern molecular epidemiologic analyses as well as our understanding of the molecular biology of the virus–host cell interaction that provides a mechanistic basis for this link. Although there was some confusion in the literature of the 1980s, some of which failed to show a strong association between HPV and cervical neoplasia, most agree that these negative findings resulted from a lack of high-quality molecular tests for HPV DNA. More recent analyses, using validated methods, confer relative risks for cervical neoplasia based on the presence of HPV on the order of hundreds to one. These are one or two orders of magnitude greater than any other epidemiologic risk factor ever described. If one controls for the presence of HPV infection, essentially all other risk factors "drop out." In epidemiologic terms, HPV infection confers 85% to 90% of the attributable risk for the development of cervical dysplasia. Cohort studies have shown that in cytologically normal women, HPV infection precedes the development of dysplasia, and that infection with HPV 16 or 18 confers the highest risk for dysplasia, particularly high-grade dysplasia. For example, in a study of 241 cytologically normal women recruited in a sexually

transmitted disease clinic, the cumulative incidence of HSIL at 2 years was 28% in HPV-positive women compared with 3% in HPV-negative women.[73] In a study of more than 200 hundred "atypical" Papanicolaou smears that were reread by five expert cytopathologists, it was shown that the HPV prevalence increased from 21% in smears classified as normal to 100% in smears unanimously classified as squamous intraepithelial lesions.[74] The prevalence of HPV in a population varies with the population and the method of HPV detection.[75] Tests using highly sensitive amplification methods capable of detecting many viral types demonstrate the highest prevalence. For instance, when a cohort of college women was studied using L1 consensus primer polymerase chain reaction in parallel with the commercially available Virapap dot blots that only had probes for seven viral types, the HPV prevalence was 46% for the polymerase chain reaction assay compared with 11% for the dot blot assay.[76,77] A conservative estimate of genital HPV prevalence in the general United States population is probably on the order of 15% to 20%, making papillomavirus infection the most common viral sexually transmitted disease. Serial sampling over time leads to a higher estimate of prevalence, but also suggests that these infections may resolve spontaneously.[78,79] We know from long experience with cytologic observation that the rate of all cytologic abnormalities is much less than the rate of HPV infection. Even a child knows from common experience that most warts regress over a period of months to 2 years. Similarly, it is also clear that most cytologic abnormalities regress, with only rare cases progressing to HSIL and even rarer cases progressing to invasive cancer.[30,80–85] The concept of a pyramid of viral infection in the population with cervical cancer at the peak and asymptomatic subclinical infection at the base is quite applicable to HPV (Fig. 5-5).

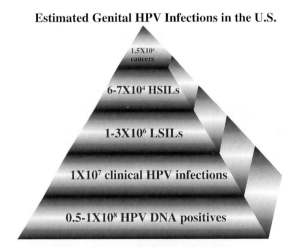

Estimated Genital HPV Infections in the U.S.

1.5X10⁴ cancers

6-7X10⁴ HSILs

1-3X10⁶ LSILs

1X10⁷ clinical HPV infections

0.5-1X10⁸ HPV DNA positives

FIG. 5-5. Pyramid representing the estimated genital human papillomavirus infections in the United States. *LSIL,* low-grade squamous intraepithelial lesion; *HSIL,* high-grade squamous intraepithelial lesion.

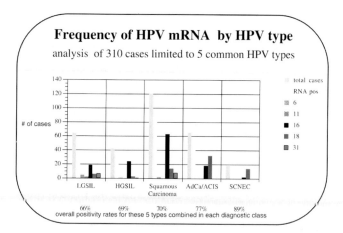

FIG. 5-6. Cervical biopsy specimens analyzed by in situ hybridization for whole genomic mRNA expression of just five human papillomavirus (HPV) types, using tritium-labeled riboprobes.[89] The proportion of positive results agrees well with the expected proportion based on larger epidemiologic studies. *LGSIL,* low-grade squamous intraepithelial lesion; *HGSIL,* high-grade squamous intraepithelial lesion; *AdCa/ACIS,* adenocarcinoma/adenocarcinoma in situ; *SCNEC,* small-cell neuroendocrine carcinoma.

MOLECULAR BIOLOGY OF HUMAN PAPILLOMAVIRUSES

These epidemiologic and pathologic insights have been greatly bolstered by data derived from modern molecular biologic techniques. Molecular detection methods can be applied in a variety of ways. Most commonly, a cellular sample is analyzed for the presence of HPV DNA by dot blot, Southern blot, or some analogous technique, and the sensitivity of the method is improved by combining it with an amplification technique such as the polymerase chain reaction.[22,86–88] Inherent in these

methods is the destruction of the morphology; hence, the results are usually correlated with some other, independent morphologic observation. These types of studies have been strongly complemented by many direct analyses that have used in situ hybridization to demonstrate directly the presence of HPV DNA or messenger RNA in defined groups of pathologies.[89,90]

As noted earlier, there are more than two dozen HPV types that infect the genital tract. All can be found in LSILs or in samples from cytologically "normal" women, and although no single type predominates, HPV 16 is probably the single most common virus at the cervix[22,91] (Figs. 5-6 and 5-7). Whereas the prevalence of HPV DNA in LSILs is in excess of 90%, the same can be said for HSILs and invasive squamous carcinomas of the cervix. However, the type spectrum in the high-grade lesions is much more restricted, with HPV types 16, 18, 31, and 45 accounting for almost 80% of the invasive cancers. Squamous cell carcinomas account for only 80% of cervical cancers, the remainder being made up of primarily endocervical adenocarcinomas and a small number of the rare but deadly small-cell neuroendocrine carcinomas.[92] Studies using sensitive methods to analyze these nonsquamous cancers and their precursors also demonstrate a very high prevalence of HPV DNA.[93–96] The virus most closely related to progressive cervical squamous neoplasia is HPV 16.[97] Although it accounts for fewer cervical infections, HPV 18 is associated more consistently with adenocarcinomas and small-cell neuroendocrine cancers of the cervix and less frequently with invasive squamous cancers (Fig. 5-8). The absolute prevalence of some of the more recently described types (eg, HPVs 31, 33, 35, 39, 42 through 45, 51, 52, 56) may be underestimated because they have not been generally available for large-scale screening.[98] Thus, HPV genetic material is present in more than 90% of premalignant

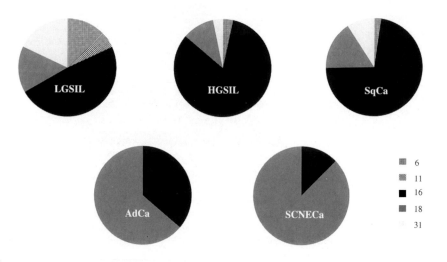

Relative proportion of common HPV types based on In situ analysis of HPV mRNA expression in 310 cervical specimens

FIG. 5-7. In low-grade squamous intraepithelial lesions, if more probes were used, the pie would be sliced many more times.[91] In contrast, there is a restricted human papillomavirus (HPV)—type spectrum in high-grade lesions that also varies with histologic cell type. *LGSIL,* low-grade squamous intraepithelial lesion; *HGSIL,* high-grade squamous intraepithelial lesion; *SqCa,* invasive squamous cell carcinoma; *AdCa,* in situ or invasive endocervical adenocarcinoma; *SCNECa,* small-cell neuroendocrine carcinoma.

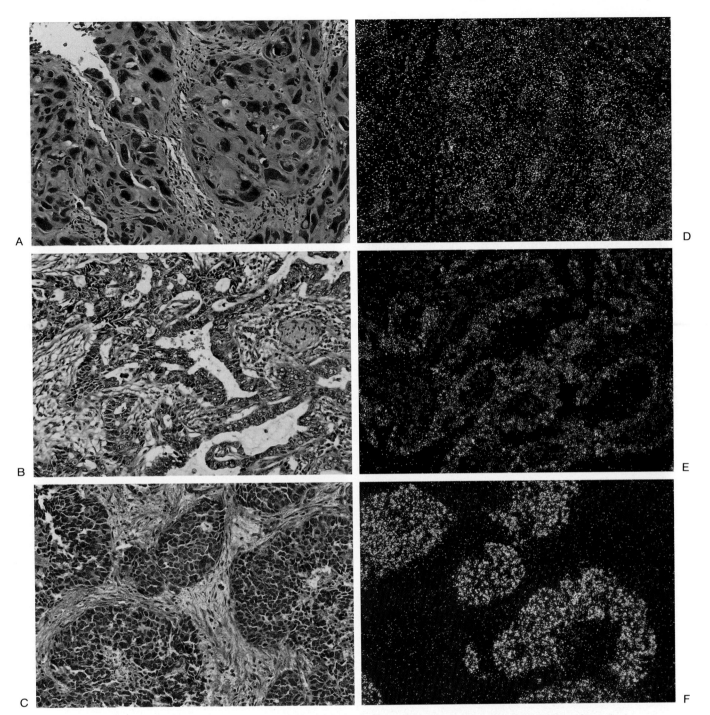

FIG. 5-8. Human papillomavirus (HPV) is present and expressed in most histologic types of cervical cancer. (**A**) Poorly differentiated squamous cell carcinoma. Hematoxylin and eosin, 50×. (**B**) Moderately differentiated endocervical adenocarcinoma. Hematoxylin and eosin, 50×. (**C**) Small-cell neuroendocrine carcinoma. Hematoxylin and eosin, 50×. (**D**) Poorly differentiated squamous cell carcinoma, with HPV 16 expression highlighting the tumor cells over the stroma. (**E**) Moderately differentiated endocervical adenocarcinoma, with HPV 18 mRNA expression. (**F**) Small-cell neuroendocrine carcinoma, with HPV 18 mRNA expression.

and malignant squamous lesions of the uterine cervix. The association of HPVs with squamous cell carcinomas at other body sites (eg, vagina, vulva, anus, penis, larynx, skin) and in a variety of genetic or induced immunodeficiency states is also well recognized.[70,99,100] Animal models for the progression from benign papilloma to carcinoma exist, and a number of well-described progressive cases have been reported in humans.[70,101–104]

Detractors of the HPV–cancer link point out that the finding of HPV DNA in a lesion is insufficient to explain pathogenicity. However, unlike any other candidate agent, it is clear not only that HPV DNA is present in every pathology linked to HPV, but that HPV messenger RNA is expressed in these lesions.[105,106] The presence of viral RNA and protein expression provides the essential pathogenic link. The patterns of viral messenger RNA expression vary with the morphologic diagnosis in a tightly regulated and differentiation-dependent manner (see later).[89,105,107,108] Thus, in low-grade lesions, all viral genes are expressed as a manifestation of vegetative viral replication (see Fig. 5-2). In contrast, in HSILs and invasive cancers, there is a restricted pattern of viral gene expression involving primarily E6 and E7 (Fig. 5-9). Just as naturally occurring malignant lesions have been found to contain HPV DNA and express viral E6 and E7 mes-

senger RNAs, so too have many long-established cervical carcinoma cell lines, such as HeLa, SiHa, and CaSki, been found to harbor integrated HPV 16 or 18 DNAs from which the transforming E6 and E7 regions are actively transcribed.[109–114] These observations further strengthen the relationship between these HPVs and carcinogenesis.

Although the presence of actively transcribed HPV DNA within lesions establishes a strong molecular association between HPV and cervical neoplasia, in vitro cell transformation experiments have pointed to an active role for these viruses in carcinogenesis. DNA from high-risk HPV types, such as 16, 18, 31, and 33, but not 6 or 11, are capable of transforming primary baby rat kidney epithelial cells in collaboration with an activated cellular oncogene, Ha-*ras*, thus mirroring general concepts of multistep carcinogenesis.[115–119] HPV 16 DNA alone can immortalize cultured primary foreskin keratinocytes or primary cervical cells in culture.[120–123] Although not inhibitory to the stratification of keratinocytes cultured on collagen rafts, HPV 16 can prevent cellular differentiation, thus inducing in these artificial epithelia a morphologic transformation that mimics CIN.[124,125] It is noteworthy that in this system, the transformed phenotype is not apparent until the cells have been passaged many

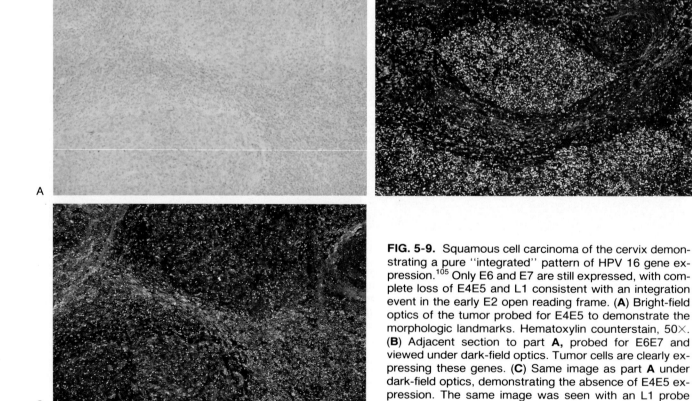

FIG. 5-9. Squamous cell carcinoma of the cervix demonstrating a pure "integrated" pattern of HPV 16 gene expression.[105] Only E6 and E7 are still expressed, with complete loss of E4E5 and L1 consistent with an integration event in the early E2 open reading frame. **(A)** Bright-field optics of the tumor probed for E4E5 to demonstrate the morphologic landmarks. Hematoxylin counterstain, 50×. **(B)** Adjacent section to part **A**, probed for E6E7 and viewed under dark-field optics. Tumor cells are clearly expressing these genes. **(C)** Same image as part **A** under dark-field optics, demonstrating the absence of E4E5 expression. The same image was seen with an L1 probe (data not shown).

generations, again suggesting the need for additional genetic events and mimicking the long progression times seen in naturally occurring lesions.

Because there seems to be a correlation between specific HPV types and the potential for clinical malignancy, there also may be an association between the physical state of HPV DNA within the cell and the malignant potential of the associated epithelial proliferation.[126-131] In benign HPV-infected lesions, the viral DNAs exist as extrachromosomal plasmids, mostly as monomeric circular molecules. However, in some cancers, HPV DNAs are found as multimeric circular molecules, sometimes with deletions, or integrated into host chromosomes.[132] Viral integration most frequently disrupts the E2 ORF, which encodes the transcription regulatory proteins. Loss of these regulatory proteins is thought to be the basis for potential dysregulation of the expression of the transforming E6 and E7 ORFs[133] (Fig. 5-10).

Concurrent with the revelation of HPV biology, there has been an explosion of information about the roles of cellular oncogenes in carcinogenesis.[134-137] Several classes of oncogenes, including growth factors, growth factor receptors, guanosine triphosphate binding proteins, protein kinases, and DNA binding proteins, have been shown to be relevant to the control of cell growth. Amplification of c-*myc* as well as c-Ha-*ras* can be documented in some cervical cancers and correlates with advanced clinical stage at the time of analysis.[138-141] In cervical cancer cell lines, HPV integration sites have been found in the same general region as some of the known oncogenes, including c-*myc*, suggesting the possibility of transcriptional activation by the virus, although this has not been directly documented.[142,143] In other cases, HPV DNA integrates near fragile sites.[144] The significance of this observation is not clear at the present time, but again suggests the potential for multiple genetic or chromosomal events in neoplastic progression.

As in other tumor systems, the inactivation of tumor suppressor genes, or *antioncogenes* as they are called now, may also be highly significant. The fusion of HPV 18–expressing HeLa cells with normal human fibroblasts or keratinocytes results in repression of the malignant phenotype of the HeLa cell.[145] Upon transplantation into nude mice, the loss of chromosome 11 from the hybrid cells results in reversion to the malignant phenotype, suggesting the presence of another tumor suppressor gene at this site. This experiment has been extended by Schwarz and colleagues, who proposed that the ability of a cellular product to suppress the expression of the

Viral Integration

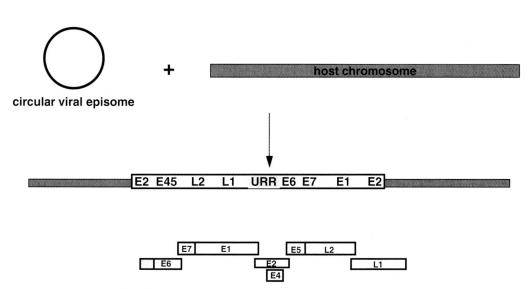

FIG. 5-10. Integration of the human papillomavirus viral episome into the host chromosome is a random event in terms of the location in the host genome. However, the viral genome usually is disrupted in the E2 open reading frame, which can lead to loss of the E2 transregulatory functions of the E2 proteins.

HPV 18 oncogene requires a humoral factor.[146-148] Therefore, the interaction of several gene products is involved in eliciting or inhibiting transformation (Fig. 5-11). The first of the antioncogenes to be characterized was the human retinoblastoma gene.[149] It is either completely absent or has significant deletions in tumors from patients with retinoblastoma, breast cancer, and some other epithelial tumors, such as squamous cell carcinoma of the head and neck.[150-154] It has been reported that the transforming E7 protein of HPV 16 has structural and functional similarities to the E1A antigen of adenovirus, the large T antigen of simian vacuolating virus 40, and the host cellular protein cyclin D1.[156-159] The importance of this finding stems from experiments demonstrating the ability of E7 and related transforming proteins to form inactivating complexes with the retinoblastoma antioncoprotein by competitive binding to the "retinoblastoma pocket." This functional inactivation causes the release of a potent host transcription factor, E2F, which is capable of activating the transcription of a variety of host genes, many of which are involved in DNA synthesis and cell-cycle progression like cyclin D1. Similar complexing and inactivation of the p53 suppressor gene by high-risk viruses such as HPV 16 E6 has been demonstrated.[160-166] E6 binds to p53 via an E6-associated host protein. This binding promotes the ubiquitin-dependent degradation of p53, the functional equivalent of mutational inactivation. Among its many functions, p53 regulates cell proliferation and, hence, tumor growth via transcriptional transactivation. For instance, p53 activates the transcription of p21 (waf 1 or cip 1), a potent inhibitor of cyclin-dependent kinase. Therefore, either mutation or E6-mediated degradation of p53 can lead to derepression of cell-cycle regulation. In rare instances in which a cervical cancer has been shown not to contain HPV, p53 mutation has been found, whereas mutation is absent in the usual cases.[167-170] Interestingly, the E6 proteins from low-risk HPVs are incapable of causing this degradation. Therefore, E6 undoubtedly has roles in the virus–host interac-

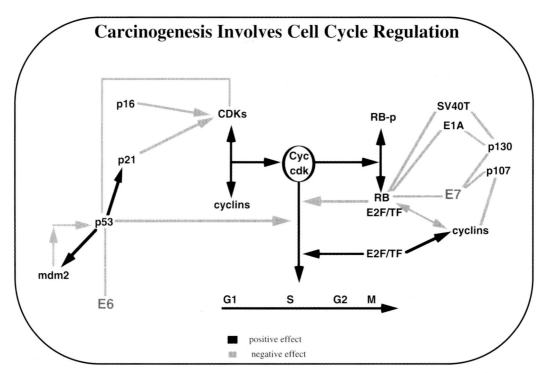

FIG. 5-11. A subset of HPV viral host protein interactions involved in the regulation of the cell cycle. Progression through the cell cycle is obviously essential to cell divison. Many of the proteins listed are members of protein families and also have more than one function, so the diagram could be much more complex. Cyclins (of which there are many) complex with their corresponding cyclin-dependent kinases (CDKs, also many) to influence progression through various cell cycle stages. For instance, the D-cyclins act during G1-to-S transition. The cyclin/CDK complexes in part influence the phosphorylation state of RB. Phosporylated RB releases a transcription factor E2F, which can have wide ranging effects on cellular transcription including activation of many of the genes involved in DNA synthesis including cyclins. Some cyclins, like D1 competively bind to the RB pocket as do viral oncoproteins, like HPV E7, simulating or complementing the effect of phosporylation of RB. p130 and p107 are other "RB like" protein. Cellular p53 also acts as a repressor or controller of cell division. It does this in part by stimulating expression of p21, an inhibitor of CDK expression. p16 is also a CDK inhibitor. Thus viral oncoprotein (like HPV 16 E6)–mediated degradation of p53 removes some of the functional brakes on cell division.

TABLE 5-3. *Human papillomaviruses (HPVs) and cervical neoplasia: summary of molecular evidence*

>90% of precursors contain and *express* HPV DNA
>90% of cancers contain and *express* HPV DNA
Different HPV types have different biologic potential
Most high-grade lesions contain only a few types
These high-risk types (HPV 16 and 18 are prototypes)
   Integrate into host DNA more frequently
   Integration disrupts the E2 transregulatory domain
   Are more capable in in vitro transformation assays
E6 and E7 are expressed consistently in all HPV-associated
   lesions
E6 interacts with p53; E7 with pRb; these interactions are
   more efficient with high-risk types
HPV transfection or multipassage systems mimic natural
   morphogenesis

tion other than p53 inactivation, such as direct effects as a transcription factor.[161,171] Thus, a molecular model for HPV-induced carcinogenesis is beginning to emerge, involving the interaction of HPV gene products with what is recognized to be a tightly controlled network of cellular oncogenes and antioncogenes that control cell proliferation and DNA synthesis (Table 5-3).

A MODEL OF HUMAN PAPILLOMAVIRUS–INDUCED CARCINOGENESIS

Consider the following model of HPV-induced carcinogenesis. It is clear that papillomaviruses must infect the reserve, basal, or stem cell population of the cervical transformation zone, cells that have the potential to differentiate along squamous, glandular, or neuroendocrine lines (Fig. 5-12). In cells committed to squamous differentiation, there is an orderly program of matura-

tion throughout the epithelial thickness at both the morphologic and molecular levels (Fig. 5-13).

The only cells capable of cell division are the basal or parabasal cells. If HPV DNA is present in morphologically normal basal cells, papillomavirus gene expression is inhibited in such cells to essentially maintenance levels because productive HPV gene expression is tightly regulated and permitted only in cells that have begun squamous differentiation, which concurrently have lost the ability to divide.[105,107,108,172–174] The eventual outcome of this coordination between host and virus is the production of a histologic LSIL, the only demonstrated source of infectious virions (Figs. 5-14 and 5-15). Such lesions can regress or maintain themselves for extended periods. Implicit in this program of differentiation-linked expression is an explanation for some of our morphologic criteria. The nuclear enlargement and hyperchromasia that we recognize as atypia is a direct result of E6- or E7-mediated activation of host DNA synthesis. In a low-grade lesion, this is regulated to occur in cells that can no longer divide (ie, intermediate squamous cells) and is primarily directed at the production of viral DNA.[173] However, given the small size of the viral genome, the several thousand copies of the virus present in a productively infected cell clearly cannot account for the twofold to fourfold nuclear enlargement that is observed. It is a fortunate coincidence that there is also ineffective (in the sense of cell division) host DNA synthesis so that we recognize these cells with enlarged nuclei and a increased nuclear-to-cytoplasmic ratio as abnormal. If the process is not fully developed or is perhaps regressing, the cells derived are morphologically classified as atypical (ie, having less nuclear abnormality than seen in classic dysplasia; see Chap. 6), whereas in the fully developed case, they are classified as being derived from mild dysplasia,

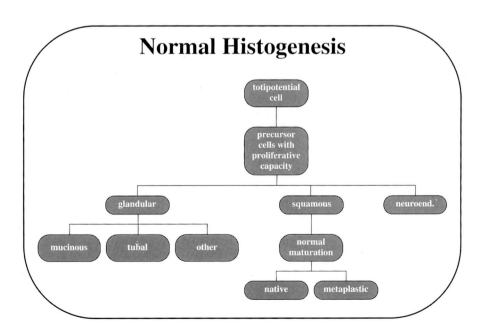

FIG. 5-12. Normal histogenesis.

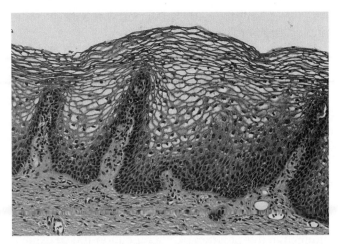

FIG. 5-13. Normal ectocervix, Hematoxylin and eosin 40×. Orderly squamous maturation. The only dividing cells are in the basal/immediate parabasal zone.[172] Note the progressive shrinkage of the nuclei as they approach the surface. Contrast with Fig 5-14.

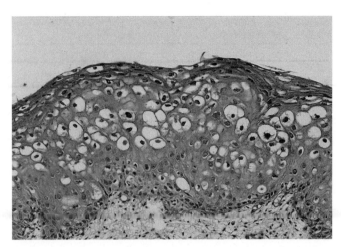

FIG. 5-14. Low-grade squamous intraepithelial lesion with minimal parabasal hyperplasia and well-developed human papillomavirus cytopathic effect, Hematoxylin and eosin 40×. Orderly maturation is relatively preserved and cell division is is still limited to the parabasal zone.

CIN 1, or LSIL. If the cells also have the correct amount and form of the cytokeratin binding protein, HPV E4, expressed, then they appear as koilocytes. As noted earlier, the absence of koilocytosis does not imply the absence of HPV gene expression. Morphologic progression to higher-grade lesions, which is correlated with cellular hyperproliferation, can occur if the coordinate link between differentiation and viral early gene expression is lost (Figs. 5-16 and 5-17). Potential mechanisms might include viral integration or mutation in E2 such that E2-controlled regulation of E6 or E7 expression is lost. In such cases, the viral oncogenes E6 and E7 are inappropriately expressed in a population of cells that retain the capacity to divide, thereby initiating cell proliferation and morphologic progression. These changes could be promoted (albeit with relatively low frequency) by smoking, other viruses, or random mutation, and are biologically manifest by the latency and relative rarity of high-

grade compared with low-grade lesions. This clearly occurs most frequently, albeit not exclusively, with high-risk viral types, and results most often in a moderate or severe squamous dysplasia. The hyperproliferative basaloid cells of these lesions are now at much greater risk for the acquisition of additional genetic errors (perhaps under the influence of the same external mutagens or host genetic predisposition), which further promotes the development of the fully malignant phenotype, most often an invasive squamous cell carcinoma. The different subtypes of squamous cancer are undoubtedly related to the multistep and somewhat random nature of the process, and the proportion of different types just reflects the relative likelihood of different genetic pathways to a "successful" cancer. For glandular neoplasms, similar considerations apply. Reserve cells that are already committed to glandular differentiation are not going to be productive of virions because they lack an appropriate

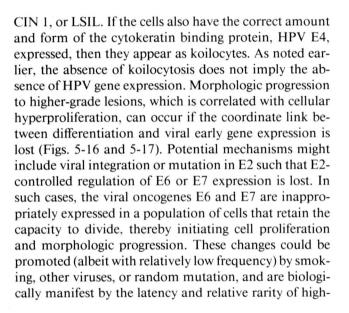
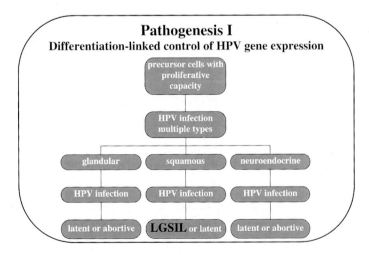

Pathogenesis I
Differentiation-linked control of HPV gene expression

precursor cells with proliferative capacity

HPV infection multiple types

glandular — squamous — neuroendocrine

HPV infection — HPV infection — HPV infection

latent or abortive — **LGSIL** or latent — latent or abortive

FIG. 5-15. Pathogenesis I. *LGSIL*, low-grade squamous intraepithelial lesion.

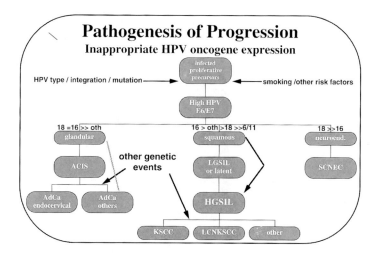

Pathogenesis of Progression
Inappropriate HPV oncogene expression

FIG. 5-16. Pathogenesis of progression II. *ACIS*, adenocarcinoma in situ; *AdCa*, adenocarcinoma; *LGSIL*, low-grade squamous intraepithelial lesion; *HGSIL*, high-grade squamous intraepithelial lesion; *KSCC*, keratinizing squamous cell carcinoma; *LCNKSCC*, large-cell nonkeratinizing squamous cell carcinoma; *neuroend*, neuroendocrine; *SCNEC*, small-cell neuroendocrine carcinoma.

differentiation environment. The usual result is probably an abortive or latent infection of endocervical cells. Much less frequently, dysregulation of viral early gene expression occurs in these nonpermissive cells. This leads to hyperproliferative lesions of glandular cells, which we morphologically recognize as adenocarcinoma in situ. It seems that HPV 18 is more successful at inducing this in glandular cells than is HPV 16. Depending upon the genetic switches that accompany this class of cell proliferation, the outcome may be an invasive adenocarcinoma, again most often endocervical but less frequently of another type (eg, endometrioid, clear-cell). Some of these lesions may not pass through a recognizable in situ phase. Essentially identical arguments can be made for the development of small-cell neuroendocrine carcinomas, tumors that are almost always associated with HPV 18 and whose low incidence probably reflects

the relative abundance of a susceptible neuroendocrine-committed precursor cell population and the rarity of "successful" viral induction of cell proliferation in such cells. None of this precludes alternative pathways of carcinogenesis unrelated to HPV. For example, in the post-diethylstilbestrol era, many clear-cell cancers of the cervix in young women may have developed along an HPV-independent path. And certainly, morphologically and biologically similar clear-cell tumors occur in the upper female genital tract without any obvious relationship to HPV. As noted earlier, cellular antioncogene mutations have been shown to be capable of substituting for the genetic effects of the viral oncogenes E6 and E7 in the rare HPV-negative cervical cancer.[141,173,175] But in the susceptible uterine cervix, the ubiquity of HPV infection makes it highly likely that the initiating steps in cervical carcinogenesis are the direct result of an HPV infection. Fortunately, progression is a relatively rare occurrence when compared with the high prevalence of the virus. Although some of this is speculative, all of it is entirely consistent with the wealth of scientific data that continues to accumulate regarding HPV-induced neoplasia.

THE CLINICAL UTILITY OF HUMAN PAPILLOMAVIRUS TESTING ON ABNORMAL CERVICAL SPECIMENS

When confronted with a cervical biopsy or Papanicolaou smear, the basic question for the pathologist is whether the morphologic changes present warrant a diagnosis within the spectrum of cervical neoplasia. In our experience, many pathologists have difficulty recognizing lesions in this continuum. Particularly challenging is separating normal or equivocal changes from diagnostic lesions, or in current terms, changes of undetermined significance from true squamous intraepithelial lesions. In particular, there is a tendency to "overcall" any cell with nonspecific halos around the nucleus as a koilocyte.

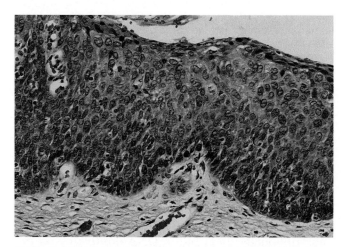

FIG. 5-17. High-grade squamous intraepithelial lesion/severe dyspalsia/Carcinoma in situ III. There has been a switch from the "differentiated" to the "proliferative" phenotype. The vast majority of such lesions express human papillomavirus mRNA but because of the lack of differentiation are not productive of virus. Hematoxylin and eosin 60×.

A common mindset seems to be that because HPV infections are ubiquitous, one should try to be as diagnostically sensitive as possible. The danger, of course, is the overdiagnosis of lesions, which can lead to overtreatment. Another argument for a confirmatory HPV test might be that by diagnosing an HPV-associated lesion, one has diagnosed a sexually transmitted disease, and this should be confirmed by an independent method for medicolegal reasons. In addition, HPV typing information might be clinically useful for prognosis and therapy. For instance, HPV 18 may be associated with rapidly progressive neoplasia and some aggressive forms of cervical cancer.[176] In contrast, HPVs 6 and 11 are almost never associated with cancer. Such a distinction might argue for differential therapy based on the presence of high-risk versus low-risk viruses.

Do the currently available tests help us with these problems? In the setting of unequivocal morphologic abnormality, a pathologic lesion within the spectrum under discussion must be assumed to be HPV-related unless proven otherwise. (To prove otherwise is not simple, given the issues of test sensitivity and the great heterogeneity of viruses.) Thus, the pathologist's problem is reduced to the application of morphologic criteria that will allow the histologic diagnosis to correlate with clinical reality. For example, koilocytosis is highly correlated with the finding of viral DNA only when well-defined perinuclear halos (koilocytosis) are present, together with definite nuclear enlargement, alteration of the nuclear-to-cytoplasmic ratio, and hyperchromasia (ie, atypia). If such strict criteria are used, then much of the need for in situ hybridization testing is obviated. Furthermore, the question of using HPV testing as an aid in borderline or low-grade cases is confounded by the limitations of the current molecular technology. In randomly selected material, roughly 40% to 70% of borderline lesions that are truly HPV-associated will be positive with these assays (Fig. 5-18). This low sensitivity is a function of several factors. It is now recognized that there is tremendous HPV type heterogeneity in low-grade lesions, yet most kits are limited in terms of their probe repertoire. In addition, even when a viral type is homologous to an available probe, the viral DNA needs to be present in sufficient concentration as well as in a chemical state that permits hybridization to occur. In high-grade lesions, there are fewer types present, so DNA heterogeneity is less of a problem. However, here, DNA copy number is often greatly reduced such that assay sensitivity is still a major issue.

In the setting of equivocal morphologic changes (atypical squamous cells of undetermined significance), a different set of problems apply. Under the best of conditions, approximately 25% to 50% of equivocal lesions are HPV-positive, and with lower-sensitivity assays, this figure is even less.[74] To argue that an equivocal lesion is clinically significant because it is HPV-positive by in situ

Clinical Condylomata
Frequency of ISH Positivity by Diagnostic Specificity

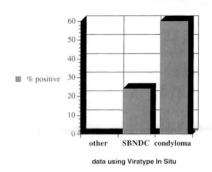

data using Viratype In Situ

Rate of Virapap Positivity vs Cytologic Diagnosis

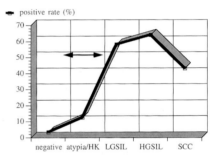

FIG. 5-18. Rates of human papillomavirus positivity for vulvar condylomata by nonradioactive in situ hybridization on formalin-fixed biopsies (**A,** Viratype In Situ, Digene Diagnostics) or dot blot analysis of DNA collected by cervical swab (**B,** Virapap, Digene Diagnostics). Both assays have a limited probe repertoire and a somewhat lower sensitivity. Importantly, the slope of the curve is steep. If strict criteria are used, definite abnormal histology (eg, condyloma, low-grade squamous intraepithelial lesion [LGSIL]) has a high human papillomavirus positivity rate. In contrast, equivocal lesions (suggestive, but not diagnostic, of condyloma [SBNDC], atypical squamous cells of undetermined significance) are positive for human papillomavirus much less often, and normal or unrelated lesions are positive even less often.[23,74,177] *HK,* hyperkeratosis; *HGSIL,* high-grade squamous intraepithelial lesion; *SCC,* squamous cell carcinoma.

hybridization or some other technique is to deny the significance of the weak morphologic findings. Conversely, the presence of a negative HPV test only provides false assurance that the lesion is truly HPV-negative because of previously cited issues of DNA heterology, copy number, and latency. For example, consider a biopsy demonstrating nonspecific halos or parakeratosis that is HPV transcriptionally silent but is DNA-positive by an extremely sensitive amplification technique. The morphologic abnormality might be due to the presence of virus, but may just as likely be a nonspecific reaction to some other stimulus (ie, DNA positivity alone does not prove pathogenetic involvement; see earlier).

TABLE 5-4. *Comparison of cytology classifications*

PAP	PAP translation	Dysplasia/CIS	CIN	Bethesda
I	Normal	Normal	Normal	Normal
II	Mild "atypia"	Squamous atypia	Atypical	ASCUS
III	Suspicious	Mild dysplasia	CIN I	LGSIL
IV	Probably malignant	Moderate dysplasia	CIN II	HGSIL
V	Malignant	Severe dysplasia	CIN III	HGSIL
		Carcinoma in situ	CIN III	HGSIL
		Cancer	Cancer	Cancer

PAP, Papanicolaou; *CIS,* carcinoma in situ; *CIN,* cervical intraepithelial neoplasia; *ASCUS,* atypical squamous cells of undetermined significance; *LGSIL,* low-grade squamous intraepithelial lesion; *HGSIL,* high-grade squamous intraepithelial lesion.

What about the prognostic significance of HPV type? In general terms, the often-quoted high-risk versus low-risk dogma may make some sense, but under scrutiny, it does not hold up very well. HPV 16 is the virus that most commonly infects the cervix. Yet, the high frequency of HPV infection relative to clinical, particularly high-grade, disease dilutes the significance of an infection by a high-risk type in a low-grade lesion. More significantly, the reservoir of high-risk viruses is undoubtedly in patients without lesions, and the factors triggering cycling between asymptomatic or latent infection and abnormal pathology are largely unknown. The overall frequency of lesion progression and regression is probably no different today than it was before we knew anything about HPVs. Although it seems clear that the high-risk viruses are the ones that more frequently progress, the fact is that the majority of lesions do not progress. The pathogenetic mechanisms discussed earlier support the concept that although strongly linked to neoplastic development, HPV infection and expression are probably only two of several steps necessary for production of the full malignant phenotype. Furthermore, occasional cases of high-grade lesions with low-risk viruses do occur. In the individual case, one has no way of knowing which lesions will progress. Hence, it would seem prudent to design treatment based on lesion grade and clinical extent without regard for HPV type.[177-181] This is especially true because there are no specific antiviral therapies for papillomaviruses, either in general or by type. Therapy is largely ablative and there is no evidence that ablative therapy effects a virologic cure. Rather, ablation eradicates clinical lesions, which then allows the patient to be placed under long-term surveillance.

HUMAN PAPILLOMAVIRUS CLASSIFICATION SYSTEMS

The pathologic spectrum of HPV-associated neoplasia can be defined essentially as those lesions in which HPV DNA is both present and expressed, so as to make the link between the presence of viral DNA and abnormal morphology pathogenetically feasible. The revised WHO histologic classification of tumors of the uterine cervix and the Bethesda system both recognize the importance of these concepts.[92,182]

The WHO reformulation utilizes the traditional dysplasia or carcinoma in situ terminology, which can easily be translated into the CIN or Bethesda terminology (Table 5-4). The Bethesda system was introduced to improve communication and increase reproducibility between pathologists. Its classification of epithelial abnormalities presents a practical approach to cytologic diagnosis that is equally applicable to histologic interpretation. It is the first classification to take into account more recent knowledge of interobserver reproducibility, the distribution of HPV types, and the clinical behavior and management of these lesions.

The Bethesda system, as it has become known, has gained reasonably wide acceptance despite some controversy. One of the most controversial points of the Bethesda classification of squamous lesions is the grouping of cellular changes associated with HPV (variously called koilocytotic atypia, condylomatous atypia, or HPV cytopathic effect) in the group designated LSIL (ie, essentially equivalent to mild dysplasia or CIN 1). Besides the pathogenetic rationale presented earlier, there is a strong scientific basis for including smears classified as koilocytotic atypia with CIN 1 in the category of LSIL, as recommended in the Bethesda system: interobserver agreement in distinguishing koilocytotic atypia from CIN 1 in smears is no better than predicted by chance[182]; the rate of HPV detection and the HPV types observed in patients with these findings is similar in cases classified as koilocytotic atypia or CIN 1[183]; patients with koilocy-

TABLE 5-5. *Koilocytotic atypia = mild dysplasia = low-grade squamous intraepithelial lesion*

Same biologic potential
Same heterogeneous human papillomavirus profile
Require similar clinical management
Overlapping morphologic criteria

TABLE 5-6. *Koilocytotic atypia: diagnostic criteria (diagnostic human papillomavirus cytopathic effect)*

Nuclear area 2–3 times a normal intermediate cell nucleus, or more
Increased nuclear-to-cytoplasmic ratio
Usually mild hyperchromasia
Sometimes degenerative nuclear changes
Well-defined cave-like cytoplasmic vacuole
Condensation of the ectocytoplasm

totic atypia and those with CIN 1 are demographically similar and have the same risk factors for squamous intraepithelial lesions[45,48]; and most studies have shown that the progression rate of koilocytotic atypia is the same as that of CIN 1 (Table 5-5).[83,85,184–186]

Our knowledge regarding cervical carcinoma and its pathogenesis has grown markedly. Research using molecular methods for the detection and analysis of HPVs has been instrumental in improving our understanding to the point that today we can clearly refocus our morphologic criteria. These lesions should be classified and reported according to the degree of specific morphologic abnormality present, regardless of the presence or absence of histologic or other evidence of HPV infection. The descriptive reporting systems for precancerous lesions of the cervix, dysplasia or carcinoma in situ, or CIN remain appropriate. The presence or absence of morphologic evidence of viral infection (ie, koilocytosis) may be mentioned as part of the diagnosis, but should not modify the clinical management of the patient. On the basis of currently available information, women with any of the lesions in this disease spectrum should receive appropriate clinical evaluation, treatment, and follow-up, irrespective of evidence of the presence or absence of HPV or a specific viral genotype. The current challenge for the diagnostic pathologist is to use established morphologic criteria that facilitate specific diagnosis. Those criteria are presented in the remainder of this text (Tables 5-6, 5-7, 5-8).

TABLE 5-7. *Cytohistologic criteria for low-grade squamous intraepithelial lesion*

Parabasal hyperplasia confined to the lower third of the epithelium
Superficial cell cytoplasm is mature, with distinct cytoplasmic borders
Superficial cell nuclear enlargement at least 3–4 times the nuclear area of a reference intermediate squamous cell nucleus
Mild nuclear hyperchromasia, uniform chromatin distribution
Nucleoli absent
Mild irregularity of nuclear outline
Binucleation common
Human papillomavirus cytopathic effect often present but not required

TABLE 5-8. *Histologic criteria for high-grade versus low-grade squamous intraepithelial lesions*

Parabasal cell proliferation extending into the middle third of the epithelium
Greater cellular disorganization or altered nuclear polarity
Increased mitotic figures
Mitotic figures in upper layers
Atypical mitoses
Unusual degrees of one or more criteria (eg, marked atypia and pleomorphism in an otherwise low-grade squamous intraepithelial lesion) may cause one-step upgrade in diagnosis

REFERENCES

1. Shope RE, Hurst EW. Infectious papillomatosis of rabbits: with a note on the histopathology. J Exp Med 1933;58:607.
2. Rous P, Kidd JG. The carcinogenic effect of a virus on tarred skin. Science 1936;83:468.
3. Kidd JG, Rous P. A transplantable rabbit carcinoma originating in a virus induced papilloma and containing the virus in masked or altered form. J Exp Med 1940;71:813.
4. Blank H, Davis C, Collins C. Electron microscopy for the diagnosis of cutaneous viral infections. Br J Dermatol 1970;83:69.
5. Boyle WF, Riggs JL, Oshiro LS, et al. Electron microscopic identification of papova virus in laryngeal papilloma. Laryngoscope 1973;83:1102.
6. Hills E, Laverty CR. Electron microscopic detection of papilloma virus particles in selected koilocytotic cells in a routine cervical smear. Acta Cytol 1979;23:53.
7. Smith J, Coleman DV. Electron microscopy of cells showing viral cytopathic effects in Papanicolaou smears. Acta Cytol 1983;27:605.
8. Rowson KEK, Mahy BWJ. Human papova (wart) virus infection. Bacteriol Rev 1967;31:110.
9. Gissmann L, Pfister H, zur Hausen H. Human papilloma viruses (HPV): characterization of four different isolates. Virology 1977;76:569.
10. Gissmann L, deVilliers EM, zur Hausen H. Analysis of human genital warts (condylomata acuminata) and other genital tumors for human papillomavirus type 6 DNA. Int J Cancer 1982;29:143.
11. de Villiers EM. Human pathogenic papillomavirus types: an update. Curr Top Microbiol Immunol 1994;186:1.
12. Koutsky LA, Galloway DA, Holmes KK. Epidemiology of genital human papillomavirus infection. Epidemiol Rev 1988;10:122.
13. Wingo PA, Tong T, Bolden S. Cancer statistics, 1995. CA Cancer J Clin 1995;45:8.
14. Brinton LA. Epidemiology of cervical cancer—an overview. In Munoz N, Bosch FX, Shah KV, et al (eds). The epidemiology of human papillomavirus and cervical cancer. New York: Oxford University Press, 1992:3.
15. Herbst AL. The Bethesda system for cervical/vaginal cytologic diagnoses. Clin Obstet Gynecol 1992;35:22.
16. Broker TR. Structure and genetic expression of papillomaviruses. Obstet Gynecol Clin North Am 1987;14:329.
17. Howley PM. Papillomavirinae and their replication. In Field BN, Knipe DM (eds). Field's virology, vol 2. New York: Raven Press, 1990:1625.
18. Howley PM. Papillomaviruses and their replication. In Field BN, Knipe DM (eds). Field's virology, vol 2. New York: Raven Press, 1995.
19. Van Ranst M, Kaplan JB, Burk RD. Phylogenetic classification of human papillomaviruses: correlation with clinical manifestations. J Gen Virol 1992;73:2653.
20. Ho GY, Burk RD, Fleming I, et al. Risk of genital human papillomavirus infection in women with human immunodeficiency virus-induced immunosuppression. Int J Cancer 1994;56:788.

21. Bernard HU. Coevolution of papillomaviruses with human populations. Trends Microbiol 1994;2:140.
22. Lorincz AT, Reid R, Jenson AB, et al. Human papillomavirus infection of the cervix: relative risk associations of 15 common anogenital types. Obstet Gynecol 1992;79:328.
23. Wilbur DC, Reichman RC, Stoler MH. Detection of infection by human papillomavirus in genital condylomata. A comparison study using immunocytochemistry and in situ nucleic acid hybridization. Am J Clin Pathol 1988;89:505.
24. Van Ranst MA, Tachezy R, Delius H, et al. Taxonomy of the human papillomaviruses. Papillomavirus Report 1993;3:61.
25. Koss LG, Durfee GR. Unusual patterns of squamous epithelium of the uterine cervix: cytologic and pathologic study of koilocytotic atypia. Ann NY Acad Sci 1956;63:1245.
26. Meisels A, Morin C, Casas CM, et al. Human papillomavirus (HPV) venereal infections and gynecologic cancer. Pathol Annu 1983;2:277.
27. Winkler B, Crum CP, Fujii T, et al. Koilocytotic lesions of the cervix. The relationship of mitotic abnormalities to the presence of papillomavirus antigens and nuclear DNA content. Cancer 1984;53:1081.
28. Ayre JE. The vaginal smear: "precancer" cell studies using a modified technique. Am J Obstet Gynecol 1949;58:1205.
29. Ayre JE. Role of the halo cell in cervical carcinogenesis: a virus manifestation in premalignancy? Obstet Gynecol 1960;17:175.
30. Patten SF. Diagnostic cytopathology of the uterine cervix (Vol. 3, 2nd ed), in Weid GR (ed) Monographs in Clinical Cytology. Basel: S Karger, 1978.
31. Meisels A, Fortin R. Condylomatous lesions of the cervix and vagina. I. Cytologic patterns. Acta Cytol 1976;20:505.
32. Meisels A. The story of a cell. The George N. Papanicolaou Award lecture. Acta Cytol 1983;27:584.
33. Purola E, Savia E. Cytology of gynecologic condyloma acuminatum. Acta Cytol 1977;21:26.
34. Kurman RJ, Shah KH, Lancaster WD, et al. Immunoperoxidase localization of papillomavirus antigens in cervical dysplasia and vulvar condylomas. Am J Obstet Gynecol 1981;140:931.
35. Kurman RJ, Sanz LE, Jenson AB, et al. Papillomavirus infection of the cervix I. Correlation of histology with viral structural antigens and DNA sequences. Int J Gynecol Pathol 1982;1:17.
36. Kurman RJ, Jenson AB, Lancaster WD. Papillomavirus infection of the cervix. II. Relationship to intraepithelial neoplasia based on the presence of specific viral structural proteins. Am J Surg Pathol 1983;7:39.
37. Laverty C. Noncondylomatous wart virus infection of the cervix: cytologic, histologic and electronmicroscopic features. Obstet Gynecol Surv 1979;34:820.
38. Sato S, Okagaki T, Clark BA, et al. Sensitivity of koilocytosis, immunocytochemistry, and electron microscopy as compared to DNA hybridization in detecting human papillomavirus in cervical and vaginal condyloma and intraepithelial neoplasia. Int J Gynecol Pathol 1986;5:297.
39. Toki T, Oikawa N, Tase T, et al. Immunohistochemical and electron microscopic demonstration of human papillomavirus in dysplasia of the uterine cervix. Tohoku J Exp Med 1986;149:163.
40. Munoz N, Bosch FX, Shah KV, et al. The epidemiology of human papillomavirus and cervical cancer. IARC Scientific Publication No. 119. New York: Oxford University Press, 1992.
41. Rigoni-Stern. Fatti statistici relativi alle malattie cancerose che servirono di base alle poche coso dette dal dott. Gior Servire Progr Path Therap 1842;2:507.
42. Towne JE. Carcinoma of the cervix in nulliparous and celibate women. Am J Obstet Gynecol 1955;69:606.
43. Roitkin ID. A comparison review of key epidemiological studies in cervical cancer related to current searches for transmissible agents. Cancer Res 1973;33:1353.
44. Munoz N, Bosch FX, de Sanjose S, et al. The causal link between human papillomavirus and invasive cervical cancer: a population-based case-control study in Colombia and Spain. Int J Cancer 1992;52:743.
45. Schiffman MH, Bauer HM, Hoover RN, et al. Epidemiologic evidence showing that human papillomavirus infection causes most cervical intraepithelial neoplasia (see comments). J Natl Cancer Inst 1993;85:958.
46. Schiffman MH. Recent progress in defining the epidemiology of human papillomavirus infection and cervical neoplasia. J Natl Cancer Inst 1992;84:394.
47. von Knebel Doeberitz M. Papillomaviruses in human disease: part I. Pathogenesis and epidemiology of human papillomavirus infections. Eur J Med 1992;1:415.
48. Schiffman MH. Epidemiology of cervical human papillomavirus infections. Curr Top Microbiol Immunol 1994;186:55.
49. Kjaer SK, Brinton LA. Adenocarcinomas of the uterine cervix: the epidemiology of an increasing problem. Epidemiol Rev 1993;15:486.
50. Bosch FX, Munoz N, de Sanjose S, et al. Importance of human papillomavirus endemicity in the incidence of cervical cancer: an extension of the hypothesis on sexual behavior. Cancer Epidemiol Biomarkers Prev 1994;3:375.
51. Venuti A, Badaracco G, Sedati A, et al. Determinants of human papillomavirus types 16 and 18 infections in the lower female genital tract in an Italian population. Eur J Gynaecol Oncol 1994;15:205.
52. Reeves WC, Gary HE Jr, Johnson PR, et al. Risk factors for genital papillomavirus infection in populations at high and low risk for cervical cancer. J Infect Dis 1994;170:753.
53. Brisson J, Morin C, Fortier M, et al. Risk factors for cervical intraepithelial neoplasia: differences between low- and high-grade lesions. Am J Epidemiol 1994;140:700.
54. Singer A, Reid R, Coppelson M. A hypothesis: the role of the high risk male in the etiology of cervcial carcinoma. A correlation of epidemiology and molecular biology. Am J Obstet Gynecol 1976;126:110.
55. Roitkin ID. Relation of adolescent coitus to cervical cancer risk. JAMA 1962;179:486.
56. Moscicki AB, Palefsky J, Gonzales J, et al. Human papillomavirus infection in sexually active adolescent females: prevalence and risk factors. Pediatr Res 1990;28:507.
57. Stewart HL, Dunham LJ, Casper J, et al. Epidemiology of cancers of the uterine cervix and corpus, breast and ovary in Israel and New York City. J Natl Cancer Inst 1966;37:1.
58. Davesa SS. Descriptive epidemiology of cancer of the uterine cervix. Obstet Gynecol 1984;63:605.
59. Pridan H, Lilienfeld AM. Carcinoma of the cervix in Jewish women in Israel (1960-67). An epidemiological study. J Med Sci Israel 1971;7:1465.
60. Kjaer SK, Engholm G, Teisen C, et al. Risk factors for cervical human papillomavirus and herpes simplex virus infections in Greenland and Denmark: a population-based study. Am J Epidemiol 1990;131:669.
61. Kjaer SK, de Villiers EM, Haugaard BJ, et al. Human papillomavirus, herpes simplex virus and cervical cancer incidence in Greenland and Denmark. A population-based cross-sectional study. Int J Cancer 1988;41:518.
62. Munoz N, Bosch FX, de Sanjose S, et al. Risk factors for cervical intraepithelial neoplasia grade III/carcinoma in situ in Spain and Colombia. Cancer Epidemiol Biomarkers Prev 1993;2:423.
63. Glew SS, Duggan-Keen M, Ghosh AK, et al. Lack of association of HLA polymorphisms with human papillomavirus-related cervical cancer. Hum Immunol 1993;37:157.
64. Apple RJ, Erlich HA, Klitz W, et al. HLA DR-DQ associations with cervical carcinoma show papillomavirus-type specificity. Nature Genetics 1994;6:157.
65. Becker TM, Wheeler CM, McGough NS, et al. Sexually transmitted diseases and other risk factors for cervical dysplasia among southwestern Hispanic and non-Hispanic white women. JAMA 1994;271:1181.
66. Melnick JL, Adam E, Rawls WE. The causative role of herpesvirus type 2 in cervical cancer. Cancer 1974;34:1375.
67. Kessler II. Perspectives on the epidemiology of cervical cancer with special reference to the herpes virus hypothesis. Cancer Res 1974;34:1091.
68. Vonka V, Kanta J, Hirsch I, et al. Prospective study on the relationship between herpes simplex type-2 virus. II. Herpes simplex type-2 antibody prevalence taken at enrollment. Int J Cancer 1984;33:61.
69. zur Hausen H, Gissmann L, Steiner W, et al. Human papilloma viruses and cancer. Bibliotheca Haematologica 1975;43:569.

70. zur Hausen H. Human papillomaviruses and their possible role in squamous cell carcinomas. Curr Top Microbiol Immunol 1977;78:1.

71. zur Hausen H. Herpes simplex virus in human genital cancer. Int Rev Exp Pathol 1983;25:307.

72. zur Hausen H, Gissmann L, Schlehofer JR. Viruses in the etiology of human genital cancer. Prog Med Virol 1984;30:170.

73. Koutsky LA, Holmes KK, Critchlow CW, et al. A cohort study of the risk of cervical intraepithelial neoplasia grade 2 or 3 in relation to papillomavirus infection. N Engl J Med 1992;327:1272.

74. Sherman ME, Schiffman MH, Lorincz AT, et al. Toward objective quality assurance in cervical cytopathology. Correlation of cytopathologic diagnoses with detection of high-risk human papillomavirus types. Am J Clin Pathol 1994;102:182.

75. de Villiers E, Wagner D, Schneider A, et al. Human papillomavirus DNA in women without and with cytological abnormalities: results of a 5-year follow-up study. Gynecol Oncol 1992;44:33.

76. Bauer HM, Ting Y, Greer CE, et al. Genital human papillomavirus infection in female university students as determined by a PCR-based method (see comments). JAMA 1991;265:472.

77. Bauer HM, Hildesheim A, Schiffman MH, et al. Determinants of genital human papillomavirus infection in low-risk women in Portland, Oregon. Sex Transm Dis 1993;20:274.

78. Schneider A, Kirchhoff T, Meinhardt G, et al. Repeated evaluation of human papillomavirus 16 status in cervical swabs of young women with a history of normal Papanicolaou smears. Obstet Gynecol 1992;79:683.

79. Hildesheim A, Schiffman MH, Gravitt PE, et al. Persistence of type-specific human papillomavirus infection among cytologically normal women. J Infect Dis 1994;169:235.

80. Nasiell K, Nasiell M, Vaclavinkova V. Behavior of moderate cervical dysplasia during long term follow up. Obstet Gynecol 1983;61:609.

81. Nasiell K, Roger B, Nasiell M. Behavior of mild cervical dysplasia during long term follow up. Obstet Gynecol 1986;67:669.

82. Syrjanen K, Mantyjarvi R, Vayrynen M, et al. Evolution of human papillomavirus infections in the uterine cervix during a long-term prospective follow-up. Applied Pathology 1987;5:121.

83. Syrjanen K, Mantyjarvi R, Saarikoski S, et al. Factors associated with progression of cervical human papillomavirus (HPV) infections into carcinoma in situ during a long-term prospective follow-up. Br J Obstet Gynaecol 1988;95:1096.

84. Syrjanen K, Hakama M, Saarikoski S, et al. Prevalence, incidence, and estimated life-time risk of cervical human papillomavirus infections in a nonselected Finnish female population. Sex Transm Dis 1990;17:15.

85. Syrjanen K, Kataja V, Yliskoski M, et al. Natural history of cervical human papillomavirus lesions does not substantiate the biologic relevance of the Bethesda system. Obstet Gynecol 1992;79:675.

86. Lorincz A. The detection of genital human papillomavirus infection using polymerase chain reaction. (Letter) JAMA 1991;265:2809.

87. Lorincz AT. Detection of human papillomavirus infection by nucleic acid hybridization. Obstet Gynecol Clin North Am 1987;14:451.

88. Lorincz A. Detection of human papillomavirus DNA without amplification: prospects for clinical utility. IARC Sci Publ 1992;119:135.

89. Stoler MH, Broker TR. In situ hybridization detection of human papillomavirus DNAs and messenger RNAs in genital condylomas and a cervical carcinoma. Hum Pathol 1986;17:1250.

90. Stoler MH. In situ hybridization. A research technique or routine diagnostic test? (Review). Arch Pathol Lab Med 1993;117:478.

91. Bergeron C, Barrasso R, Beaudenon S, et al. Human papillomaviruses associated with cervical intraepithelial neoplasia: great diversity and distinct distribution in low-grade and high-grade lesions. Am J Surg Pathol 1992;16:641.

92. Kurman RJ, Norris HJ, Wilkinson EJ. Tumors of the cervix, vagina and vulva. In Rosai J (ed). Atlas of tumor pathology, vol 4. Washington DC: Armed Forces Institute of Pathology, 1990.

93. Duggan MA, Benoit JL, McGregor SE, et al. The human papillomavirus status of 114 endocervical adenocarcinoma cases by dot blot hybridization (see comments). Hum Pathol 1993;24:121.

94. Farnsworth A, Laverty C, Stoler MH. Human papillomavirus messenger RNA expression in adenocarcinoma in situ of the uterine cervix. Int J Gynecol Pathol 1989;8:321.

95. Tase T, Sato S, Wada Y, et al. Prevalence of human papillomavirus type 18 DNA in adenocarcinoma and adenosquamous carcinoma of the uterine cervix occurring in Japan. Tohoku J Exp Med 1988;156:47.

96. Stoler MH, Mills SE, Gersell DJ, et al. Small-cell neuroendocrine carcinoma of the cervix. A human papillomavirus type 18-associated cancer. Am J Surg Pathol 1991;15:28.

97. Campion MJ, McCance DJ, Cuzick J, et al. Progressive potential of mild cervical atypia: prospective cytological, colposcopic, and virological study. Lancet 1986;2:237.

98. Kiviat NB, Koutsky LA, Critchlow CW, et al. Prevalence and cytologic manifestations of human papilloma virus (HPV) types 6, 11, 16, 18, 31, 33, 35, 42, 43, 44, 45, 51, 52, and 56 among 500 consecutive women. Int J Gynecol Pathol 1992;11:197.

99. Lutzner MA. Papillomavirus lesions in immunodepression and immunosuppression. Clin Dermatol 1985;3:165.

100. Schneider A, de Villiers EM, Schneider V. Multifocal squamous neoplasia of the female genital tract: significance of human papillomavirus infection of the vagina after hysterectomy. Obstet Gynecol 1987;70:294.

101. Campo MS, Jarrett WF. Papillomavirus infection in cattle: viral and chemical cofactors in naturally occurring and experimentally induced tumours. Ciba Found Symp 1986;120:117.

102. Campo MS. Papillomas and cancer in cattle. Cancer Surv 1987;6:39.

103. Rous P, Beard JW. The progression to carcinoma of virus induced rabbit papilloma (Shope). J Exp Med 1935;62:523.

104. zur Hausen H. Human genital cancer: synergism between two virus infections or synergism between a virus infection and initiating events? Lancet 1982;2:1370.

105. Stoler MH, Rhodes CR, Whitbeck A, et al. Human papillomavirus type 16 and 18 gene expression in cervical neoplasias. Hum Pathol 1992;23:117.

106. Crum CP, Barber S, Symbula M, et al. Coexpression of the human papillomavirus type 16 E4 and L1 open reading frames in early cervical neoplasia. Virology 1990;178:238.

107. Stoler MH, Wolinsky SM, Whitbeck A, et al. Differentiation-linked human papillomavirus types 6 and 11 transcription in genital condylomata revealed by in situ hybridization with message-specific RNA probes. Virology 1989;172:331.

108. Stoler MH, Whitbeck A, Wolinsky SM, et al. Infectious cycle of human papillomavirus type 11 in human foreskin xenografts in nude mice. J Virol 1990;64:3310.

109. Smotkin D, Wettstein FO. Transcription of human papillomavirus type 16 early genes in a cervical cancer and a cancer-derived cell line and identification of the E7 protein. Proc Natl Acad Sci U S A 1986;83:4680.

110. Baker CC, Phelps WC, Lindgren V, et al. Structural and transcriptional analysis of human papillomavirus type 16 sequences in cervical carcinoma cell lines. J Virol 1987;61:962.

111. Boshart M, Gissmann L, Ikenberg H, et al. A new type of papillomavirus DNA, its presence in genital cancer biopsies and in cell lines derived from cervical cancer. EMBO J 1984;3:1151.

112. Schwarz E, Freese UK, Gissmann L, et al. Structure and transcription of human papillomavirus sequences in cervical carcinoma cells. Nature 1985;314:111.

113. Yee C, Krishnan HI, Baker CC, et al. Presence and expression of human papillomavirus sequences in human cervical carcinoma cell lines. Am J Pathol 1985;119:361.

114. Schneider-Gadicke A, Schwarz E. Different human cervical carcinoma cell lines show similar transcription patterns of human papillomavirus type 18 early genes. EMBO J 1986;5:2285.

115. Land H, Parada LF, Weinberg RA. Cellular oncogenes and multistep carcinogenesis. Science 1983;222:771.

116. Matlashewski G, Schneider J, Banks L, et al. Human papillomavirus type 16 DNA cooperates with activated ras in transforming primary cells. EMBO J 1987;6:1741.

117. Matlashewski G, Osborn K, Banks L, et al. Transformation of primary human fibroblast cells with human papillomavirus type 16 DNA and EJ-ras. Int J Cancer 1988;42:232.

118. Storey A, Pim D, Murray A, et al. Comparison of the in vitro

transforming activities of human papillomavirus types. EMBO J 1988;7:1815.

119. Storey A, Banks L. Human papillomavirus type 16 E6 gene cooperates with EJ-ras to immortalize primary mouse cells. Oncogene 1993;8:919.

120. Pirisi L, Yasumoto S, Feller M, et al. Transformation of human fibroblasts and keratinocytes with human papillomavirus type 16 DNA. J Virol 1987;61:1061.

121. Pirisi L, Batova A, Jenkins GR, et al. Increased sensitivity of human keratinocytes immortalized by human papillomavirus type 16 DNA to growth control by retinoids. Cancer Res 1992;52:187.

122. Woodworth CD, Doniger J, DiPaolo JA. Immortalization of human foreskin keratinocytes by various human papillomavirus DNAs corresponds to their association with cervical carcinoma. J Virol 1989;63:159.

123. Woodworth CD, Waggoner S, Barnes W, et al. Human cervical and foreskin epithelial cells immortalized by human papillomavirus DNAs exhibit dysplastic differentiation in vivo. Cancer Res 1990;50:3709.

124. McCance DJ, Kopan R, Fuchs E, et al. Human papillomavirus type 16 alters human epithelial cell differentiation in vitro. Proc Natl Acad Sci U S A 1988;85:7169.

125. Laimins LA. The biology of human papillomaviruses: from warts to cancer. Infect Agents Dis 1993;2:74.

126. El-Awady MK, Kaplan JB, O'Brien SJ, et al. Molecular analysis of integrated human papillomavirus 16 sequences in the cervical cancer cell line SiHa. Virology 1987;159:389.

127. Choo KB, Pan CC, Liu MS, et al. Presence of episomal and integrated human papillomavirus DNA sequences in cervical carcinoma. J Med Virol 1987;21:101.

128. Choo KB, Pan CC, Han SH. Integration of human papillomavirus type 16 into cellular DNA of cervical carcinoma: preferential deletion of the E2 gene and invariable retention of the long control region and the E6/E7 open reading frames. Virology 1987;161:259.

129. Matsukura T, Koi S, Sugase M. Both episomal and integrated forms of human papillomavirus type 16 are involved in invasive cervical cancers. Virology 1989;172:63.

130. Shirasawa H, Tomita Y, Kubota K, et al. Detection of human papillomavirus type 16 DNA and evidence for integration into the cell DNA in cervical dysplasia. J Gen Virol 1986;67:2011.

131. Shirasawa H, Tomita Y, Sekiya S, et al. Integration and transcription of human papillomavirus type 16 and 18 sequences in cell lines derived from cervical carcinomas. J Gen Virol 1987;68:583.

132. Cullen AP, Reid R, Campion M, et al. Analysis of the physical state of different human papillomavirus DNAs in intraepithelial and invasive cervical neoplasm. J Virol 1991;65:606.

133. Chin MT, Hirochika R, Hirochika H, et al. Regulation of human papillomavirus type 11 enhancer and E6 promoter by activating and repressing proteins from the E2 open reading frame: functional and biochemical studies. J Virol 1988;62:2994.

134. Bishop JM. Viral oncogenes. Cell 1985;42:23.

135. Goustin AS, Leof EB, Shipley GD, et al. Perspectives in cancer research: growth factors and cancer. Cancer Res 1986;46:1015.

136. Weinberg RA. The actions of oncogenes in the cytoplasm and nucleus. Science 1985;230:770.

137. Weinberg RA. The integration of molecular genetics into cancer management. Cancer 1992;70:1653.

138. Ocadiz R, Sauceda R, Salcedo M, et al. Occurrence of human papillomavirus type 16 DNA sequences and c-myc oncogene alterations in uterine-cervix carcinoma. Archivos de Investigacion Medica 1989;20:355.

139. Riou GF. Proto-oncogenes and prognosis in early carcinoma of the uterine cervix. Cancer Surv 1988;7:441.

140. Riou GF, Bourhis J, Le MG. The c-myc proto-oncogene in invasive carcinomas of the uterine cervix: clinical relevance of overexpression in early stages of the cancer. Anticancer Res 1990;10:1225.

141. Riou G, Le MG, Favre M, et al. Human papillomavirus-negative status and c-myc gene overexpression: independent prognostic indicators of distant metastasis for early-stage invasive cervical cancers. J Natl Cancer Inst 1992;84:1525.

142. Durst M, Croce CM, Gissmann L, et al. Papillomavirus sequences integrate near cellular oncogenes in some cervical carcinomas. Proc Natl Acad Sci U S A 1987;84:1070.

143. Durst M, Kleinheinz A, Hotz M, et al. The physical state of human papillomavirus type 16 DNA in benign and malignant genital tumours. J Gen Virol 1985;66:1515.

144. Cannizzaro LA, Durst M, Mendez MJ, et al. Regional chromosome localization of human papillomavirus integration sites near fragile sites, oncogenes, and cancer chromosome breakpoints. Cancer Genet Cytogenet 1988;33:93.

145. Stanbridge EJ, Der CJ, Doerson CJ, et al. Human cell hybrids: analysis of transformation and tumorigenicity. Science 1982;215:252.

146. zur Hausen H. Papillomaviruses in human cancer. Cancer 1987;59:1692.

147. Bosch FX, Schwarz E, Boukamp P, et al. Suppression in vivo of human papillomavirus type 18 E6-E7 gene expression in nontumorigenic HeLa X fibroblast hybrid cells. J Virol 1990;64:4743.

148. Bosch FX, Durst M, Schwarz E, et al. The early genes E6 and E7 of cancer associated human papilloma viruses as targets of tumor suppression? Behring Inst Mitt 1991;89:108.

149. Lee W-H, Bookstein R, Hong F, et al. Human retinoblastoma gene: cloning, identification and sequence. Science 1987;235:1394.

150. Lee W-H, Shew J-Y, Hong FD, et al. The retinoblastoma susceptibility gene encodes a nuclear phosphoprotein associated with DNA binding activity. Nature 1987;329:642.

151. Dowdy SF, Hinds PW, Louie K, et al. Physical interaction of the retinoblastoma protein with human D cyclins. Cell 1993;73:499.

152. Cryns VL, Thor A, Xu H-J, et al. Loss of the retinoblastoma tumor-suppressor gene in parathyroid carcinoma. N Engl J Med 1994;330:757.

153. Ewen ME, Sluss HK, Sherr CJ, et al. Functional interactions of the retinoblastoma protein with mammalian D-type cyclins. Cell 1993;73:487.

154. Munger K, Phelps WC, Bubb V, et al. The E6 and E7 genes of the human papillomavirus type 16 together are necessary and sufficient for transformation of primary human keratinocytes. J Virol 1989;63:4417.

155. Phelps WC, Yee CL, Munger K, et al. Functional and sequence similarities between HPV16 E7 and adenovirus E1A. Curr Top Microbiol Immunol 1989;144:153.

156. Dyson N, Howley PM, Munger K, et al. The human papilloma virus-16 E7 oncoprotein is able to bind to the retinoblastoma gene product. Science 1989;243:934.

157. Munger K, Werness BA, Dyson N, et al. Complex formation of human papillomavirus E7 proteins with the retinoblastoma tumor suppressor gene product. EMBO J 1989;8:4099.

158. Howley PM, Munger K, Werness BA, et al. Molecular mechanisms of transformation by the human papillomaviruses. Int Symp Princess Takamatsu Cancer Res Fund 1989;20:199.

159. Phelps WC, Yee CL, Munger K, et al. The human papillomavirus type 16 E7 gene encodes transactivation and transformation functions similar to those of adenovirus E1A. Cell 1988;53:539.

160. Scheffner M, Werness BA, Huibregtse JM, et al. The E6 oncoprotein encoded by human papillomavirus types 16 and 18 promotes the degradation of p53. Cell 1990;63:1129.

161. Werness BA, Levine AJ, Howley PM. Association of human papillomavirus types 16 and 18 E6 proteins with p53. Science 1990;248:76.

162. Huibregtse JM, Scheffner M, Howley PM. A cellular protein mediates association of p53 with the E6 oncoprotein of human papillomavirus types 16 or 18. EMBO J 1991;10:4129.

163. Werness BA, Munger K, Howley PM. Role of the human papillomavirus oncoproteins in transformation and carcinogenic progression. Important Adv Oncol 1991;1991:3.

164. Scheffner M, Munger K, Byrne JC, et al. The state of the p53 and retinoblastoma genes in human cervical carcinoma cell lines. Proc Natl Acad Sci U S A 1991;88:5523.

165. Munger K, Scheffner M, Huibregtse JM, et al. Interactions of HPV E6 and E7 oncoproteins with tumour suppressor gene products. Cancer Surv 1992;12:197.

166. Scheffner M, Takahashi T, Huibregtse JM, et al. Interaction of the human papillomavirus type-16 E6 oncoprotein with wild-type and mutant human p53 proteins. J Virol 1992;66:5100.

167. Crook T, Wrede D, Tidy JA, et al. Clonal p53 mutation in primary cervical cancer: association with human-papillomavirus-negative tumours (see comments). Lancet 1992;339:1070.

168. Crook T, Wrede D, Vousden KH. p53 point mutation in HPV negative human cervical carcinoma cell lines. Oncogene 1991;6:873.

169. Fujita M, Inoue M, Tanizawa O, et al. Alterations of the p53 gene in human primary cervical carcinoma with and without human papillomavirus infection. Cancer Res 1992;52:5323.

170. Kessis TD, Slebos RJ, Han SM, et al. p53 Gene mutations and MDM2 amplification are uncommon in primary carcinomas of the uterine cervix. Am J Pathol 1993;143:1398.

171. Lechner MS, Laimins LA. Inhibition of p53 DNA binding by human papillomavirus E6 proteins. J Virol 1994;68:4262.

172. Demeter LM, Stoler MH, Broker TR, et al. Induction of proliferating cell nuclear antigen in differentiated keratinocytes of human papillomavirus-infected lesions. Hum Pathol 1994;25:343.

173. Dollard SC, Wilson JL, Demeter LM, et al. Production of human papillomavirus and modulation of the infectious program in epithelial raft cultures. Gene Develop 1992;6:1131.

174. Demeter LM, Stoler MH, Sobel ME, et al. Expression of high-affinity laminin receptor mRNA correlates with cell proliferation rather than invasion in human papillomavirus-associated cervical neoplasms. Cancer Res 1992;52:1561.

175. Higgins GD, Davy M, Roder D, et al. Increased age and mortality associated with cervical carcinomas negative for human papillomavirus RNA. Lancet 1991;338:910.

176. Kurman RJ, Schiffman MH, Lancaster WD, et al. Analysis of individual human papillomavirus types in cervical neoplasia: a possible role for type 18 in rapid progression. Am J Obstet Gynecol 1988;159:293.

177. Masih AS, Stoler MH, Farrow GM, et al. Human papillomavirus in penile squamous cell lesions. A comparison of an isotopic RNA and two commercial nonisotopic DNA in situ hybridization methods. Arch Pathol Lab Med 1993;117:302.

178. Kurman RJ, Henson DE, Herbst AL, et al. Interim guidelines for the management of abnormal cervical cytology. JAMA 1994;271:1866.

179. Bonfiglio TA, Stoler MH. Human papillomavirus and cancer of the uterine cervix. (Editorial) Hum Pathol 1988;19:621.

180. National Coordinating Network (National Cervical Screening Programme), British Society for Clinical Cytology, and Royal College of Pathologists' Working Party. Borderline nuclear changes in cervical smears: guidelines on their recognition and management. J Clin Pathol 1994;47:481.

181. Dalence CR. Diagnostic and therapeutic technology assessment (DATTA): human papillomavirus testing in the management of cervical neoplasia. JAMA 1993;270:2975.

182. Kurman RJ, Malkasian GJ, Sedlis A, et al. From Papanicolaou to Bethesda: the rationale for a new cervical cytologic classification. Obstet Gynecol 1991;77:779.

183. Sherman ME, Schiffman MH, Erozan YS, et al. The Bethesda system. Arch Pathol Lab Med 1992;116:1155.

184. Willett GD, Kurman RJ, Reid R, et al. Correlation of the histologic appearance of intraepithelial neoplasia of the cervix with human papillomavirus types. Emphasis on low grade lesions including so-called flat condyloma. Int J Gynecol Pathol 1989;8:18.

185. Kataja V, Syrjanen K, Mantyjarvi R, et al. Prospective follow-up of cervical HPV infections: life table analysis of histopathological, cytological and colposcopic data. Eur J Epidemiol 1989;5:1.

186. Kataja V, Syrjanen K, Syrjanen S, et al. Prospective follow-up of genital HPV infections: survival analysis of the HPV typing data. Eur J Epidemiol 1990;6:9.

Gynecologic Cytopathology. Edited by
Thomas A. Bonfiglio and Yener S. Erozan.
Lippincott–Raven Publishers, Philadelphia, © 1997.

CHAPTER 6

The Cytopathology of Squamous Epithelial Lesions of the Cervix and Vagina

Thomas A. Bonfiglio

The squamous epithelial lesions of the cervix encompass a broad spectrum of abnormalities, including the most common of the clinically significant lesions detected in cytologic samples taken from the uterine cervix and vagina. Also included are invasive squamous carcinoma and its intraepithelial precursor lesions, and those cytologic abnormalities involving squamous cells whose significance cannot be unequivocally determined on the basis of their morphologic appearance. The latter group encompasses those cellular changes that are morphologically intermediate between benign reactive changes and true intraepithelial lesions.

As we consider these squamous lesions, including those that are clearly within the spectrum of preinvasive cervical neoplasia, certain important considerations about the biology of the process of carcinogenesis in the uterine cervix should be emphasized. Much has been learned in recent years regarding the etiology and pathogenesis of this disease, particularly in respect to the role of human papillomavirus (HPV) in the process. This, in large part, began with the landmark publications of Meisels and Fortin and Purola and Savia in the mid-1970s,[1–3] and has led to a better understanding of the biology behind the complexities of the behavior of these lesions and the molecular alterations leading to the structural changes that are evident in the tissue and the individual cells. The details of HPV biology in relation to the neoplastic process are discussed in Chapter 5. This chapter will emphasize the morphologic manifestations of the process in cytologic samples, the differential diagnostic criteria, and the relationship of these features to clinical behavior.

At the outset, it is important to consider some points about the biologic potential of the various lesions under discussion. These are graphically outlined in Figure 6-1. It can be noted from the chart that the changes at any point are not necessarily progressive, and that the majority of cases of slight dysplasia, for example, do not progress, but either persist at that stage or regress. The chart also points out that not all cases of carcinoma in situ (CIS) would necessarily progress to outspoken invasive carcinoma. This reflects the very likely possibility that not all cases currently called CIS are true intraepithelial cancer. It also suggests that in some patients, the host response to the early invasive lesions may be successful in destroying the cancer. It must be pointed out at this juncture that although the morphologic criteria for classifying these lesions at each step in this spectrum are defined, the biologic behavior or potential of the stages is not. Indeed, many cases of moderate dysplasia have the same biologic potential as cases of severe dysplasia, and most cases that are classified as severe dysplasia have the same biologic potential as those classified as CIS. These facts, of course, support the utilization of the terminology specified in the Bethesda system for the reporting of results because it most closely corresponds to our current understanding of the biology of these lesions and, therefore, relates to treatment approaches.

ATYPICAL SQUAMOUS CELLS OF UNDETERMINED SIGNIFICANCE

The category of the Bethesda classification known as *atypical squamous cells of undetermined significance* (ASCUS) encompasses those cytologic changes that although clearly abnormal, are not severe enough to meet the criteria for establishing a diagnosis of an intraepithelial lesion and yet are more severe than those changes that are classified in the *benign cellular changes* category.

T. A. Bonfiglio: Department of Pathology and Laboratory Medicine, University of Rochester Medical Center, Rochester, New York 14642.

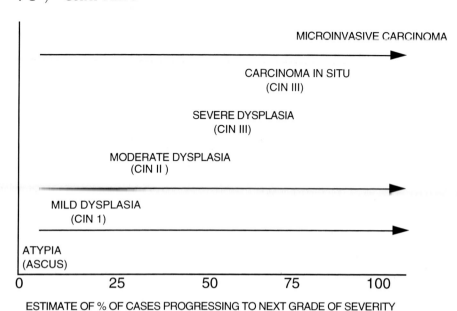

FIG. 6-1. Chart comparing the overall biologic potential of squamous intraepithelial lesions of varying degrees of severity. *CIN*, Cervical Intraepithelial Neoplasia; *ASCUS*, atypical squamous cells of undetermined significance.

In this sense, the diagnosis of ASCUS is one of exclusion (ie, the changes neither fall into the definitively benign category nor meet the established definition for squamous intraepithelial lesions). It is important to point out that the description of this category by the Bethesda committee stresses that this group should not be considered the equivalent of the old "class 2" designation of the Papanicolaou system or of any other uses of the term *atypia* in the past, such as reactive atypia or inflammatory atypia. These cellular changes are included in the category of the current system termed *benign reactive changes*.[4] There are specific criteria that have been established for the inclusion of cellular changes in the ASCUS category. These are summarized in Table 6-1. The use of this category, however, may vary somewhat between pathologists. This has caused some to be concerned that the overuse of this classification may lead to unnecessary follow-up or diagnostic procedures in some situations, or to the underdiagnosis of true intraepithelial lesions in others. To date, there is little evidence that this has occurred, although it is undoubtedly true that not all laboratories were using the term in a consistent and similar fashion, particularly during the early stages of the use of this terminology. The prevalence of this diagnosis, even if used consistently from laboratory to laboratory, will vary, of course, with the population being screened. In general, however, no more than about 5% of cases would be expected to fall into this category. As a general rule, the frequency of the ASCUS diagnosis should not exceed two or three times that of the squamous intraepithelial lesion diagnosis in an individual laboratory.[4]

The specific criteria used for this diagnosis per the Bethesda system terminology are nearly identical to those that were well described by Patten in his monograph published in 1978.[5] In summary, the most common cells in this category resemble normal superficial or intermediate squamous cells in configuration and size. Their cytoplasm is abundant, polygonal, and eosino-

TABLE 6-1. *Summary of differential diagnostic features of atypical squamous cells of undetermined significance (ASCUS)*

Cytoplasmic areas and configuration approximate those of normal intermediate squamous cells in most cases; less often like those of squamous metaplastic cells

Nuclei 2–3 times the size of normal intermediate squamous cell nuclei

Normochromatic to mildly hyperchromatic nuclei

Round nuclei with no or minimal nuclear envelope irregularities

Absence of definitive human papillomavirus effect

Cells usually isolated (except atypical repair)

Relative Nuclear Sizes

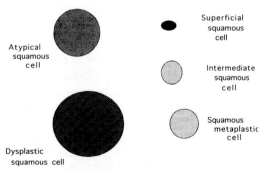

FIG. 6-2. Diagramatic representation of comparative nuclear size of various normal and abnormal squamous epithelia.

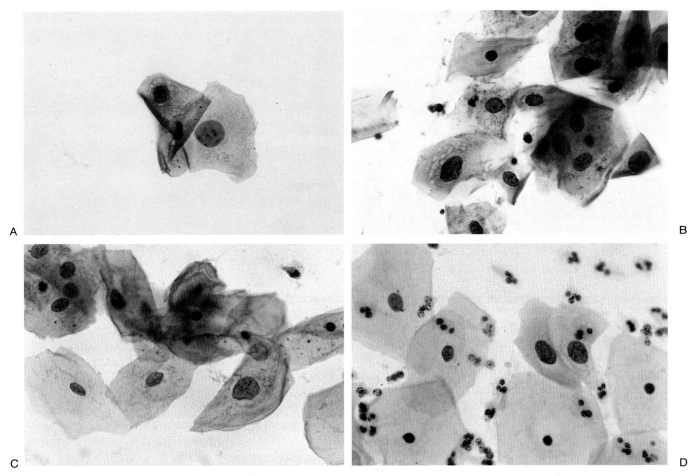

FIG. 6-3. (A–D) Atypical squamous cells of undetermined significance (ASCUS). Note the moderate nuclear enlargement and minimal hyperchromasia in these several examples of atypia in mature appearing squamous cells.

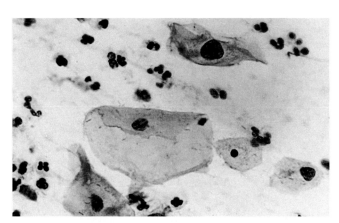

FIG. 6-4. Atypical squamous cells of undetermined significance. There is a single atypical cell in the upper portion of the photograph and normal intermediate cells for comparison.

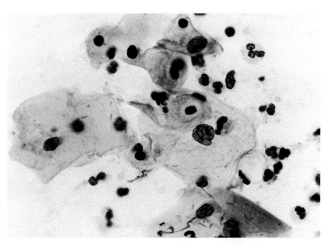

FIG. 6-5. Atypical squamous cells of undetermined significance, probably reactive. This field contains two cells with atypical nuclei probably representing a reactive change. The small perinuclear halo in the center is a nonspecific finding often seen with inflammation.

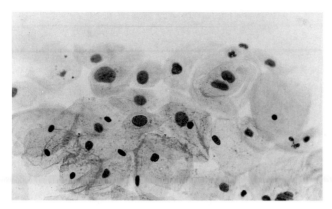

FIG. 6-6. Atypical squamous cells of undetermine significance. The abnormal cells are in upper half of illustration. Note the increase in nuclear size and binucleation.

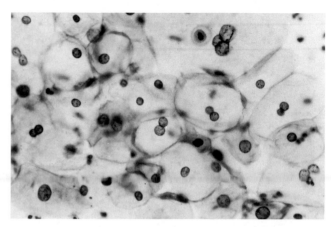

FIG. 6-8. Atypical squamous cells of undetermined significance. These cells show changes that are suggestive but not diagnostic of human papillomavirus cytopathic effect.

philic, but may also be cyanophilic in staining character. They are distinguished from normal, however, by the fact that they have enlarged nuclei, which are generally two or three times the size of normal intermediate squamous cell nuclei, or 70 to 120 μm^2 in surface area (Fig. 6-2). These nuclei have finely granular, evenly distributed chromatin and are normochromatic or, at most, slightly hyperchromatic. Binucleation and nonspecific, small, perinuclear halos may also be present (Figs. 6-3 through 6-8).

Similar changes may also occur in more immature-appearing squamous cells of metaplastic type. This type of ASCUS, also referred to as *atypical cells of squamous metaplastic type,* has similar abnormally enlarged nuclei (70 to 120 μm^2 in surface area) and finely granular, evenly distributed chromatin. Their cytoplasm tends to be less abundant and more cyanophilous, with cell shapes that are generally rounder. Their nuclear-to-cytoplasmic ratios are higher than those in the more common type of ASCUS[5,6] (Figs. 6-9 and 6-10).

Even more immature-appearing "atypical" squamous cells may be identified in cytologic samples. In these cases, the differential diagnosis often is difficult. These cells resemble very immature squamous metaplastic cells and have been referred to as *atypical cells of immature squamous metaplastic type.* Although they may be considered a subgroup of ASCUS, their frequent association with high-grade intraepithelial lesions suggests that they should be considered separately, at least in terms of patient management.

Atypical cells of immature squamous metaplastic type have nuclei that are generally much smaller than the size range mentioned earlier for other atypical squamous cells, but their nuclear-to-cytoplasmic ratio is much higher. Their cytoplasm is scant, generally amphophilic, and has a round to oval configuration. The nuclei tend to be mildly hyperchromatic and the nuclear chromatin

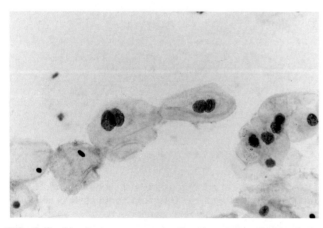

FIG. 6-7. Atypical squamous cells of undetermined significance. Both abnormal squamous cells in the center are binucleated.

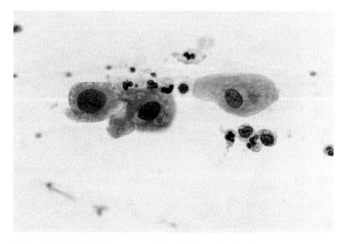

FIG. 6-9. Atypical squamous cells of undetermined significance. (Atypical cells are of squamous metaplastic type.) Note: Atypical metaplastic cell on left, compared to normal immature metaplastic cell on right.

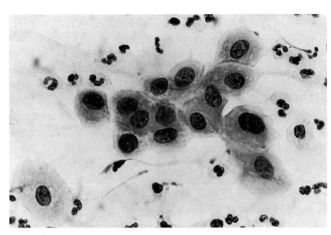

FIG. 6-10. Atypical squamous metaplastic cells of undetermined significance. The nuclei are enlarged but there are no significant irregularities of the nuclear envelope.

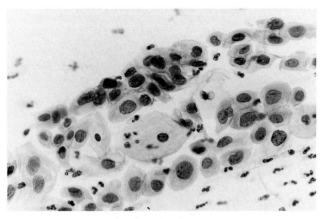

FIG. 6-12. Atypical immature squamous metaplastic cells suggestive of high-grade squamous intraepithelial lesion. This field contains a mixture of atypical metaplastic cells of varying degrees of maturity. Although not diagnostic of a high-grade lesion the small atypical cells in the top half of the field are particularly worrisome and warrant recommending a colposcopic examination.

remains finely granular and evenly distributed (Figs. 6-11 through 6-13). These cells resemble the so-called *third-type cells* derived from CIS described by Graham[7,8] and others, and this presents the diagnostic dilemma. The cells originating from CIS, however, usually show significant hyperchromasia as well as nuclear envelope irregularities. If these features are present, a diagnosis of high-grade squamous intraepithelial lesion (HSIL) is likely and the interpretation should be as such. In other instances where the nuclear changes are not such that a definitive diagnosis of a high-grade lesion can be made, the most appropriate interpretation may be as follows: ASCUS (atypical cells of immature squamous metaplastic type); HSIL cannot be excluded.

The fact that these atypical immature metaplastic cells closely resemble the small cells that are associated with some HSILs has led to considerable controversy as to the legitimacy of this category, with some arguing that all cells of this type are derived from HSILs. Indeed, one

possibility is that some of these cells may be degenerating cells shed from an HSIL. In fact, as has been noted in a study performed in our laboratory, a significant proportion of such cells are related to high-grade lesions. In that study, performed by Dressel and Wilbur, the authors reviewed 294 cases of atypical cells of immature squamous metaplastic type diagnosed between 1980 and 1990. In this group of patients, progression or association with a squamous intraepithelial lesion or carcinoma was noted in 37% of cases.[9] However, it was apparent that there is an appreciable group of patients with very small atypical metaplastic–like cells of this type who do not appear to have an HSIL.

As mentioned earlier, hyperchromasia and nuclear en-

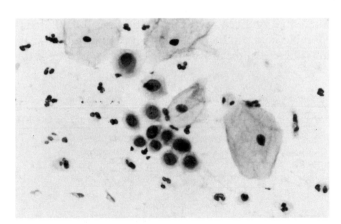

FIG. 6-11. Atypical immature squamous metaplastic cells. These immature cells have a very high nuclear/cytoplasmic ratio but have uniformly round nuclei and finely granular chromatin.

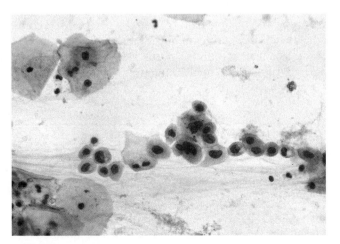

FIG. 6-13. Atypical immature squamous metaplastic cells. These cells have hyperchromatic nuclei, some of which are also mildly irregular in shape. The nuclear/cytoplasmic ratio, however, is not as high as is seen in high-grade lesions.

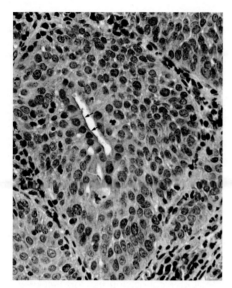

FIG. 6-14. Atypical immature squamous metaplasia involving an endocervical gland. Note the relative uniformity, regular arrangement and lack of mitoses in this immature epithelial proliferation. The arrows designate residual mucinous endocervical glandular epithelium overlying the metaplastic epithelium. (Reproduced with permission from Kurman RJ, Norris HJ, Wilkinson EJ: Tumors of the cervix, vagina and vulva. Washington, DC, Armed Forces Institute of Pathology, 1992.)

velope irregularities appear to be the best indicators of origin from a significant lesion. There is, however, uncertainty in many cases, and a definite potential to undercall a significant lesion exists if these types of cells are simply classified as ASCUS in those cases where there is doubt.

The histologic counterpart of this cytologic group is uncertain, but may well be a well-described but often unrecognized entity that has been termed *immature squamous metaplasia with atypia*.[10,11] This lesion, which histologically may simulate an HSIL, is distinguished from the more serious lesion in tissue sections by the lack of crowding and disorganization, and by the fact that component cells have uniform, round nuclei with less hyperchromasia than is found in a true HSIL. In addition, abnormal mitoses and nuclear membrane irregularities are

not present. Like its proposed cytologic counterpart, the biologic significance of this histologic lesion is not well understood (Fig. 6-14). Fu and Reagan reported that this lesion coexists with 34% of condylomata and 16% of cervical intraepithelial neoplasia. The association with HPV-related lesions and the fact that HPV capsid antigens have been identified in some of these lesions by immunohistochemistry suggests that, like the squamous intraepithelial lesion, this may represent an HPV-related lesion.[11]

The cytologic significance of these small atypical cells remains unclear. The differential diagnosis in these cases is an HSIL versus a histologic lesion, atypical immature metaplasia, which itself is of uncertain significance. Until this cytologic category of atypical cells of immature squamous metaplastic type is better elucidated to determine whether there is a subgroup that is associated with an HSIL and another that represents an immature but benign process, it remains appropriate to recommend colposcopic examination and biopsy (if indicated) in all instances where this type of cytologic abnormality is encountered.

Atypical Repair

The cytologic manifestations of atypical reparative reactions are also included in the ASCUS category per the Bethesda system. This category is characterized by the presence of markedly atypical cells in sheets or syncytium-like aggregates. Although some of these aggregates resemble squamous cells, others suggest endocervical differentiation. The cells differ from those of typical repair in that they tend to be more irregularly arranged within the aggregates, to demonstrate anisonucleosis and nuclear hyperchromasia, and to have coarsely granular chromatin. Nucleoli may be multiple and vary in both size and configuration. In short, the abnormal cells demonstrate many of the features associated with malignancy. In those severe cases where differentiation from invasive carcinoma is difficult, considerable help can be obtained by keeping in mind certain differential diagnostic features (Table 6-2). Cells de-

TABLE 6-2. *Comparison of Cytologic Features of Repair Versus Squamous Carcinoma and Adenocarcinoma*

Cytologic feature	Repair	Squamous carcinoma	Endocervical cell adenocarcinoma
Slide background	Inflammatory	Diathesis	Clean or diathesis
Cytoplasm	Variable	Polygonal, pleomorphic	Columnar, cuboidal
Cell arrangement	Sheets	Syncytium-like, single cells	Sheets, syncytia, single cells
Nuclei	Enlarged, normochromatic to mildly hyperchromatic	Variable size, hyperchromatic	Variable size, hyperchromatic
Nuclear envelope	Smooth	Irregular	Irregular
Chromatin	Finely granular, evenly distributed	Coarsely granular, uneven distribution	Finely to coarsely granular, uneven distribution
Nucleoli	Macronucleoli; may be multiple	Macronucleoli; usually single	Macronucleoli; may be multiple
Mitoses	Commonly evident, normal; may be many	Few; may be abnormal	Few

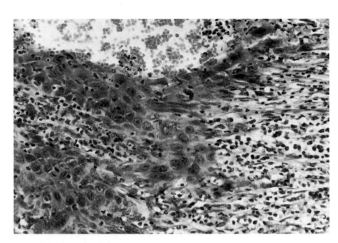

FIG. 6-15. Tissue section showing atypical repair in a cervical biopsy specimen. The nuclear enlargement and prominent nucleoli correspond to the cytologic features noted in smears of such lesions. (Reproduced with permission from Bonfiglio TA: Cytopathology of cervical dysplasia, carcinoma in situ and invasive carcinoma. *In* Astarita R: *Basic Cytopathology,* New York, Churchill Livingstone, 1989.)

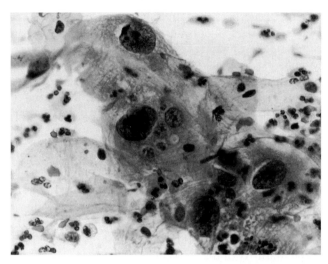

FIG. 6-17. Atypical repair. There are mild irregularities of the nuclear envelopes of some of these cells and large nucleoli are evident but the nuclear cytoplasmic ratio is low.

rived from reparative reactions occur in sheets. Isolated cells with the characteristics of malignancy are not commonly found. Generally, a lower nuclear-to-cytoplasmic ratio is maintained. Furthermore, a true tumor diathesis does not occur in association with reparative reactions. Finally, significant alterations of nuclear chromatin distribution are generally not seen in cells derived from repair.[12] Nevertheless, in very severe atypical reparative reactions, clear-cut distinction from a serious process cannot always be made. In those situations, it is best to report the findings as atypical repair, state that a more serious process (ie, invasive carcinoma) cannot be excluded, and recommend appropriate clinical evaluation (Figs. 6-15 through 6-18).

Follow-up Studies of Patients With Atypical Squamous Cells of Undetermined Significance

Many studies have shown that the rate of occurrence of a diagnosis of an intraepithelial lesion in a patient after a diagnosis of atypia ranges from as low as 10.1% to as high as 57%.[13–21] The total rate of association of an AS-CUS diagnosis with a subsequent or concurrent diagnosis of a squamous intraepithelial lesion for this author's laboratory patient cohort falls at the low end of this broad range (13.5%), and compares favorably with the rate established in some early studies of approximately 10% association between "squamous atypia" and a subsequent diagnosis of an intraepithelial lesion. These rates, from a recent study in our laboratory, where the

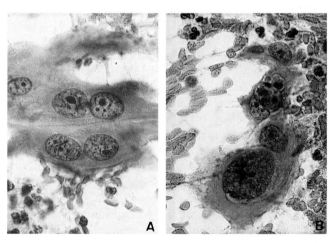

FIG. 6-16. Atypical repair. Note prominent nucleoli, hyperchromais, and coarse chromatin. The cells in frame **B** also show variation in nuclear size.

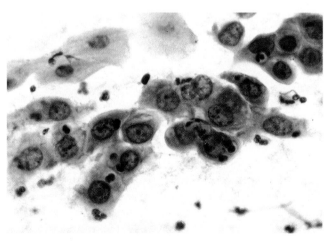

FIG. 6-18. Atypical repair. Macronucleoli are seen but the chromatin abnormalities, which are more marked than those seen in the usual repair are the most atypical feature.

cytologic criteria of the Bethesda system are utilized and factors placing patients in differential risk groups are eliminated (eg, histories of prior dysplasia, samples from patients being seen in colposcopy clinics), might be judged to represent reasonable estimations of the frequency of association of ASCUS with intraepithelial lesions.[22] A rate of association with the diagnosis of an intraepithelial lesion in the range of 10% to 15% is also supported by long-term follow-up data generated by Syrjanen and colleagues in an untreated population in Finland.[23]

In addition, the results of a study of ASCUS by Shiels and Wilbur at Rochester suggest that there is value in subclassifying the types of squamous atypia based on defined morphologic criteria.[22] These authors reported that as the maturity of the atypical cells decreases, their association with intraepithelial lesions increases substantially, as does the percentage of cases associated with HSILs. In their study, ASCUS with mature cytoplasm were associated with intraepithelial lesions in 10% of cases, whereas those with metaplastic-type cytoplasm were associated in 24% of cases. Atypical immature squamous metaplastic cells, discussed earlier, were associated with intraepithelial lesions in 42% of cases. In addition, 42% of patients with atypia involving metaplastic-type squamous cells and 60% of those with the most immature type of atypical squamous cells who were subsequently diagnosed with intraepithelial lesions had high-grade processes, compared with only 30% of those with the more common, mature type of ASCUS.

In summary, the overall findings of the studies at Rochester and other sites show that in an unselected population of patients with the cytologic diagnosis of ASCUS, the overall rate of association with a subsequent diagnosis of dysplasia ranges from 10% to 15%. In addition, when attempts are made to distinguish morphologically between atypia based on the maturation of the involved cells, distinct differences between the groups are noted. With decreasing maturity levels of the atypical cells, an increasing overall association with the concurrent presence or future development of dysplasia is noted.

Management of Atypical Squamous Cells of Undetermined Significance

Whenever possible in a case of ASCUS, a statement as to whether origin of the cells from an intraepithelial process or a benign reactive process is favored should be made, along with a recommendation regarding follow-up. However, although this is desirable, in practice, it is seldom feasible because this category was designed for use when the significance of the cytologic alterations is unclear. In the majority of patients, the finding of AS-CUS appears to be of no clinical significance, with the atypia being the result of unknown but apparently transient and benign alterations in the cells. However, in a distinct minority of patients, the changes appear to be the only cytologic manifestation of a true intraepithelial process existing in the cervix; in others, they may be a manifestation of a potential for the future development of such a process.

One controversy surrounding the ASCUS category concerns the clinical management of the patient with this diagnosis. In certain situations, specific recommendations for follow-up are indicated. In the postmenopausal patient with an atrophic smear and scattered atypical squamous cells, a short course of estrogen therapy followed by a second cytologic examination often resolves the problem. In the absence of a significant lesion, the smear should revert to normal, with a cellular pattern of superficial squamous cells and no atypical forms. In the presence of a true intraepithelial lesion, abnormal cells would be expected to persist. In the case of highly atypical repair, where an invasive carcinoma is in the differential diagnosis and cannot be excluded on the basis of the cytologic findings, an immediate colposcopic examination and biopsy may be needed. Likewise, as discussed earlier, ASCUS composed of atypical cells of immature squamous metaplastic type warrants a recommendation of colposcopic examination and biopsy to exclude the presence of an HSIL.

On the other hand, the relatively low rate of association with a significant abnormality of the usual type of ASCUS composed of squamous cells with mature cytoplasm resembling normal intermediate or superficial squamous cells suggests that patients with these findings can be followed up much more conservatively. A 3- to 6-month follow-up Papanicolaou smear is recommended in our laboratory. In the absence of other confounding factors, colposcopic examination is recommended only in those cases with persisting atypia (ie, similar abnormalities on one or two more smears).

A conference involving a number of experts in the field held at the National Institutes of Health in 1992 resulted in the publication of interim guidelines for the management of patients with the diagnosis of ASCUS or low-grade squamous intraepithelial lesions (LSILs). The recommendations are basically similar to those described earlier. In particular, the guidelines point out that follow-up Papanicolaou smears are acceptable for an unqualified diagnosis of ASCUS. They state that a smear should be obtained every 4 to 6 months until there are three consecutive negative smears, at which point the patient can be monitored by routine screening. They also recommend that colposcopy should be considered if a second ASCUS report occurs in the 2-year follow-up period. They further note that if the patient's history places her at high risk, the option of colposcopy could be considered after the initial ASCUS report. The reader is referred to the original publication for details of the recommendations.[24]

SQUAMOUS INTRAEPITHELIAL LESIONS

A wide diversity of histologic patterns are included under the broadly descriptive term, *squamous intraepithelial lesions.* This spectrum of changes contributes a variety of abnormal cells to the cellular sample obtained from the cervix. A careful consideration of the morphologic aspects of this cellular material will permit the cytopathologist not only to determine the presence of an abnormality, but also to predict with a high degree of accuracy the histologic appearance of the tissue of origin.

Histology of Squamous Intraepithelial Lesions

The intraepithelial phase of the neoplastic process in the cervix is characterized by a disordered development of the squamous epithelium that is manifest histologically by a proliferation of primitive cells, beginning in the lower portions of the epithelial layer. This is accompanied by nuclear abnormalities, including hyperchromasia, increased nuclear size, increased numbers of mitoses, and the presence of abnormal mitotic forms. In general, the more severe is the process, the more the appearance of the epithelium deviates from the normal patterns of cervical squamous maturation. Representative examples of the histologic spectrum of squamous intraepithelial lesions are depicted in Figures 6-19 through 6-28.

In the classic nomenclature, the term *mild dysplasia* is applied when the proliferation of primitive cells is confined to the lower one third of the epithelium. *Moderate dysplasia* refers to those lesions in which primitive cells involve the middle one third of the epithelium, and as the upper one third of the epithelium becomes involved

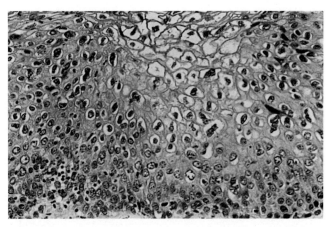

FIG. 6-20. Mild dysplasia with human papillomavirus cytopathic effect (low-grade squamous intraepithelial lesion).

by primitive cells, the dysplasia is considered to be *severe.* If the entire thickness of the epithelium is replaced by the proliferation, the lesion is termed *CIS.* As the process increases in severity, the degree of nuclear abnormality of the component cells increases. In addition, mitoses are found at higher and higher levels in the epithelium, and increased numbers of abnormal mitoses are identified. Fu and colleagues have shown that the presence of abnormal mitoses correlates with the presence of an aneuploid cell population, and that this is predictive of those lesions that are most likely to progress.[25,26] It is of significant interest that the presence of abnormal mitoses also correlates with the identification of high-risk papillomavirus type DNA in these lesions.[27]

In addition to subclassifying intraepithelial neoplasia according to its stage of development, as described earlier, it can also be subdivided on the basis of the two basic morphologic tissue patterns observed. The first and most common pattern is characteristic of the usual type of lesion that arises in the transformation zone. This is referred to as the *nonkeratinizing* type and, as used here, also includes those lesions termed *metaplastic dysplasia*

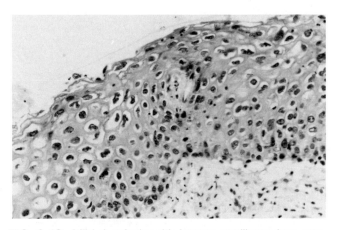

FIG. 6-19. Mild dysplasia with human papillomavirus cytopathic effect (low-grade squamous intraepithelial lesion).

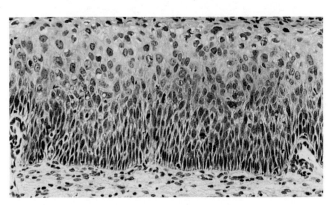

FIG. 6-21. Moderate dysplasia (high-grade squamous intraepithelial lesion).

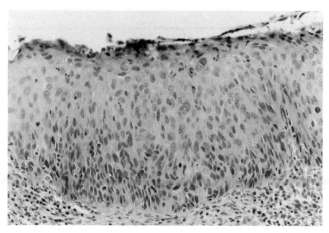

FIG. 6-22. Moderate dysplasia (high-grade squamous intra-epithelial lesion).

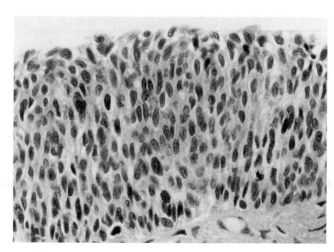

FIG. 6-25. Carcinoma in situ (high-grade squamous intraepi-thelial lesion).

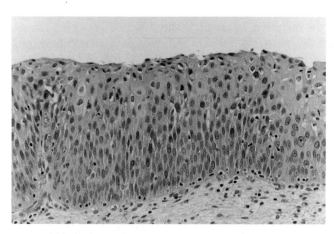

FIG. 6-23. Moderate to severe dysplasia (high-grade squa-mous intraepithelial lesion).

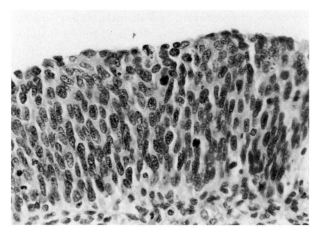

FIG. 6-26. Carcinoma in situ (high-grade squamous intraepi-thelial lesion).

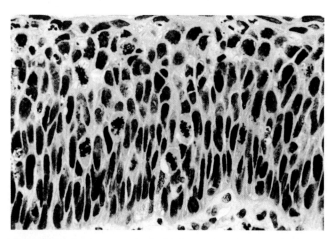

FIG. 6-24. Severe dysplasia (high-grade squamous intraepi-thelial lesion).

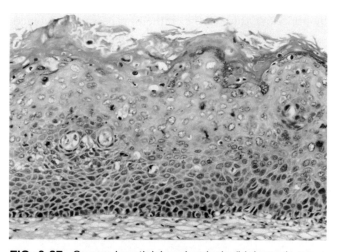

FIG. 6-27. Severe keratinizing dysplasia (high-grade squa-mous intraepithelial lesion). (Reproduced with permission from Bonfiglio TA: Cytopathology of cervical dysplasia, carci-noma in situ and invasive carcinoma. *In* Astarita R: *Basic Cy-topathology,* New York, Churchill Livingstone, 1989.)

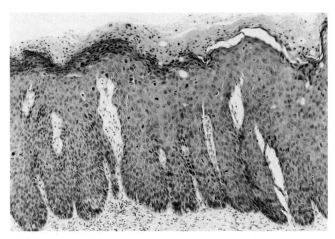

FIG. 6-28. Severe keratinizing dysplasia (high-grade squamous intraepithelial lesion).

by Patten.[5] The second type of lesion, termed *keratinizing* because of the marked keratinization of many of the component cells, is much less common. It usually occurs on the portio of the cervix (see Figs. 6-27 and 6-28). Marked cellular pleomorphism is also a characteristic of this lesion, and has led some to refer to the process as *pleomorphic dysplasia.* With keratinizing dysplasia, morphologic subclassification according to the severity of the process is less precise than with the more common patterns of intraepithelial lesions. Although the degree of pleomorphism and the number of mitoses, especially atypical forms, have been used to quantify severity, the results of such grading are not as predictive of biologic behavior as they are in the nonkeratinizing intraepithelial lesions. Keratinizing invasive cancers commonly arise from an overlying surface epithelium that may be classified as only a mild dysplasia if the extent of epithelial replacement by primitive cells is the only criterion used. Therefore, any keratinizing intraepithelial lesion should be considered high-grade insofar as its potential to advance to invasive carcinoma, and should be treated as such.

When the histology is considered in relation to the cytologic findings of this whole group of squamous intraepithelial lesions, it is important to emphasize that there is a full-thickness epithelial abnormality even in mild cases. Although the proliferation of primitive cells does not involve the full thickness of the epithelium in lesions of less severity than CIS, all cases of dysplasia demonstrate nuclear abnormalities, including increased size and hyperchromasia, even in the superficial portions of the reaction. In addition, the degree of nuclear abnormality observed and the number of abnormal mitoses noted are important indicators of the degree of severity of a lesion, apart from simple evaluation of the level of primitive cells in the abnormal epithelium. In low-grade lesions, it is interesting to note that the cytologically most atypical-appearing cells are usually observed in the middle and upper third of the epithelium. Although these cells are not primitive in their appearance (they show clear-cut evidence of mature squamous differentiation of the cytoplasm), their nuclei are markedly enlarged and hyperchromatic, and often show degenerative changes related to the cytopathic effect of the HPV. This is in contrast to the relatively bland-appearing nuclei of the immature cells that are seen in the deeper layers. In higher-grade lesions, the cells of the deep epithelial layers do not exhibit an HPV cytopathic effect, but often show more significant nuclear alterations.

The cytologic manifestations of the squamous intraepithelial lesions reflect the morphologic appearances of these processes as seen in tissue samples. The patterns of the cellular samples derived from the various epithelial processes under consideration can be predicted from a study of the appearance of the cells in tissue biopsies taken from involved areas. The cells sampled by the cervical scrape and brush techniques are generally derived from the superficial cell layers of the epithelium and represent the cells seen in the more superficial portions of the epithelium of the proliferations.

THE BETHESDA SYSTEM AND HISTOLOGIC TERMINOLOGY

Although the Bethesda classification has gained wide usage, the dysplasia or CIS and cervical intraepithelial neoplasia terminologies still are most commonly applied to histologic material, and are the terms used in the most recent World Health Organization classification of tumors of the female genital system.[28]

It is important to note that the terms *koilocytotic atypia, flat condyloma,* and *condylomatous atypia* are not included as diagnostic categories in either the Bethesda system or the current World Health Organization histologic classification system. These terms really represent descriptive rather than diagnostic entities. The changes represented by these terms are now considered to be part of the spectrum of LSILs (ie, mild dysplasia). This categorization and the resultant revision of thought regarding the spectrum of mild dysplasia represents one of the more controversial aspects of the Bethesda system. The concern revolves around the fact that prior to the development of this new classification, these changes were thought of as representing something less than cervical intraepithelial neoplasia 1 or mild dysplasia and, therefore, did not require the same follow-up or treatment as a "true intraepithelial neoplastic process." However, there is little evidence to support this distinction. In fact, the rationale for placing those lesions showing simply the cytopathic effect of HPV in the same category as those demonstrating classic criteria for mild dysplasia or cervical intraepithelial neoplasia 1 is compelling. The HPV profile for both groups of lesions is identical,[29] their biologic behavior is similar (a relatively low progression rate to HSIL in the range of 14% to 16%),[30] and their distinction on histologic and cytologic grounds is not clearly defined and not very reproducible.[4] Because classic mild dysplasia and koilocytotic atypia both appear to have similar progression rates, demonstrate similar HPV types, and are poorly separated on morphologic grounds, it seems unreasonable, at least on the basis of current knowledge, to advocate differences in treatment or to classify them separately (see Chap. 5).

However, this has resulted in some expansion of the number of cases included in the mild dysplasia (LSIL) category and, if all these patients are referred for colposcopy, will cause a significant increase in the number of procedures performed and a concomitant rise in related costs. In this regard, there is considerable ongoing discussion as to the appropriate management of patients with LSILs on cytology. Interim guidelines, as noted earlier, suggest that it is not necessary to refer all patients with a cytologic diagnosis of LSIL for immediate colposcopy.[24] In addition, a national study currently in progress should provide the information necessary to establish firm guidelines on the most reasonable approach to the management of these low-grade lesions.

There has also been controversy regarding the elimination of the three-tier classification of the histologic system in the Bethesda cytologic system, placing moderate and severe dysplasia along with CIS (cervical intraepithelial neoplasia 2 and 3) in the high-grade category. In this regard, it is important to point out that from a practical patient management perspective, a three-tier versus a two-tier cytologic system makes little difference. Currently, all patients with cytologic diagnoses of moderate dysplasia or above (all HSILs) are generally handled in the same manner (ie, biopsy confirmation followed by appropriate treatment). It should also be emphasized that there is no proscription in the Bethesda system from reporting cytologic findings using both the Bethesda terminology and the more traditional histologic terms (eg, HSIL [moderate dysplasia or cervical intraepithelial neoplasia 2]).

GENERAL CYTOLOGIC FEATURES OF SQUAMOUS INTRAEPITHELIAL LESIONS

Detailed studies of the morphologic features of the cells derived from squamous intraepithelial lesions can be found in the earlier cytopathology literature. The contributions of Reagan and Patten in particular emphasize a detailed qualitative as well as quantitative analysis of the cellular features of these lesions as reflected in cervical samples.[5,31–36] More recent publications summarize the details of the cytologic characteristics of intraepithelial lesions in relation to modern morphologic classifications and current knowledge of the biology of disease.[4,37,38]

Abnormal cells derived from squamous intraepithelial lesions generally appear in cytologic samples in environments that can be described as "clean." There may be evidence of infection, trichomonads, or mucus, but there is no evidence of the cellular debris and broken-down blood that is seen in the presence of tissue necrosis and is referred to as a tumor diathesis. The cells derived from the lower-grade lesions (ie, mild dysplasia) are most commonly found as isolated single cells, but small sheet-like aggregates are occasionally seen. The cells in such aggregates are arranged in the form of a sheet. The cells derived from high-grade lesions may also be isolated, but in the most advanced lesion of this group (ie, CIS), they frequently appear as aggregates in a syncytium-like arrangement. The presence of such syncytium-like aggregates of abnormal cells implies the presence of a high-grade intraepithelial lesion in the sampled cervix.

The number of abnormal cells in the cytologic sample varies with the collection technique used and the extent of the lesion. Although counts of abnormal cells vary from one case to another, in general, lesser degrees of dysplasia are associated with fewer abnormal cells per slide, whereas more severe lesions are reflected by a markedly increased abnormal cell count. As reported in studies by Reagan and Patten, cells derived from dysplasia have nuclear areas ranging from 150 to 200 μm^2. The size varies somewhat with the differentiation of the dysplastic process. Nuclei from CIS may range from 75 to 200 μm^2, again depending on the subclass of CIS that is present.[33,39]

In general, three chromatin patterns are associated with dysplasia (Fig. 6-29). The nuclei of cells derived from dysplastic reactions may have a finely granular, evenly distributed chromatin; a finely granular, evenly distributed chromatin with some chromatin clumping; or, in keratinizing lesions, very dense, deeply staining, opaque chromatin. A finely granular, evenly distributed chromatin pattern may also be seen in cells derived from CIS. In some cases of CIS however, different chromatin patterns consisting of evenly distributed, coarsely granular chromatin or evenly distributed, coarsely granular chromatin with interrupted nuclear membranes are seen. Irregular chromatin distribution and so-called areas of nuclear clearing are generally not seen in the intraepithelial reactions, but are characteristic of invasive processes. Prominent nucleoli are also not a typical feature of cells derived from intraepithelial lesions.

The degree of severity of an intraepithelial neoplastic process is evaluated on a cytologic sample by a consideration of the morphologic characteristics of the constituent cells. Of less importance is the number of abnormal cells present. The morphologic features related to severity include those involving both the nucleus and the cytoplasm, although the nuclear features are the most significant.

CHROMATIN PATTERNS IN CERVICAL NEOPLASIA

CHROMATIN PATTERN	CONDITIONS
Finely granular, evenly distributed	Dysplasia, atypia, carcinoma in situ
Finely granular, evenly distributed with clumping	Dysplasia
Finely granular, irregular distribution, nuclear clearing (with nucleoli)	Microinvasive carcinoma
Dense, opaque	Keratinizing dysplasia Keratinizing invasive carcinoma
 Coarsely granular, evenly distributed	Carcinoma in situ
Coarsely granular with interrupted nuclear envelope	Carcinoma in situ
Coarsely granular, irregular distribution, nuclear clearing (with nucleoli)	Microinvasive cancer Invasive squamous cell carcinoma (with macronucleoli)

FIG. 6-29. Chromatin patterns of squamous lesions of cervix. (Reproduced with permission from Bonfiglio TA: Cytopathology of cervical dysplasia, carcinoma in situ and invasive carcinoma. *In* Astarita R: *Basic Cytopathology,* New York, Churchill Livingstone, 1989.)

CYTOLOGY OF LOW-GRADE SQUAMOUS INTRAEPITHELIAL LESIONS

Low-grade squamous intraepithelial lesions are characterized by the presence of cells with mature, well-defined cytoplasm similar to that of normal intermediate or superficial squamous cells. Their nuclei are four to six times the size of intermediate squamous cell nuclei, hyperchromatic, and often display irregularities of the nuclear envelope. Binucleation is common. The cells typically appear singly or, less commonly, as sheets (Figs.

6-30 through 6-33). Koilocytotic changes, the morphologic hallmark of an HPV cytopathic effect, are most commonly associated with these lower-grade lesions. Intraepithelial lesions demonstrating koilocytotic features but having nuclei slightly smaller than those described earlier for classic dysplasia have previously been termed *koilocytotic atypia,* as discussed earlier. The same term or synonymous terms (eg, warty atypia, condylomatous atypia) have been used in the past as cytologic diagnoses in cell samples characterized by these features. As noted

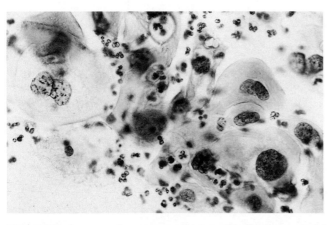

FIG. 6-30. Low-grade squamous intraepithelial lesion (mild dysplasia). These cells have mature appearing cytoplasm but the nuclei are hyperchromatic and markedly enlarged.

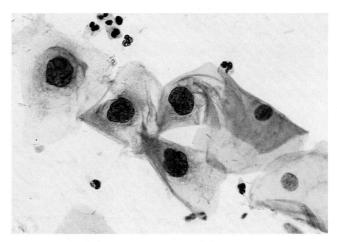

FIG. 6-31. Low-grade squamous intraepithelial lesion (mild dysplasia). Note the nuclear hyperchromasia and mild nuclear envelope irregularities.

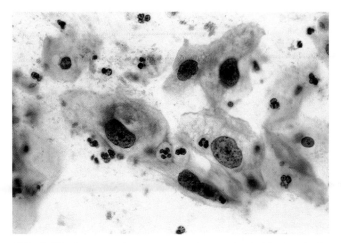

FIG. 6-32. Low-grade squamous intraepithelial lesion (mild dysplasia).

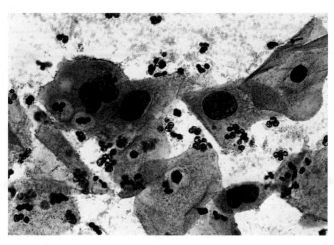

FIG. 6-33. Low-grade squamous intraepithelial lesion (mild dysplasia).

earlier, in the Bethesda system, these lesions are classified as LSIL along with mild dysplasia. This is quite appropriate because, as also discussed earlier, the biologic behavior of koilocytotic atypia and mild dysplasia are similar, as are the HPV types involved with both lesions.[29]

Indeed, mild dysplasia and koilocytotic atypia can be considered identical for purposes of patient management, treatment, and follow-up.

With this in mind, it is important, therefore, to distinguish true koilocytotic changes from the cytologic alter-

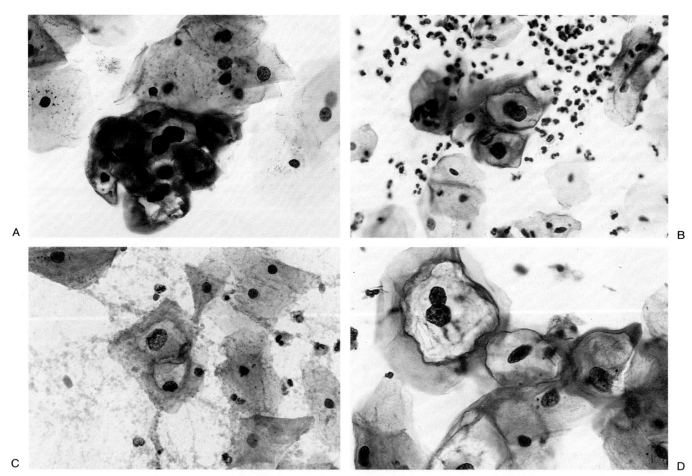

FIG. 6-34. (A–D) Low-grade squamous intraepithelial lesion (mild dysplasia) with classical human papillomavirus cytopathic effect characterized by large sharply delineated perinuclear halo and atypical nuclei.

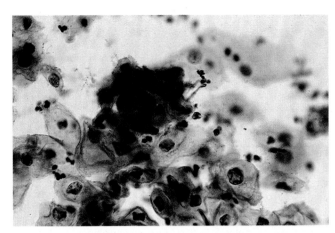

FIG. 6-35. Low-grade squamous intraepithelial lesion (mild dysplasia) with human papillomavirus cytopathic effect. In addition to the koilocytotic cells there is a cluster of "dyskeratotic" cells with deep red cytoplasm and pyknotic nuclei.

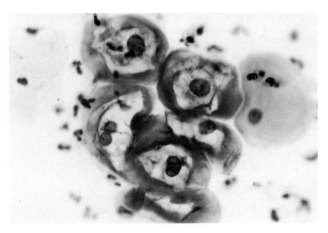

FIG. 6-37. Low-grade squamous intraepithelial lesion (mild dysplasia) with human papillomavirus cytopathic effect. These cells have features similar to those in Fig. 6-36.

ations that may mimic them. The true "koilocyte" is a cell with an atypical nucleus and a clearly defined, sharply delineated, perinuclear halo. The nuclear atypia is characterized by hyperchromasia, nuclear enlargement, and, in some cases, wrinkling of the nuclear envelope or more advanced degenerative changes such as smudging of the chromatin and pyknosis (Figs. 6-34 through 6-37). A simple perinuclear halo alone is not diagnostic and is a nonspecific finding that may occur as a variation of normal or as a reactive change (Fig. 6-38). Cytoplasmic glycogen can sometimes give an appearance of a perinuclear clear zone, particularly in tissue sections (Fig. 6-39). Perinuclear halos, generally smaller or less well defined than those of koilocytes, are also seen as nonspecific manifestations of inflammation (Fig.

6-40). Smears with these characteristics should not be classified as dysplasia or squamous intraepithelial lesions.

CYTOLOGY OF HIGH-GRADE SQUAMOUS INTRAEPITHELIAL LESIONS

As the squamous intraepithelial lesion becomes more severe, the amount of cytoplasm of the constituent cells in the sample decreases and appears progressively more immature (metaplastic cell–like), and the nuclear-to-cytoplasmic ratio increases. The extreme of cellular immaturity is reached in cells derived from CIS. The nucleus reflects the severity of the process by changes that involve a progressive increase in chromatin abnormalities, including clumping and coarseness

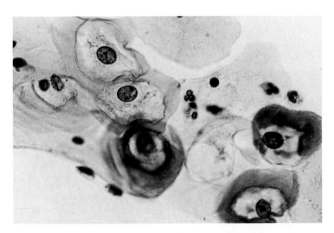

FIG. 6-36. Low-grade squamous intraepithelial lesion (LSIL), (mild dysplasia) with human papillomavirus (HPV) cytopathic effect. The nuclei of these cells are smaller than those seen in classic dysplasia (See Figs. 6-31–6-33) but the features are diagnostic of HPV cytopathic effect and therefore are diagnostic of LSIL.

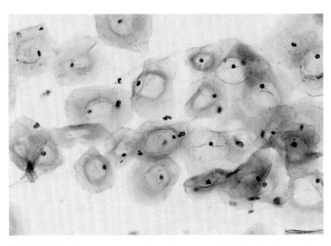

FIG. 6-38. Squamous cells with pseudokoilocytotic perinuclear halos. This is a nonspecific change unassociated with human papillomavirus effect and should not be confused with viral induced changes.

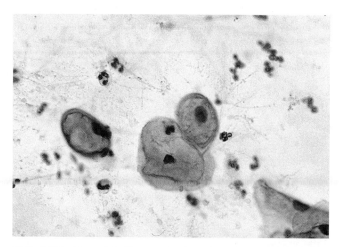

FIG. 6-39. Pseudokoilocytosis. Cytoplasmic "vacuoles" due to glycogen.

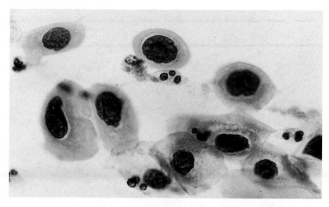

FIG. 6-41. High-grade squamous intraepithelial lesion (HSIL) (moderate dysplasia). The nuclear/cytoplasmic ratio is greater than that noted in low-grade squamous intraepithelial lesions (LSIL). Nuclear hypercromasia and irregularities of the nuclear envelope are also more prominent.

of the chromatinic material, and increasing nuclear envelope irregularities.

HSIL, in the Bethesda terminology, encompasses the spectrum of lesions ranging from moderate dysplasia through CIS. Although for purposes of ensuring that patients receive appropriate follow-up and treatment, classification of all these lesions in the HSIL category is appropriate, more specific classification of the cytologic sample is often possible, providing additional information as to the estimated severity of the process and improved histologic correlation.

In moderate dysplasia, although cells similar to those described for mild dysplasia are often found, there are also more immature-appearing abnormal cells. These cells have an increased nuclear-to-cytoplasmic ratio and less abundant cytoplasm, which is dense and resembles, in texture and configuration, that of immature metaplastic cells (Figs. 6-41 through 6-44). Nuclei are hyperchro-

matic, may demonstrate increased clumping of chromatinic material, and typically exhibit more irregularities of the nuclear envelope than are evident in LSILs. Like the cells of mild dysplasia, the cells of moderate dysplasia are usually found singly or, when in tissue aggregates, as sheets with well-defined cell borders.

Severe dysplasia is usually characterized by the presence of more abnormal cells than are found in less advanced intraepithelial lesions. The nuclear-to-cytoplasmic ratio is also significantly increased over that seen in lesser grades of disease, but the actual size of the nuclei may be considerably less than in LSILs. The cells tend to be round to oval, with relatively little cytoplasm. The cytoplasm, however, remains well-defined, resembling that of very immature metaplastic cells. Nuclei tend to be considerably hyperchromatic, and marked irregularities of the nuclear envelope may be present. The cells, when present as tissue aggregates, may be seen as less well

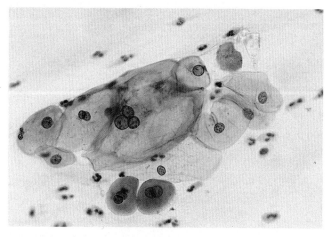

FIG. 6-40. Atypical squamous cells of undetermined significance. Very mild nuclear enlargement and indistinct perinuclear halos suggestive, but not diagnostic of human papillomavirus effect.

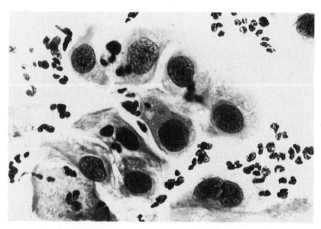

FIG. 6-42. High-grade squamous intraepithelial lesion (HSIL) (moderate dysplasia). Moderate hyperchromasia, finely granular chromatin, and significant nuclear enlargement characterize these cells.

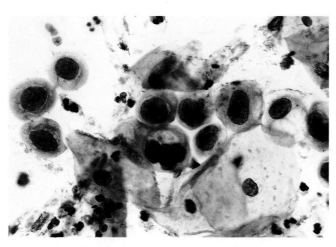

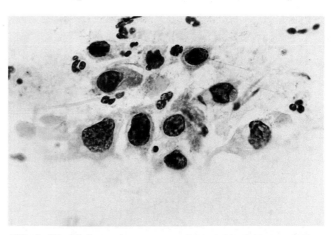

FIG. 6-43. High-grade squamous intraepithelial lesion (HSIL) (moderate dysplasia). The dense rounded cytoplasm of these cells resembles that of metaplastic cells but the nuclei are significantly enlarged and hyperchromatic. (Reproduced with permission from Bonfiglio TA: Cytopathology of cervical dysplasia, carcinoma in situ and invasive carcinoma. *In* Astarita R: *Basic Cytopathology,* New York, Churchill Livingstone, 1989.)

FIG. 6-45. High-grade squamous intraepithelial lesion (HSIL) (severe dysplasia). Note the markedly increased nuclear/cytoplasmic ratio, coarse chromatin, and irregularities of the nuclear outline.

defined sheets or, less commonly, in syncytium-like aggregates (Figs. 6-45 through 6-47B).

CIS in cytologic samples is manifest by large numbers of primitive-appearing cells that may vary in size from case to case. Large-, intermediate-, and small-cell variants of CIS have been described, but no biologic significance has been definitively associated with this size-based distinction.[5,33] The cells again may appear as single, isolated units or as syncytium-like aggregates with indistinct cell borders and a disordered, irregular arrangement of the nuclei in relation to one another. The cytoplasmic margins of the cells in the groups often have an indistinct, wispy appearance that appears to fade into the background of the slide (Figs. 6-48 through 6-55). On the other hand, single, isolated cells originating in CIS

may have only a small rim of cytoplasm around a very atypical, small nucleus (Figs. 6-56 through 6-58). The chromatin patterns observed range from finely to coarsely granular. The nuclear envelope is irregular and may have an interrupted appearance suggesting impending mitosis. Mitotic figures are not frequently identified, but some, including atypical forms, may be noted (Fig. 6-59).

The small, single cells derived from HSILs (CIS) are among the abnormal cells that are most difficult to detect in routine screening. It has been documented in several reports that it is these cells that are most commonly missed when false-negative examinations occur because of screening errors in patients with high-grade intraepithelial lesions.[40,41] This is undoubtedly related to their small size and the difficulty in detecting them, particularly in the presence of inflammation in the slide background, where they are easily obscured.

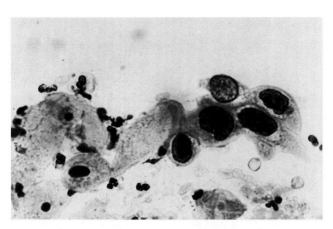

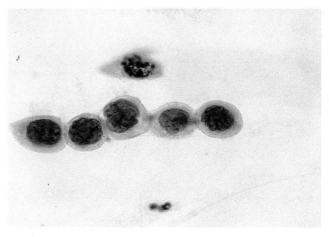

FIG. 6-44. High-grade squamous intraepithelial lesion (HSIL). (moderate to severe dysplasia). These cells have a very high nuclear/cytoplasmic ratio and irregular nuclear outlines.

FIG. 6-46. High-grade squamous intraepithelial lesion (HSIL). These cells are derived from severe dysplasia. Irregularities of the nuclear outline are particularly evident. One cell is undergoing karyorrhexis.

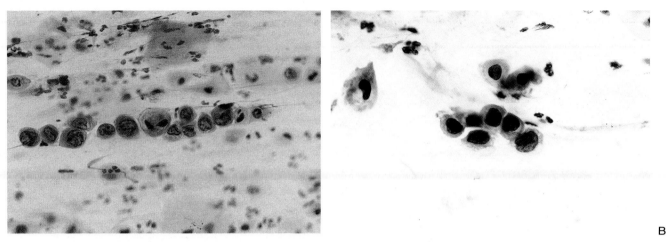

A   B

FIG. 6-47. (A, B) High-grade squamous intraepithelial lesion (HSIL). Taken at slightly lower magnification than fig. 6-46 these slides also depict groups of cells derived from severe dysplasia.

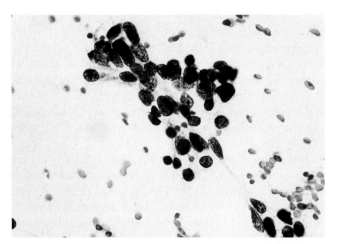

FIG. 6-48. High-grade squamous intraepithelial lesion (HSIL) (carcinoma in situ, large cell type). Cells are arranged in a syncytial like aggregate. (Reproduced with permission from Bonfiglio TA: Cytopathology of cervical dysplasia, carcinoma in situ and invasive carcinoma. *In* Astarita R: *Basic Cytopathology,* New York, Churchill Livingstone, 1989.)

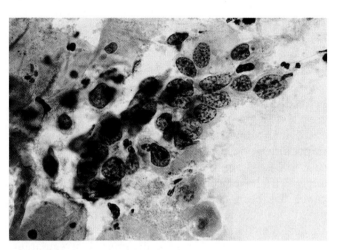

FIG. 6-50. High-grade squamous intraepithelial lesion (HSIL) (carcinoma in situ, large cell type).

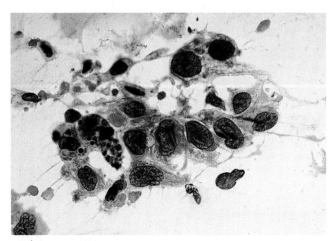

FIG. 6-49. High-grade squamous intraepithelial lesion (HSIL) (carcinoma in situ, large cell type). Note nuclear irregularities and indistinct cell borders.

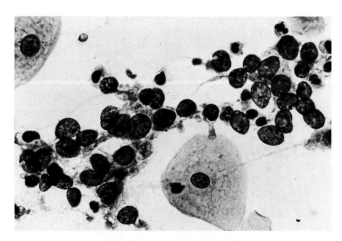

FIG. 6-51. High-grade squamous intraepithelial lesion (HSIL) (carcinoma in situ). Note the scant amount of "wispy" cytoplasm in this syncytial like aggregate of cells.

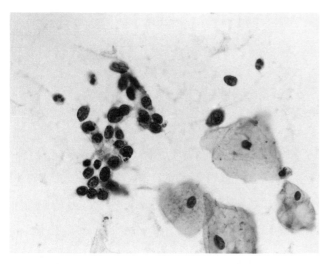

FIG. 6-52. High-grade squamous intraepithelial lesion (HSIL). Syncytial aggregate and single cells derived from a small cell carcinoma in situ.

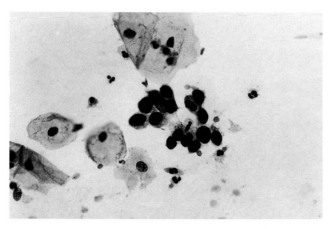

FIG. 6-53. High-grade squamous intraepithelial lesion (HSIL) (carcinoma in situ).

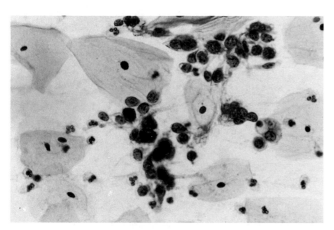

FIG. 6-54. High-grade squamous intraepithelial lesion (HSIL) (carcinoma in situ).

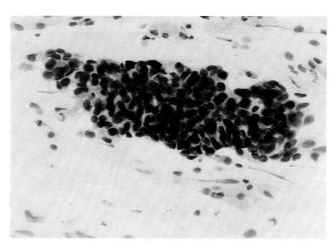

FIG. 6-55. High-grade squamous intraepithelial lesion (HSIL). Large syncytial aggregate of small cell carcinoma in situ cells. Almost no cytoplasm is evident in this group.

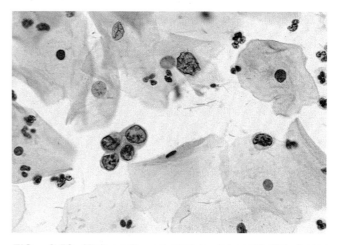

FIG. 6-56. High-grade squamous intraepithelial lesion (HSIL). Small cluster of cells derived from carcinoma in situ. Note the scant cytoplasm and clumped chromatin.

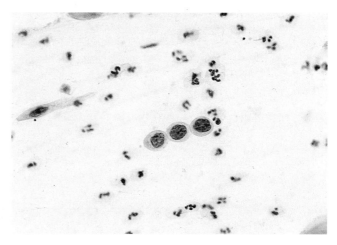

FIG. 6-57. High-grade squamous intraepithelial lesion (HSIL). Group of small cells derived from carcinoma in situ. Such cells can easily be overlooked, particularly in an inflammatory background.

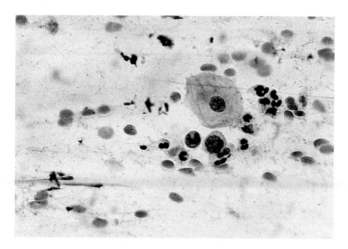

FIG. 6-58. Single cells derived from small cell type of high-grade squamous intraepithelial lesion (carcinoma in situ). The normal intermediate squamous cell in the field provides a good size comparison.

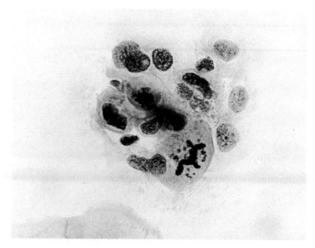

FIG. 6-59. Note the atypical mitotic figure in this group of cells derived from a high-grade squamous intrepithelial lesion. Although common in biopsy specimens, this is an unusual finding on cervical smears.

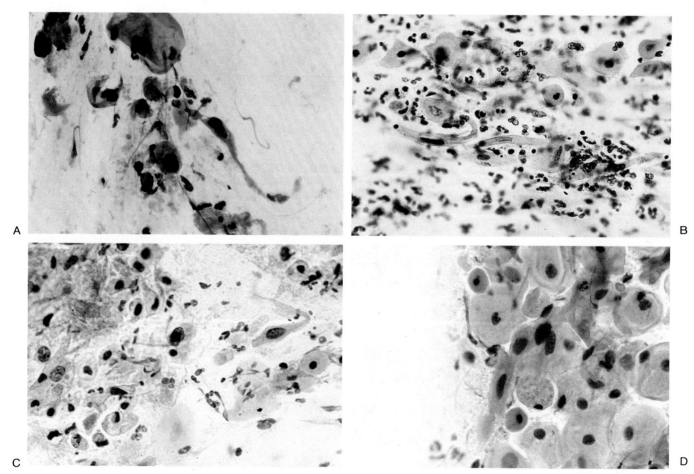

A

B

C

D

FIG. 6-60. (A–D) Pleomorphic dysplastic cells derived from high-grade squamous intraepithelial lesion (Keratinizing or pleomorphic dysplasia). The spindled and caudate forms are characteristic of this type of lesion.

TABLE 6-3. *Summary of the criteria for the diagnosis of squamous intraepithelial lesions*

LOW-GRADE SQUAMOUS INTRAEPITHELIAL LESIONS

Cells occur singly or in sheets
Cells demonstrate cytoplasmic maturation with distinct borders
Nuclei are 4–6 times the size of normal intermediate cell nuclei
Moderate variation in nuclear size
Binucleation may be present
Mild hyperchromasia of nuclei
Mild nuclear envelope irregularities
Uniformly distributed, usually finely granular chromatin
Absent nucleoli
Human papillomavirus cytopathic effect often prominent

HIGH-GRADE SQUAMOUS INTRAEPITHELIAL LESIONS

Cells arranged singly or in syncytium-like arrangements (carcinoma in situ)
Smaller cells with cytoplasm resembling that of immature squamous metaplastic cells or pleomorphic keratinized cells
Decreased nuclear size, but markedly increased nuclear-to-cytoplasmic ratio
Increased hyperchromasia
Increased nuclear envelope irregularities
Increased chromatin clumping
Nucleoli absent

The keratinizing intraepithelial processes discussed earlier are generally all considered to represent high-grade lesions. These lesions are characterized by a variety of cellular forms, including spindle-shaped and elongated cells, and caudate or "tadpole" forms. Nuclei also vary widely in shape and frequently have a dense, often opaque degenerated appearance. Anucleate, keratinized, pleomorphic cells are also present. In general, the more severe is the reaction, the greater is the proportion of pleomorphic forms (Figs. 6-60A through 6-60D).

The criteria for the diagnosis of squamous intraepithelial lesions are summarized in Table 6-3 and charted in relation to the degree of severity of the process in Table 6-4.

DIFFERENTIAL DIAGNOSIS OF SQUAMOUS INTRAEPITHELIAL LESIONS

The differential diagnosis of squamous intraepithelial reactions includes both benign and malignant entities. LSILs must be distinguished from benign cellular changes and ASCUS. Some of the important differentiating characteristics are presented in Table 6-5. The important distinction of LSILs with an HPV cytopathic effect from pseudokoilocytotic changes has been discussed earlier.

More severe intraepithelial processes are sometimes confused with immature squamous metaplasia, or, more commonly, with the atypia that may be associated with postmenopausal atrophy. Histologically, the atrophic epithelium in these cases is characterized by the presence of scattered cells with mildly hyperchromatic, enlarged nuclei. There is no mitotic activity or other feature of a true intraepithelial lesion (Fig. 6-61). Cytologically, a careful evaluation of nuclear characteristics is usually the most helpful consideration in the differential diagnostic process because marked hyperchromasia, chromatin abnormalities, and irregularities of the nuclear envelope are usually absent in these nondysplastic cells (Figs. 6-62 and 6-63). In certain cases, however, atypical cells may be present that cannot be readily distinguished from those originating from a true squamous lesion (Figs. 6-64 and 6-65). The differential diagnostic problem with these smears, which are generally classified in the ASCUS category, in some instances may need to be resolved through colposcopic examination and biopsy. However, in many cases, the differential diagnosis can be resolved as discussed earlier in the section on the management of patients with a diagnosis of ASCUS by treating the patient with a short course of estrogen, then performing a second Papanicolaou smear. The estrogen will result in a maturation of the epithelium and a temporary reversal of the atrophic pattern. If the abnormal cells are related to the atrophic changes, they will disappear from the smear. If they are derived from a true epithelial lesion, they will persist.[42]

TABLE 6-4. *Summary of cytologic features of squamous intraepithelial lesions*

Cytologic features	Low-grade		High-grade	
	Mild dyspl	Mod dyspl	Sev dyspl	CIS
N/C ratio·	+	++	+++	++++
Hyperchromasia	++	++	+++	++++
Chromatin abnormality	+	++	+++	++++
Nuclear envelope irregularity	+	++	+++	++++
Number of cells	+	++	+++	++++
HPV cytopathic effect	++++	++	±	±
Background	Clean	Clean	Clean	Clean
Cell aggregates	Sheets	Sheets	Syncytia-like	Syncytia-like

Dyspl, dysplasia; *mod,* moderate; *sev,* severe; *CIS,* carcinoma in situ; *N/C,* nuclear-to-cytoplasmic; *HPV,* human papillomavirus.

TABLE 6-5. *Comparison of cellular features distinguishing normal and atypical squamous cells from those derived from squamous intraepithelial lesions (SILs)*

Normal	Atypia	SILs
Nucleus 35–50 μm^2	Nucleus 100 μm^2	Nucleus 125 + μm^2
Normochromatic	Normochromatic +	Hyperchromatic
Uniform nuclear envelope	Normal or mild irregularities	Irregular nuclear envelope
N/C = +	N/C = ++	N/C = ++++

N/C, nuclear-to-cytoplasmic ratio.

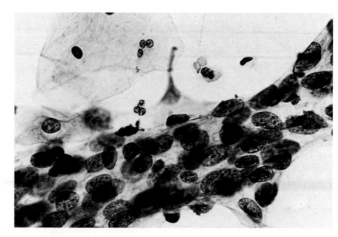

FIG. 6-63. True syncytial like aggregate in a case of carcinoma in situ.

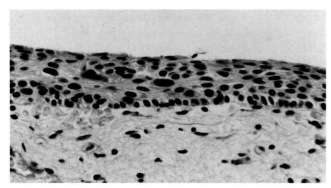

FIG. 6-61. Postmenopausal atrophy with cytologic atypia. (Hematoxylin and eosin) medium power.

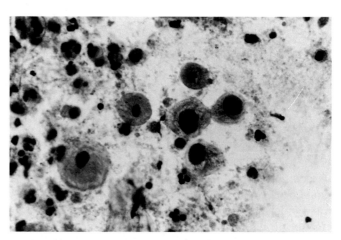

FIG. 6-64. Atypical appearing cells in an atrophic smear.

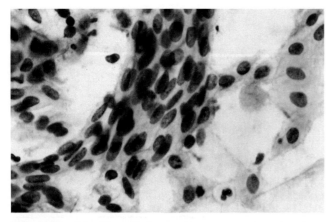

FIG. 6-62. Atrophic cells in a postmenopausal smear simulating a syncytial like arrangement.

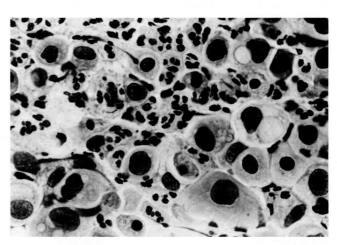

FIG. 6-65. Atypical cells in a smear from a postmenopausal woman with atrophy. This pattern would revert to normal following a short course of estrogen if the cells were not from a true intraepithelial lesion.

The differential diagnosis of high-grade intraepithelial lesions, particularly squamous CIS, also includes deep endometrial stromal cells, immature squamous metaplasia, reactive endocervical cells, tubal metaplasia, endocervical adenocarcinoma in situ, and invasive squamous carcinoma.

Deep endometrial stromal cells normally appear in cervical smears in the early phase of the menstrual cycle. They are small, hyperchromatic cells with little cytoplasm, arranged in aggregates that can resemble the syncytial aggregates of small-cell variants of CIS (Fig. 6-66). Although stromal cells are usually considerably smaller than cells derived from CIS, the most helpful distinguishing features are evident mainly in the nuclei. The nuclei of stromal cells are much more uniform in configuration and size than those of CIS. In addition, the coarse chromatin pattern and nuclear envelope irregularities of the small-cell type of CIS are not found in stromal cells (Figs. 6-67 and 6-68). Another helpful feature is the lack of any evidence of coexisting, more mature dysplastic cells, which are usually identified in cases of CIS in those cases that represent simply endometrial stromal cells.

The problem of atypical cells of immature squamous metaplastic type, and their distinction from high-grade intraepithelial lesions, was discussed in some detail earlier, in the section on ASCUS. The difficulty here is essentially one of the differential diagnosis of cells with a high nuclear-to-cytoplasmic ratio. Again, the differential features are principally related to the nuclei. The nuclei of atypical metaplastic cells (Figs. 6-69A and 6-69B) are more uniform, are normochromatic or mildly hyperchromatic, and do not have significant nuclear membrane irregularities or chromatin abnormalities, whereas cells from high-grade intraepithelial lesions demonstrate these characteristics (Figs. 6-69C and 6-69D).

Reactive endocervical cells can be confused with cells

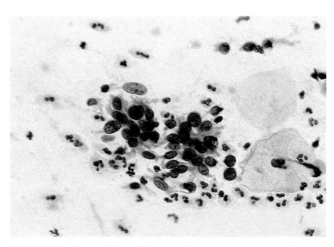

FIG. 6-67. Cells derived from high-grade squamous intraepithelial lesion (carcinoma in situ, small cell type). Note the larger nuclear size and chromatin changes as compared with the stromal cells.

derived from CIS because of their ability to mimic the appearance of syncytial aggregates of abnormal squamous cells in some circumstances. As noted in the section on reactive cellular changes, endocervical nuclei can show significant nuclear enlargement in the reactive state. This, together with the fact that the borders between the cells are often indistinct when aggregates of these cells are smeared on a slide, particularly when they are allowed to dry somewhat, can present a picture that superficially resembles the appearance of syncytial aggregates of intermediate- or large-cell variants of CIS. The lack of significant nuclear abnormalities beyond enlargement and the absence of isolated cells with the features of a high-grade intraepithelial lesion are the most helpful distinguishing features (Fig. 6-70).

Tubal metaplasia has presented a more common differential diagnostic problem in recent years because of the widespread use of devices that readily sample the

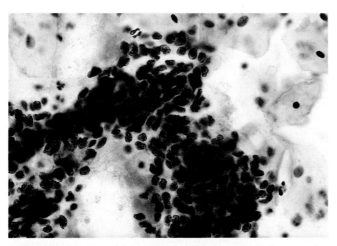

FIG. 6-66. Endometrial stromal cells in a smear taken on day 6 from a patient with a normal cycle are depicted in this slide. Compare with the cells derived from high-grade squamous epithelial lesion in figure, 6-67 and 6-68.

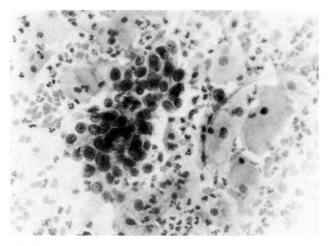

FIG. 6-68. Cells derived from high-grade squamous intraepithelial lesion (carcinoma in situ, small cell type).

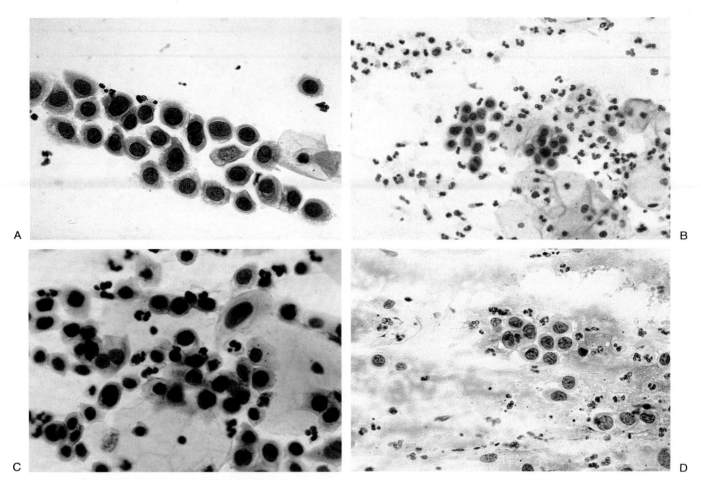

FIG. 6-69. (A–D) Atypical cells of immature squamous metaplastic type in figures 6-69**A** and 6-69**B** compared with cells derived from high-grade squamous intraepithelial lesion in figures 6-69**C** and 6-69**D**. The latter cells are more hyperchromatic, have more evident nuclear envelope irregularities and a higher nuclear/cytoplasmic ratio.

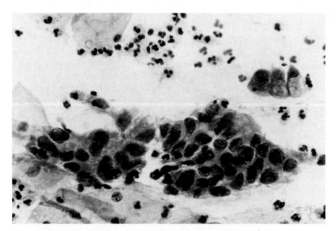

FIG. 6-70. Atypical appearing reactive endocervical cells. Such groups, particularly if poorly preserved, may resemble syncytial aggregates of high-grade squamous intraepithelial lesion. Note, however, preservation of columnar or cuboidal configuration.

higher portions of the endocervical canal. This process is more commonly confused with glandular lesions, particularly adenocarcinoma in situ (see Chap. 7), but can also present problems in the differential diagnosis of squamous CIS. This is particularly true when the slide preparations are less than ideal and air drying has occurred. Tubal metaplasia is characterized by columnar cells that are hyperchromatic and have interspersed, intercalated cells with larger, somewhat atypical-appearing nuclei. Although the presence of cilia on the cells easily identifies the process as tubal metaplasia in tissue samples, these structures frequently are not easily identified on smear preparations. This is particularly true when cell drying has occurred. In addition, as a result of the preparation process, some of the aggregates may assume configurations that resemble fragments of a high-grade lesion. Nevertheless, a careful search for cilia may be helpful in correctly identifying the origin of the cells. In addition,

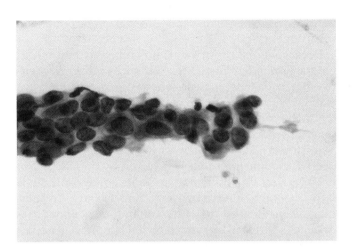

FIG. 6-71. Tubal metaplasia. No cilia are evident in this particular group, making definitive identification as tubal metaplastic cells difficult. The cells do not have well-defined borders and the nuclei are enlarged but have bland appearing chromatin and smooth nuclear envelopes.

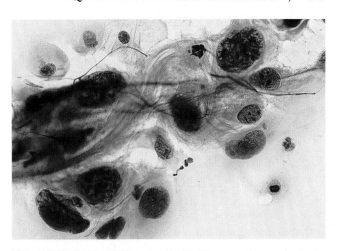

FIG. 6-72. Postradiation dysplasia. These cells are similar to those of other squamous intraepithelial lesions. The chromatin shows more prominent clumping than is seen in the usual case of low-grade squamous intraepithelial lesion.

carefully evaluating the nuclei and searching other areas of the slide for more definitive evidence of a high-grade intraepithelial process usually helps in making a definitive interpretation (Fig. 6-71).

Another differential diagnostic problem that appears to be related to the newer sampling methods is the differential diagnosis of squamous CIS with involvement of endocervical glands from adenocarcinoma in situ. The endocervical brush technique mechanically removes large aggregates of cells not only from the surface epithelium, but also from the frequently involved underlying glands. These aggregates may have attached columnar epithelial cells from adjacent or overlying epithelium, suggesting to the observer that they are of glandular rather than squamous origin. Palisading of nuclei at the periphery of the groups also suggests a glandular lesion. In a study of this problem by Selvaggi, several features were noted that were of differential diagnostic help.[43] These included the absence of strips of abnormal columnar cells and of gland or rosette formation in the smears that proved to be from squamous lesions. The smears in cases of true adenocarcinoma in situ contained abnormal cells that were characterized by the presence of "cigar-shaped" nuclei and nucleoli features not usually observed in intraepithelial squamous lesions.

POSTIRRADIATION INTRAEPITHELIAL NEOPLASIA

In some patients who have undergone irradiation for squamous cell carcinoma of the cervix, intraepithelial lesions (postirradiation dysplasia) (Figs. 6-72 through 6-73) develop after treatment. These lesions are cytologically and histologically identical to intraepithelial lesions in nonirradiated patients.[44] They must be distinguished from acute and chronic radiation changes and

from recurrent or residual cancer. Whether this type of dysplasia in an individual patient represents recurrence of the original lesion in an intraepithelial form or a new intraepithelial lesion resulting from reinfection with papillomavirus is of theoretical interest, but is not known. It would seem that both mechanisms are possible. In some studies, an association between postirradiation dysplasia and recurrent carcinoma has been made.[44–46] Although postirradiation dysplasia has been reported from a few months to many years after the completion of therapy, those lesions that occur within the first 3 years are most often associated with recurrent cancer.

SUPERFICIALLY INVASIVE SQUAMOUS CARCINOMA OF THE UTERINE CERVIX

In the early phase of squamous cell carcinoma of the cervix, superficial invasion of the underlying stroma de-

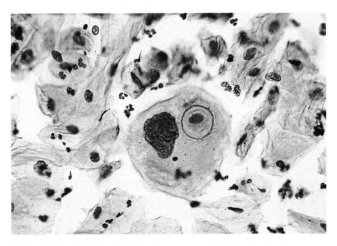

FIG. 6-73. Postradiation dysplasia. Changes of this type must be distinguished from chronic radiation effect.

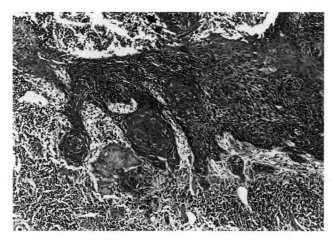

FIG. 6-74. Superficially invasive (microinvasive) squamous cell carcinoma. (Reproduced with permission from Bonfiglio TA: Cytopathology of cervical dysplasia, carcinoma in situ and invasive carcinoma. *In* Astarita R: *Basic Cytopathology,* New York, Churchill Livingstone, 1989.)

velops (Fig. 6-74). This almost always occurs in association with an overlying high-grade intraepithelial lesion. The early stage of this process has been referred to as *microinvasion,* a term first presented by Meswerdt in 1947.[47] These early carcinomas are classified as stage Ia in the 1987 FIGO staging system.[48] Since Meswerdt's time, microinvasive carcinoma of the cervix has had many definitions. The criteria utilized to include or exclude lesions from this group remain controversial. The crux of the controversy centers on defining criteria that can identify patients who are not at risk for lymph node metastases. The main points of contention involve the depth of invasion and the significance of vascular space involvement. The reported maximum depth of invasion for "microinvasive" carcinomas has varied from 1 to 5 mm. In some series, vascular invasion does not exclude a case from the diagnosis of microinvasive carcinoma, whereas in others, it does.

Microinvasive squamous cell carcinoma of the uterine cervix is perhaps best defined, however, as a carcinoma that has invaded the cervical stroma to a depth no greater than 3 mm from the site of origin and does not demonstrate lymphatic or blood vessel invasion. Other definitions have been proposed for this entity in the literature, but this is the one accepted by the Society of Gynecologic Oncologists and most commonly employed in the United States. This definition is a rather conservative one that identifies a group of patients who are at extremely low risk for the development of lymph node metastases or for dying from their disease. Although some reports have indicated that lesions with up to 5 mm of invasion should be considered microinvasive carcinomas, and that the demonstration of lymphatic invasion has no association with metastasis in these microinvasive tumors, other studies have shown that metastasis, recurrence, and death, although uncommon, do occur in patients with greater than 3 mm of invasion or lymphatic involvement.[49-53]

Because of the controversy, it is probably best not to use the term *microinvasive carcinoma* as a diagnostic entity, but to diagnose these lesions as superficially invasive carcinoma and specify the maximum depth of invasion, the method used to measure it, and the presence or absence of vascular space involvement.

In almost all cases, the invasive foci develop out of an overlying epithelium that is involved by an HSIL. The invasive foci usually appear as tongue-like projections into the underlying stroma and tend to have irregular margins, in contrast to the smooth outline of endocervical glands involved by intraepithelial neoplasia. This is a helpful feature in distinguishing such glandular involvement from early invasion. At the point of invasion, the epithelium also typically shows evidence of "paradoxical" differentiation in the form of increased and sometimes keratinized cytoplasm. In addition, there is usually a dense plasma cell and lymphocytic infiltrate present in proximity to the invasive focus, which may represent a manifestation of host response to the tumor.

Cytopathology of Superficially Invasive Carcinoma

The cytologic manifestations of superficially invasive cancer vary directly with the depth of stromal penetration. These features were described in detail by Ng and associates in 1972.[54] The cells derived from microinvasive cancer occur in isolated and aggregate form. The majority of abnormal cells occur in syncytial arrangements. The cytologic features that distinguish these cells from those arising from CIS are the presence of true nucleoli and chromatin clearing in a proportion of the cells. In the study by Ng and associates, the abnormal cells had a mean area of 219.1 μm^2. The nuclei had an average area of 88.2 μm^2. Nucleoli were observed in approximately 16% of the cells; usually, these were micronucleoli. With increasing depth of penetration, the changes began to resemble more and more those of outright cancer. The total number of abnormal cells containing nucleoli increased, as did nucleolar size. The number of cells displaying irregularities of chromatin distribution with areas of so-called *nuclear clearing* also increased. A true tumor diathesis was noted in 42.8% of the cases with stromal penetration of less than 2 mm. Among those cases with stromal penetration of more than 2 mm, more than 90% had a tumor diathesis. Early invasion of the cervical stroma may often be predicted on the basis of these characteristic cytologic findings and can be distinguished from CIS and outright cancer (Figs. 6-75 through 6-78).

An intermediate step between classic CIS and microinvasive squamous cell cancer may exist. The term *CIS* as applied to the classically described lesion is probably a misnomer, at least on a morphologic basis. The

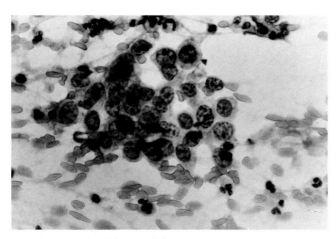

FIG. 6-75. Syncytial aggregate of cells from a patient with early superficially invasive squamous cell carcinoma. Nucleoli and coarse chromatin are present.

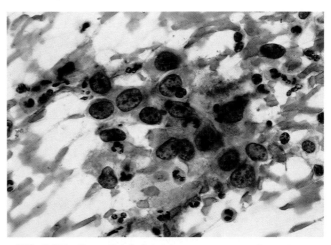

FIG. 6-77. Superficially invasive squamous cell carcinoma.

cells of CIS do not have all the features of malignant cells in that they lack the true nucleoli that are a characteristic feature of outright invasive squamous cell cancer. Morphologically, there is evidence to suggest that during the transformation of CIS to microinvasive cancer, a stage occurs wherein true nucleoli appear within the cells of the intraepithelial reaction. It may be that this change antedates the changes in chromatin distribution noted in microinvasive cancer and heralds the increased metabolic activity occurring in the cells prior to their development of the ability to invade the underlying stroma. The intraepithelial reaction at this point may then represent true intraepithelial cancer. Cells derived from this type of a reaction are sometimes seen in cytologic samples. Cytologically, these cells have all the characteristics of CIS, except that true micronucleoli are present. They lack the irregularities of chromatin distribution noted with microinvasive cancer.

Invasive Squamous Cell Carcinoma

The subclassification of invasive squamous cell carcinoma of the uterine cervix is based on histologic morphology. It differs from the popular subclassification first formulated by Broders, which is based on a grading system utilizing keratinization as the main index of differentiation.[55] The current subclassification, which has been adopted by the World Health Organization, was modified from that proposed by Wentz and Reagan in 1959.[56] It divides squamous cell carcinoma into keratinizing and nonkeratinizing types. Small-cell carcinoma, which in the original classification was included as a subtype of squamous cell carcinoma, is no longer classified as such. The majority of small-cell carcinomas are now known to be tumors of neuroendocrine differentiation and, like their counterparts in the lung, are classified as

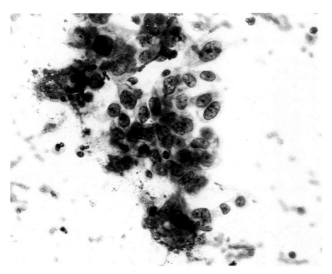

FIG. 6-76. Malignant cells from superficially invasive squamous cell carcinoma. Prominent nucleoli are seen. Note also the granular diathesis adherent to the cell aggregates.

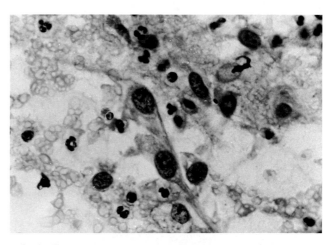

FIG. 6-78. High-power view of tumor cells in a smear from a superficially invasive squamous cell carcinoma. These cells have the features of invasive cancer, including macronucleoli and irregularly distributed coarse chromatin.

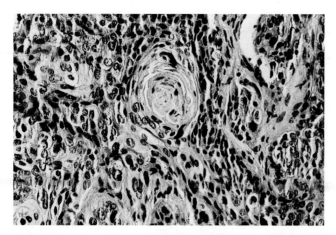

FIG. 6-79. Keratinizing invasive squamous cell carcinoma in biopsy specimen. The cellular pleomophism and well-defined keratin pearls are characteristic.

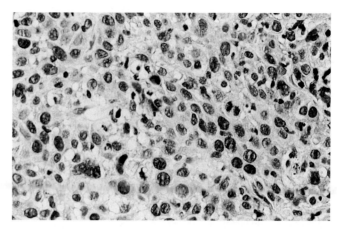

FIG. 6-81. Nonkeratinizing squamous cell carcinoma. Medium-power field showing sheet-like proliferation of polygonal malignant squamous cells.

such. These are the tumors that are generally believed to be responsible for the poor prognosis associated with the small cell tumors in the Wentz-Reagan classification. The remaining small-cell malignancies of the cervix represent variants of nonkeratinizing squamous carcinomas and can be included in that group. The subtypes of carcinomas mentioned have demonstrated a correlation between histologic type and survival after radiation therapy in some studies.[57-59] Other studies have failed to show such a correlation.[50-61] Other subclassification and grading systems, including the standard Broders grading system, have shown no evidence of a correlation between grade or tumor morphology and survival.

Histologic Characteristics of Squamous Cell Carcinoma

Keratinizing carcinomas demonstrate the histologic features that have been associated with "well-differentiated" squamous neoplasms. They are composed of sheets and nests of infiltrating squamous epithelial cells characterized by the presence of well-formed keratin "pearls" formed by concentric rings of layered keratin. Intercellular bridges are identifiable between adjacent cells and hyperchromatic, often pyknotic nuclei are characteristic. Cellular pleomorphism is a prominent feature of these tumors. Mitoses, although not numerous, are easily found, and abnormal mitotic forms are evident. These tumors often have an exophytic growth pattern and usually infiltrate the cervical stroma as irregular, sharp tongues of neoplastic cells (Figs. 6-79 and 6-80).

Nonkeratinizing carcinomas are composed of polygonal cells, usually arranged in sheets forming masses with pushing borders. Keratinization of single cells may be present, but keratin "pearls" are not found. The nuclei are enlarged and variable in size, and have prominent nuclei and coarsely granular chromatin. Mitoses are more common than in the keratinizing tumors (Figs. 6-81 and 6-82).

In both types of squamous carcinoma, the adjacent stroma frequently shows a desmoplastic response and

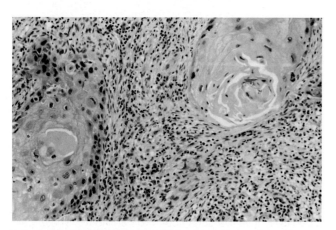

FIG. 6-80. Keratinizing invasive squamous cell carcinoma. Nests of keratinized cells invading the cervical stroma.

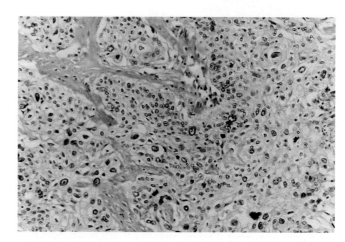

FIG. 6-82. Nonkeratinizing squamous cell carcinoma.

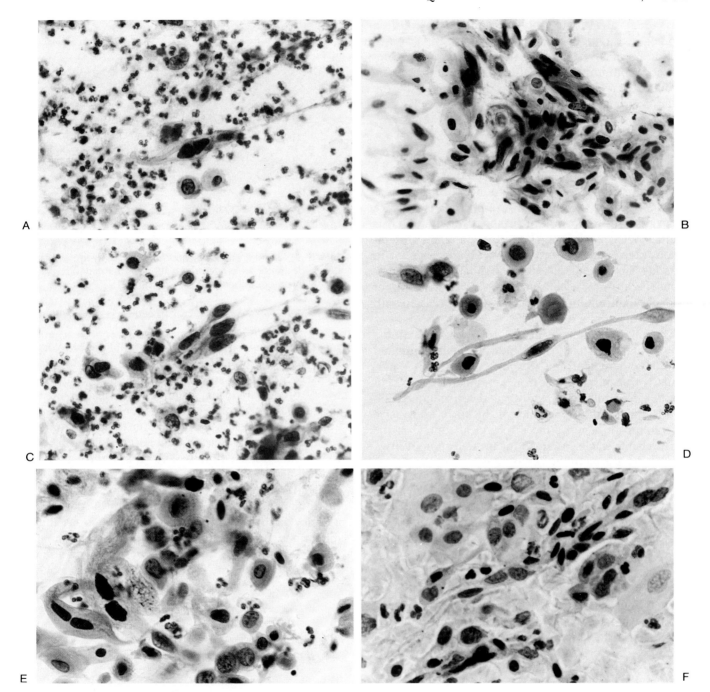

FIG. 6-83. (A–F) Keratinizing squamous cell carcinoma in cytologic samples showing the typical cellular pleomorphiosm with spindle-shaped cells, elongate and caudate forms, and frequent opacified nuclei. Note lack of a tumor diathesis.

may contain an inflammatory cell infiltrate. This is often composed of lymphocytes, but in some cases, eosinophils are numerous and may predominate. Tumor necrosis is a common finding with the nonkeratinizing carcinomas, but is seen much less frequently with the keratinizing variants.

Cytologic Features of Invasive Squamous Cell Carcinoma

Cellular samples from cases of nonkeratinizing squamous cell carcinoma almost invariably contain evidence of necrosis in the form of a tumor diathesis, which is characterized by the presence of a granular, proteinaceous precipitate and broken-down blood pigment in the slide background. Keratinizing squamous cell carcinoma, because it is usually an exophytic growth without evidence of ulceration, is not commonly associated with evidence of a tumor diathesis.

The cellular samples from cases of invasive carcinoma may contain relatively few abnormal cells compared with those derived from CIS and dysplasia. This is particularly true of specimens from keratinizing cancers. In some cases, cytologic recognition and correct interpretation is difficult in the presence of this form of invasive carcinoma. In general, the ectocervical sample is the most reliable single specimen for the detection of invasive cancer arising in the cervix, and most of the abnormal cells that are present are found in this sample.

The cells in cases of keratinizing squamous cell carcinoma are variable in size and configuration. There is often associated evidence of hyperkeratosis in the form of anucleate squames, and of pleomorphic parakeratosis in the form of miniature squamous cells with pyknotic nuclei of variable size and shape. The mean cellular area per case was described as being $274.6 \pm 106.8 \ \mu m^2$ by Reagan and colleagues.[62] About 15% of the abnormal cell population is characterized by elongated and caudate forms. These are not seen in the other varieties of squamous cell carcinoma. The cytoplasm may range from eosinophilic to cyanophilic. The nuclei have a

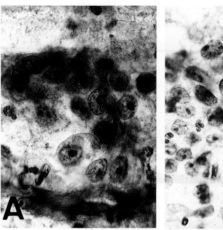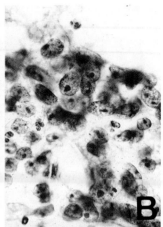

FIG. 6-84. Nonkeratinizing squamous cell carcinoma. Aggregates of tumor cells demonstrating prominent nucleoli. A granular tumor diathesis is seen in frame **B**.

mean area of approximately 80 μm^2 and are often irregular in configuration. The chromatin is hyperchromatic, coarsely granular, and often irregularly distributed. Many of the abnormal cells contain opaque nuclear masses indicative of cell degeneration. Macronucleoli are present, but are less common than in nonkeratinizing squamous cell carcinoma and are often difficult to identify in the cytologic sample (Figs. 6-83A through 6-83F Table 6-6).

Cellular samples from nonkeratinizing squamous cell carcinomas are typically characterized by the presence of a tumor diathesis in the background. Numerous abnormal cells are usually present. Individual cells are smaller than those of many intraepithelial lesions, with a mean area of $256 \pm 69 \ \mu m^2$.[62] They are arranged in isolated

---

TABLE 6-6. *Summary of diagnostic features of nonkeratinizing squamous cell carcinoma*

Slide background	Tumor diathesis
Number of abnormal cells	Many
Arrangement of cells	Syncytial aggregates and isolated
Cell configuration	Polygonal with poorly defined borders
Nuclei	1.5–3 times normal; irregular outline; coarse, irregularly distributed chromatin
Nucleoli	Many macronucleoli; irregular shape

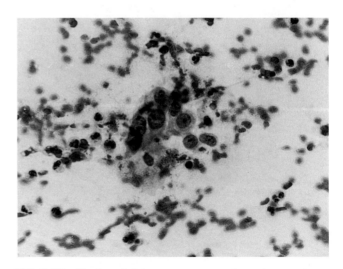

FIG. 6-85. Nonkeratinizing squamous cell carcinoma. A syncytial aggregate of tumor cells in a bloody background.

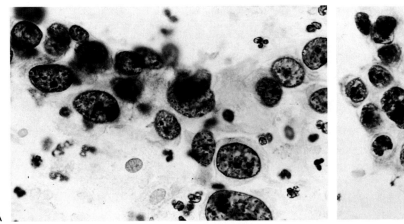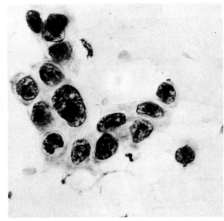

FIG. 6-86. (A, B) High-power view of tumor cells from nonkeratinizing squamous cell carcinoma showing details of nuclear structure including coarse chromatin, focal chromatin clearing, and macro nucleoli.

forms and in syncytial aggregates with ill-defined cellular borders and cyanophilic cytoplasm. The nuclei are round or oval to irregular in configuration and average approximately 90 μm^2 in area. The chromatin is coarsely granular, irregularly distributed, and hyperchromatic. Macronucleoli are common and easily identified (Figs. 6-84 through 6-87; Table 6-7).

Differential Diagnosis of Squamous Cell Carcinoma of the Uterine Cervix

The cytologic diagnosis of invasive squamous cell carcinoma is usually achieved with little difficulty. However, there are a number of different entities that may mimic the changes of invasive cancer, and these must be excluded when considering individual cases. The differential diagnosis of an intraepithelial lesion and invasive squamous carcinoma is usually straightforward. Invasive cancer is characterized by the presence of macronucleoli, irregular chromatin distribution, and a tumor diathesis. These features are absent in the intraepithelial process. In the case of keratinizing intraepithelial processes, however, the distinction is more difficult (Fig. 6-88).

Although most invasive cancers are characterized cytologically by the presence of a tumor diathesis, macronucleoli, and irregularities in nuclear chromatin distribution, these features often are not evident in smears from invasive keratinizing carcinomas. The presence of any of these features strongly suggests the presence of invasion; however, their absence does not rule out invasion, particularly in a case with numerous pleomorphic forms.

An atypical reparative process involving the cervix, as discussed earlier, can mimic invasive cancer and may be the entity most frequently confused cytologically with malignancy. Other entities that may be confused with invasive squamous cell carcinoma of the uterine cervix in the cytologic sample are viral infections, radiation or chemotherapeutic effects, decidual reactions of the cervix, poorly differentiated adenocarcinomas, and metastasis of tumors to the female genital tract, especially colonic cancers. These difficulties are usually obviated

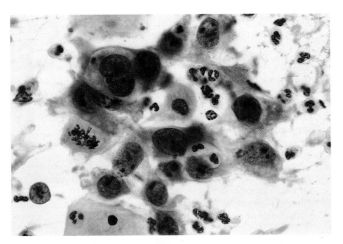

FIG. 6-87. Nonkeratinizing squamous cell carcinoma.

TABLE 6-7. *Summary of diagnostic features of keratinizing squamous cell carcinoma*

Slide background	Often clean; rare tumor diathesis
Number of abnormal cells	Few to many
Arrangement of cells	Mainly isolated; some syncytial
Cell configuration	Pronounced pleomorphism
Nuclei	1–2 times normal; pleomorphic; variable chromatin; often opaque
Nucleoli	Rare macronucleoli

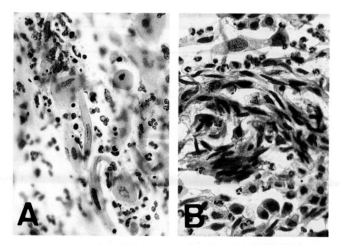

FIG. 6-88. Keratinizing dysplasia (**A**) versus Keratinizing squamous cell carcinoma (**B**). This may be a difficult differential in some cases. Keratinizing carcinomas may have more abnormal cells and greater pleomorphism as in this comparison but this is not a consistent finding. (**B** reprinted from Patten SF. Cytology of dysplexia, carcinoma in situ and invasive carcinoma of the uterine cervix. Chicago, Tutorials of Cytology, 1973.)

through a combination of good clinical history and a careful systematic approach utilizing the criteria outlined earlier. In those rare cases where differential diagnosis is impossible, it is quite appropriate and necessary for the pathologist to relate the diagnostic possibilities to the clinician so that appropriate further diagnostic procedures may be carried out.

REFERENCES

1. Meisels A, Fortin R. Condylomatous lesions of the cervix and vagina. I. Cytologic patterns. Acta Cytol 1976;20:505.
2. Meisels A, Fortin R, Roy M. Condylomatous lesions of the cervix. II. Cytologic, colposcopic and histopathologic study. Acta Cytol 1977;21:379.
3. Purola E, Savia E. Cytology of gynecologic condyloma acuminatum. Acta Cytol 1977;21:26.
4. Kurman RJ, Solomon D. The Bethesda system for reporting cervical/vaginal cytologic diagnoses. Definitions, criteria, and explanatory notes for terminology and specimen adequacy. New York: Springer-Verlag, 1994.
5. Patten SF. Diagnostic cytopathology of the uterine cervix, 2nd ed. Basel: S Karger, 1978.
6. Patten SF. Benign proliferative reactions of the uterine cervix. In Wied GL, Keebler CM, Koss LG, et al (eds). Compendium on diagnostic cytology, 7th ed. Chicago: Tutorials of Cytology, 1992:77.
7. Graham RM. The cytologic diagnosis of cancer, 3rd ed., p 62. Philadelphia: WB Saunders, 1963.
8. Graham RM. Cytomorphology of carcinoma in situ. Acta Cytol 1961;5:425.
9. Dressel DM, Wilbur DC. Atypical immature squamous metaplastic cells in cervical smears: association with high grade squamous intraepithelial lesions (HGSIL) and carcinomas of the cervix. Acta Cytol 1992;36:630.
10. Geirsson G, Woodworth F, Patten SF, et al. Epithelial repair and regeneration in the uterine cervix. I. An analysis of the cells. Acta Cytol 1977;21:371.
11. Fu YS, Reagan JW. Pathology of the uterine cervix, vulva and vagina. Philadelphia: WB Saunders, 1989:228.
12. Kurman RJ, Norris HJ, Wilkinson E. Atlas of tumor pathology: tumors of the cervix, vagina and vulva. Washington, DC: Armed Forces Institute of Pathology, 1990:41.
13. Hulka BS. Cytologic and histologic outcome following an atypical cervical smear. Am J Obstet Gynecol 1968;101:190.
14. Kaminski PF, Stevens CW, Wheelock JB. Squamous atypia on cytology. The influence of age. J Reprod Med 1989;34:617.
15. Melamed MR, Flehinger BJ. Non-diagnostic squamous atypia in cervico-vaginal cytology as a risk factor for early neoplasia. Acta Cytol 1976;20:108.
16. Noumoff JS. Atypia in cervical cytologies: a risk factor for intraepithelial neoplasia. Am J Obstet Gynecol 1987;156:628.
17. Nyirjesy I. Atypical or suspicious cervical smears: an aggressive diagnostic approach. JAMA 1972;222:691.
18. Paavonen J, Kiviat ND, Wölner-Hanssen P, et al. Significance of mild cervical cytologic atypia in a sexually transmitted disease clinic population. Acta Cytol 1989;33:831.
19. Jones DED, Creasman WT, Dombroski RA, et al. Evaluation of the atypical smear. Am J Obstet Gynecol 1987;157:544.
20. Soutter WP, Wisdom S, Brough AK, et al. Should patients with mild atypia in a cervical smear be referred for colposcopy? Br J Obstet Gynaecol 1986;93:70.
21. Spitzer M, Krumholz BA, Chernys AE, et al. Comparative utility of repeat Papanicolaou smears, cervicography and colposcopy in the evaluation of atypical Papanicolaou smears. Obstet Gynecol 1987;69:731.
22. Shiels LA, Wilbur DC. The significance of atypical cells of squamous type on cervical smears with stratification of risk based on morphology. (In press)
23. Syrjanen K, Kataaja V, Yliskoski M, et al. Natural history of cervical human papillomavirus lesions does not substantiate the biologic relevance of the Bethesda system. Obstet Gynecol 1992;79:675.
24. Kurman RJ, Henson DE, Herbst AL, et al. Interim guidelines for the management of abnormal cervical cytology. JAMA 1994;271:1866.
25. Fu YS, Reagan JW, Richart RM, et al. Nuclear DNA and histopathologic studies of genital lesions in DES exposed progeny. I. Intraepithelial squamous abnormalities. Am J Clin Pathol 1979;72:502.
26. Fu YS, Reagan JW, Richart RM. Definition of precursors. Gynecol Oncol 1981;12:S220.
27. Fu YS, Huang I, Beaudenon S, et al. Correlative study of human papillomavirus DNA: histopathology and morphometry in cervical condyloma and intraepithelial neoplasia. Int J Gynecol Pathol 1988;7:297.
28. Scully R, Bonfiglio TA, Kurman RJ, et al. Histologic typing of female genital tract tumors, p 41. New York: Springer-Verlag, 1994.
29. Willett Gd, Kurman RJ, Reid R, et al. Correlation of the histologic appearance of intraepithelial neoplasia of the cervix with human papillomavirus types. Int J Gynecol Pathol 1989;8:18.
30. Valente PT. Update on the Bethesda system for reporting cervical/vaginal diagnoses. Boston: Kluwer Academic Publishers, 1994:15.
31. Reagan JW, Bell BA, Neuman JL, et al. Dysplasia in the uterine cervix during pregnancy: an analytical study of the cells. Acta Cytol 1961;5:17.
32. Reagan JW, Hamonic MJ. Dysplasia of the uterine cervix. Ann NY Acad Sci 1956;63:1236.
33. Reagan JW, Hamonic MJ. The cellular pathology in carcinoma in situ. A cytohistopathological correlation. Cancer 1956;9:385.
34. Reagan JW, Patten SF. Analytical study of cellular changes in carcinoma in situ, squamous-cell cancer and adenocarcinoma of uterine cervix. Clin Obstet Gynecol 1961;4:1097.
35. Reagan JW, Patten SF. Dysplasia: a basic reaction to injury in the uterine cervix. Ann NY Acad Sci 1962;97:662.
36. Reagan JW, Seidemann IL, Saracusa Y. The cellular morphology of carcinoma in situ and dysplasia of atypical hyperplasia of the uterine cervix. Cancer 1953;6:244.
37. Patten SF, Bonfiglio TA. Cytopathology and morphologic subclassification of squamous intraepithelial lesions of the uterine cervix. In Wied GL, Keebler CM, Koss LG, et al (eds). Compendium on diagnostic cytology, 7th ed. Chicago: Tutorials of Cytology, 1992:91.

38. Bonfiglio TA. Cytopathology of cervical dysplasia, carcinoma in situ and invasive carcinoma. In Astarita R (ed). Basic cytopathology, p 60. New York, Churchill Livingstone, 1991.

39. Patten SF. Diagnostic cytopathology of the uterine cervix, 2nd ed. Basel: S Karger, 1978:288.

40. Sherman ME, Kelly D. High-grade squamous intraepithelial lesions and invasive carcinoma following the report of three negative Papanicolaou smears: screening failures or rapid progression? Mod Pathol 1992;5:337.

41. Hatem F, Wilbur DC. High-grade cervical lesions following negative Papanicolaou smears: false negative cervical cytology or rapid progression. Diagn Cytol 1995;12:135.

42. Keebler CM, Wied GL. Use of the estrogen test as an aid in differential diagnostic problems related to screening the cell sample from the menopausal patient. Acta Cytol 1974;18:482.

43. Selvaggi SM. Cytologic features of squamous cell carcinoma in situ involving endocervical glands in endocervical Cytobrush specimens. Acta Cytol 1994;38:687.

44. Patten SF. Postradiation dysplasia of the cervix. In Wied GL, Keebler CM, Koss LG, et al (eds). Compendium on diagnostic cytology, 7th ed. Chicago: Tutorials of Cytology, 1992:191.

45. Patten SF, Reagan JW, Obenauf M, et al. Postirradiation dysplasia of uterine cervix and vagina: an analytical study of the cells. Cancer 1963;16:173.

46. Koss LG, Melamed MR, Daniel WW. In situ epidermoid carcinoma of the cervix and vagina following radiotherapy for cervix cancer. Cancer 1961;14:353.

47. Meswerdt G. Probeexzision und kolposkopie in des fruhdiagnose des portio karcinom. Zentralbl Gynakol 1947;4:326.

48. International Federation of Gynecology & Obstetrics. Changes in definitions for clinical staging for carcinoma of the cervix and ovary. Am J Obstet Gynecol 1987;156:263.

49. Benson WL, Norris HJ. A critical review of the frequency of lymph node metastases and death from microinvasive carcinoma of the cervix. Obstet Gynecol 1977;49:632.

50. Boronow RC, Averette HE, Nelson JH Jr, et al. Defining cervical microinvasive carcinoma. Contemporary Obstetrics and Gynecology 1975;5:121.

51. Sedlis A, Sall S, Tsukada Y, et al. Microinvasive carcinoma of the uterine cervix: a clinico-pathologic study. Am J Obstet Gynecol 1979;133:64.

52. Seski JC, Abell MR, Morley GW. Microinvasive squamous carcinoma of the cervix. Definition, histologic analysis, late results of treatment. Obstet Gynecol 1977;50:410.

53. Ng ABP, Reagan JW. Microinvasive carcinoma of the uterine cervix. Am J Clin Pathol 1969;52:511.

54. Ng ABP, Reagan JW, Lindner E. The cellular manifestations of microinvasive squamous cell carcinoma of the uterine cervix. Acta Cytol 1972;6:5.

55. Broders AC. Carcinoma grading and practical application. Arch Pathol 1926;2:376.

56. Wentz WB, Reagan JW. Survival in cervical cancer with respect to cell type. Cancer 1959;12:384.

57. Wentz WB. Histological grade and survival in cervical cancer. Obstet Gynecol 1961;18:412.

58. Wentz WB, Lewis GC. Correlation of histologic morphology and survival in cervical cancer following radiation therapy. Obstet Gynecol 1965;26:228.

59. Swan DS, Roddick JW. A clinicopathologic correlation of cell type classification for cervical cancer. Am J Obstet Gynecol 1973;116:666.

60. Goellner JR. Carcinoma of the cervix. Am J Clin Pathol 1976;66:775.

61. Crissman JD, Makuch R, Budhraja M, et al. Histopathologic grading of squamous cell carcinoma of the uterine cervix. An evaluation of 71 stage Ib patients. Cancer 1985;55:1590.

62. Reagan JW, Hamonic MJ, Wentz WB. Analytical study of cells in cervical squamous-cell cancer. Lab Invest 1957;6:241.

ADDITIONAL READING

Crum CP, Nuovo GJ. Genital papillomaviruses and related neoplasms. New York: Raven Press, 1991.

Keebler CM, Somrak TM (eds). The manual of cytotechnology. Chicago: ASCP Press, 1993.

Koss LG. Diagnostic cytology and its histologic basis. Philadelphia: JB Lippincott, 1992.

Nuovo GJ. Cytopathology of the lower female genital tract: an integrated approach. Baltimore: Williams & Wilkins, 1994.

Vooijs GP. Benign proliferative reactions, intraepithelial neoplasia and invasive cancer of the uterine cervix. In Bibbo M (ed). Comprehensive cytopathology. Philadelphia: WB Saunders, 1991:153.

Gynecologic Cytopathology. Edited by
Thomas A. Bonfiglio and Yener S. Erozan.
Lippincott–Raven Publishers, Philadelphia, © 1997.

CHAPTER 7

The Cytology of the Endocervix, Endometrium, and Upper Female Genital Tract

David C. Wilbur

With the wider use of new sampling devices that provide improved cellular yields from higher in the endocervical canal, interest is increasing in the cytology of the normal endocervical canal and the benign and neoplastic processes that involve it. The Bethesda System for cervical cytology terminology and reporting has stressed the need to provide assessments of specimen adequacy for optimal sensitivity and interpretation. As part of these adequacy assessments, the presence of endocervical or squamous metaplastic cells on the slide has been stressed, in order to document transformation zone sampling. As a result of this drive to provide adequate samples for sensitive cytologic evaluation, new sampling devices have been developed that are designed to provide increased cellular yields from the transformation zone and the endocervical mucosa from higher regions of the endocervical canal.[1-7] The use of these sampling devices, most notably the endocervical brush and broom, has generated cytologic samples showing new patterns of endocervical cell presentation. These new patterns have caused significant difficulty for practicing cytologists who were trained on material derived by the traditional collection methods of spatula and cotton swab. Over the past several years, the diagnosis of *atypical endocervical cells (atypical glandular cells of undetermined significance— endocervical type [AGCUS])* has been utilized more commonly, and the cytologic differentiation of benign and reactive endocervical cells from cells derived from lesions of neoplastic origin has become a more common, and seemingly more difficult, problem.

It is the purpose of this chapter to review the normal cytology of the endocervical canal, present the neoplastic lesions that originate there, and detail the spectrum of changes that represent their benign and reactive mimickers. In addition, this chapter presents a discussion of the exfoliative cytology of the endometrium, including normal, reactive, and neoplastic processes. The ancillary findings of normal-appearing endometrial cells presenting at abnormal times and cells found on cervical smears in association with endometrial lesions also are discussed.

THE NORMAL HISTOLOGY OF THE ENDOCERVICAL CANAL

The glandular portion of the transformation zone and regions proximal to it are generally composed of a simple

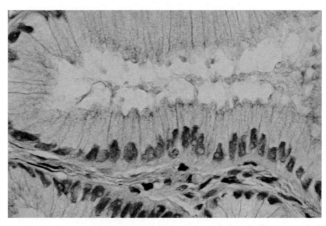

FIG. 7-1. Normal endocervical mucosal lining is illustrated. It consists of a simple columnar, mucous-producing epithelium. Nuclei are basilar within each cell (hematoxylin and eosin).

D. C. Wilbur: Department of Pathology and Laboratory Medicine, University of Rochester Medical Center, Rochester, New York 14642.

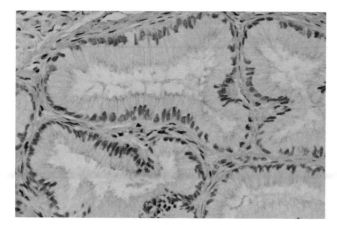

FIG. 7-2. Normal endocervical glands extend into an underlying fibromuscular stroma (hematoxylin and eosin).

columnar mucus-producing epithelium, as illustrated in Figure 7-1. The mucosa is arranged architecturally into a surface portion and glandular pouches that extend into the underlying muscular cervical stroma (Fig. 7-2). Endocervical epithelial cells may also show ciliated forms, which may combine with goblet and intercalated cells to form the pattern known as ciliated cell, or tubal, metaplasia. This process recapitulates the normal epithelium of the uterine tube and is commonly found involving the uppermost portions of the endocervical canal mucosal surface.

Histologic studies performed in this author's laboratory on normal cervices, derived from hysterectomy specimens without cervical pathology, have shown distinctive features of the endocervical canal that are important when considering the cytologic presentation of endocervical cells derived from the newer "canal-sampling" collection devices.[8] If the endocervical canal is divided into three equal portions, the lowest portion contains the fewest and most shallow endocervical glands, followed by the uppermost segment. The middle

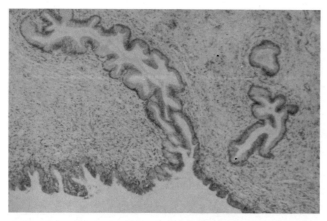

FIG. 7-3. The midportion of the endocervical canal normally contains the deepest extent of the endocervical gland crypts into the underlying stroma, as illustrated here (hematoxylin and eosin).

portion of the canal contains the most and deepest endocervical glands (Fig. 7-3). In the middle and upper portions of the canal, there can be significant crowding and pseudostratification of the "simple" columnar epithelium, and this crowding appears to be most pronounced at the openings of the mouths of the glands (Fig. 7-4). In

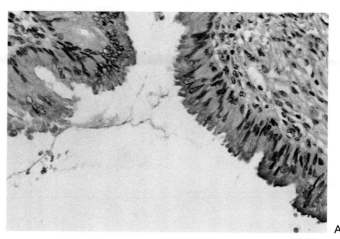

A

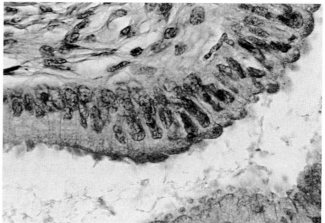

B

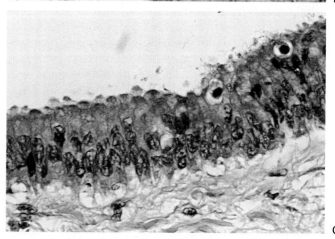

C

FIG. 7-4. **(A, B, C)** These three slides show the normally nonstratified endocervical mucosa in various degrees of nuclear pseudostratification and crowding. This phenomenon has been found to be a relatively common finding in the middle and upper portions of the endocervical canal (hematoxylin and eosin).

TABLE 7-1. *Histologic features of the normal endocervical canal*

Histologic finding	A (lower)	B (middle)	C (upper)
Mean number of endocervical glands	46	74	42
Percentage of glands crowded	39	47	50
Mean number of ciliated cells	45	210	355

the uppermost portion of the gland, tubal metaplasia is virtually always present, and overall, the endocervical cells become progressively smaller and blend gradually into the surface endometrial cells of the lower uterine segment. The normal histologic patterns found in the various endocervical regions are presented in Table 7-1.

THE NORMAL CYTOLOGY OF THE ENDOCERVICAL CANAL

The endocervical histologic pattern of a simple columnar mucus-producing epithelium is well demonstrated in most cell studies that include transformation zone sampling. Endocervical cells may present cytologically in several ways, depending on their orientation on the slide, their arrangement with other endocervical cells in a grouping, and the manner in which they were sampled. When spontaneously exfoliated, endocervical cells appear most commonly as single cells with significant rounding of the normally columnar cytoplasm (Fig. 7-5). Such rounding indicates that the cells have been truly exfoliated, free from attachment to neighboring

cells and stroma, allowing for a conformation indicative of a "fluid" environment. When traumatically sampled, as with a cell collection device, endocervical cells may appear isolated or in cohesive groups. In both cases, the cells recapitulate their "native" appearance in histologic samples. In isolation, they show a distinct columnar or rounded rectangular shape with a basilar nucleus (Fig. 7-6). The cytoplasm is frothy to granular and stains in an amphophilic fashion with the Papanicolaou stain. The nuclei of normal endocervical cells measure in the range of 50 to 60 μm^2. This is larger than the nuclei of intermediate squamous or endometrial cells, both of which measure in the range of 30 to 40 μm^2. The relative nuclear area is low, generally in the range of 30%. The nuclei are round to oval and generally regular, with finely granular chromatin that is evenly distributed. Small to medium-sized nucleoli may be seen in most cells. When present in groups, and oriented such that the epithelium is viewed from the side, the endocervical cells show the typical "picket fence" arrangement, as seen in Figure 7-7. When viewed on end, they present a "honeycomb" pattern, as illustrated in Figure 7-8. Although the nuclei of normal endocervical cells are generally uniform in appearance, there is some degree of pleomorphism of size, even in nonreactive cells. This is important in the differential diagnosis of groups of endocervical cells showing "atypia."

As was noted in the histology of the endocervical canal, ciliated columnar endocervical cells may also represent a normal variant of endocervical cells (Fig. 7-9). Such cells have thin, wavy, eosinophilic, filamentous cilia extending from one end. Typically, a thick eosinophilic terminal bar is present, which forms the anchor for the cilia. In many cases, the cilia are lost, leaving only the

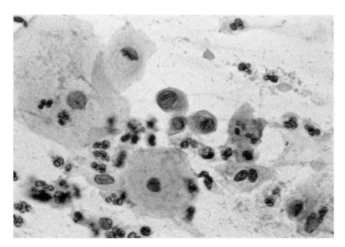

FIG. 7-5. An example of two small endocervical cells that have been spontaneously exfoliated and therefore acquired characteristics consistent with suspension in a "fluid" environment. These characteristics include round to oval configuration and isolated nature (Papanicolaou stain).

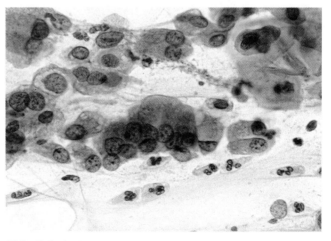

FIG. 7-6. Isolated columnar endocervical cells are seen at the periphery of the central group. The columnar presentation implies that these cells have been traumatically removed from the endocervical canal during the sampling procedure (Papanicolaou stain).

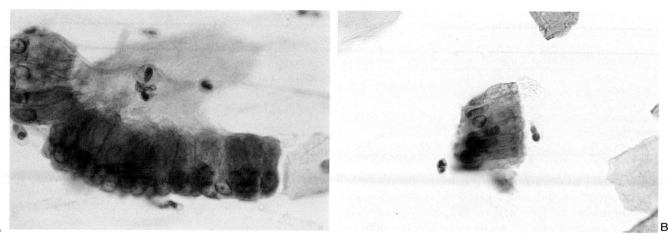

FIG. 7-7. **(A, B)** These two slides show the typical "picket-fence" arrangement of endocervical cells that have been traumatically removed from the normal epithelial lining and viewed from the side (**A,** conventional smear; **B,** Cyto-Rich; both, Papanicolaou stain).

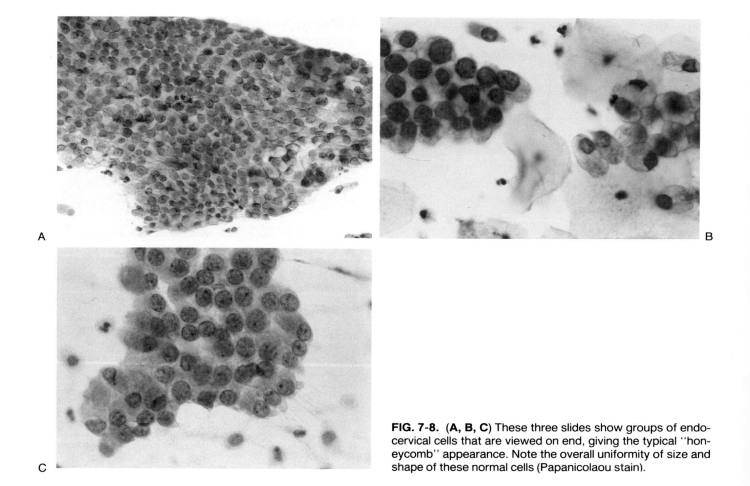

FIG. 7-8. **(A, B, C)** These three slides show groups of endocervical cells that are viewed on end, giving the typical "honeycomb" appearance. Note the overall uniformity of size and shape of these normal cells (Papanicolaou stain).

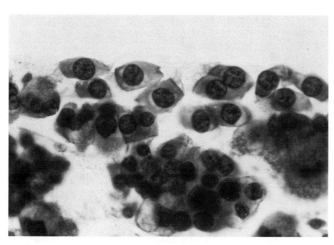

FIG. 7-9. Benign ciliated endocervical cells are shown. Note the thin, filamentous cilia projecting from the cell surface, and the terminal bar at the apex of the cell to which the cilia are attached. In ciliated endocervical cells, nuclei tend to be present in the central portions of the cell cytoplasm rather than basilar. This nuclear location most probably accounts for the appearance of pseudostratification in the endocervical epithelium when abundant ciliated cells are present (Papanicolaou stain).

terminal bar, or eosinophilic fragments of the terminal bar, present in each cell. It is also more common for the nuclei of ciliated endocervical cells to be located more centrally. This undoubtedly is partly responsible for the pseudostratification that is commonly noted in epithelia composed predominantly of ciliated cells. When true tubal metaplasia is present (typically in the upper reaches of the canal), all three cell types may be represented in the pattern, although it is not uncommon to see only one or two of the components in a particular sample. The cytologic presentation of tubal metaplasia may also be a common cause of differential diagnostic difficulties in cases of endocervical atypia, and these changes are discussed in greater detail later.

ENDOCERVICAL NEOPLASIA

The incidence of invasive endocervical adenocarcinoma has increased over the past 50 years. This increase has been a relative one because of the decrease in cervical squamous carcinoma; however, it has also been absolute. In the early 1940s, Reagan and Ng found that endocervical adenocarcinoma made up 5% of all cervical carcinoma. In the early 1970s, they found that this figure had risen to 16%.[9] More recent studies have detected incidence rates of endocervical adenocarcinoma ranging between 14% and 34% of all cervical cancer.[10–13]

Epidemiologic studies of endocervical carcinoma have shown that this lesion differs significantly when compared with its squamous counterpart in the uterine cervix. Endocervical carcinoma, although less so than en-

dometrial cancer, has been postulated to have an association with hormonal stimulation. Several studies have shown an association with a history of oral contraceptive use,[14,15] although other studies have not confirmed this finding.[16,17] This type of cancer appears to affect women of higher socioeconomic classes, with higher levels of education, lower rates of unemployment, and higher incomes, than does squamous cell carcinoma,[18] perhaps because the use of exogenous hormones probably is more common in such populations. In addition, unlike squamous carcinoma, endocervical disease shows only a weak linkage to early sexual intercourse[19,20] and to smoking.

Similar to squamous neoplasia, the association of endocervical cancer with the human papillomavirus (HPV) is strong. In cases of invasive carcinoma, studies have shown detection rates of greater than 70% for HPV nucleic acid when examined by sensitive hybridization techniques.[21] A composite of HPV nucleic acid detection results from studies of endocervical neoplastic lesions is presented in Table 7-2. Invasive endocervical adenocarcinoma contains evidence of HPV DNA in 31% to 83% of cases.[22–26] Studies predominantly have demonstrated the presence of "high-risk" virus types 16 and 18, as in squamous neoplasia. However, in contrast to squamous cancer, endocervical carcinoma generally has a higher proportion of cases (up to 80%) associated with HPV type 18[23–27] (Fig. 7-10). Cases of noninvasive adenocarcinoma in situ (AIS) have also consistently shown the presence of HPV DNA (63% to 89%), with a similar overrepresentation of type 18.[22,23,28–30] These data suggest that HPV may also play some role in the pathogenesis of endocervical neoplasia, although possible mechanisms have yet to be elucidated. Several investigators have also looked for HPV in the lesion referred to as *endocervical glandular dysplasia,* which may represent a precursor lesion to endocervical adenocarcinoma. These groups have noted significantly lower rates of HPV nucleic acid detection, ranging from 4% to 46%.[28,30,31] One of the studies found a predominance of type 18 (46% positive cases), similar to the studies of AIS and invasive le-

TABLE 7-2. *Human papillomavirus detection and typing in lesions of the endocervix*

Study	Invasive (18/16)	In situ (18/16)	Dysplasia (18/16)
Wilczynski[26]	64% (71/29)	ND	ND
Gordon[25]	83% (80/20)	ND	ND
Smotkin[24]	50% (0/100)	ND	ND
Tase[23]	64% (63/37)	70% (71/29)	ND
Griffin[22]	31% (20/80)	63% (0/100)	ND
Duggan[27]	ND	66 (65/35)	ND
Farnsworth[28]	ND	88.6% (67/33)	0%
Leary[30]	ND	70% (52/48)	46% (67/33)
Tase[31]	ND	ND	6%

ND, not done.

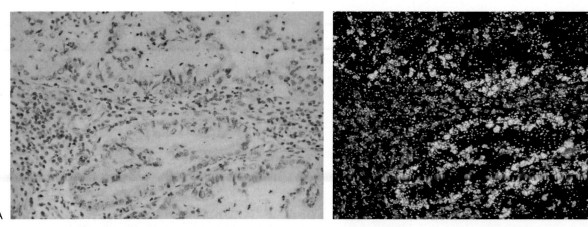

FIG. 7-10. Example of in situ hybridization for human Papillomavirus type 18, in a case of endocervical adenocarcinoma in situ. Figure (**A**) represents bright-field illumination to show the typical glandular structure of the carcinoma. Figure (**B**) represents the dark-field illumination, which shows the abundant signal present as light grains within the glands in this autoradiographic detection system (hematoxylin stain, autoradiography). (These slides courtesy of Mark H. Stoler, MD, University of Virginia Health Sciences Center, Charlottesville, VA).

sions.[30] Given the lack of agreement regarding the criteria for making a diagnosis of endocervical glandular dysplasia (see later) and, therefore, the difficulty in making a definitive diagnosis, the lack of agreement between these studies regarding the presence of HPV is not surprising. Many cases that are found to be negative for HPV nucleic acid may represent endocervical processes of a nonneoplastic, benign, or reactive nature. In the study by Leary and colleagues, endocervical glandular dysplasia is defined in a rigorous and currently acceptable manner. Based on the stringency of the definition, nearly half the cases of "dysplasia" were positive for HPV DNA.[30] This finding lends support to the belief that this entity may be a precursor lesion in the spectrum of endocervical neoplasia.

A clear-cut association exists between endocervical and squamous lesions of the cervix. Endocervical adenocarcinoma is associated with squamous neoplasia elsewhere in the cervix in as many as 50% of cases. Squamous neoplasia is, of course, a much more common lesion, and when present, is associated with concomitant glandular cervical neoplasia in approximately 4% of cases. That such an association exists at all, again provides indirect evidence to support the hypothesis that squamous and glandular neoplasia share some common features in their histogenesis, and probably arise from similar, uncommitted stem cells in the cervix. Differentiation of these transformed cells along squamous or endocervical glandular lines, therefore, may be determined by other factors, probably working in complex concert. Elements might include such factors as hormonal stimulation and HPV type, as well as other, as yet undiscovered, genetic and environmental influences.

Endocervical adenocarcinoma is more difficult to diagnose than its squamous counterpart. Endocervical neoplasia involves areas above the transformation zone or deep in the endocervical glands; hence, the sensitivity of routine cervical smears is less than that noted for the detection of squamous lesions occupying the transformation zone. Even in cases where invasive carcinoma is present, 20% to 30% of colposcopic examinations may be interpreted as benign.[32] In addition, invasive lesions may be completely asymptomatic in up to 20% of cases. When symptoms are present, abnormal vaginal bleeding is most common, with vaginal discharge or pain reported occasionally.[33] In asymptomatic cases, the tumor is generally discovered via a routine cytologic smear. However, the sensitivity of detection is low. In one series, 51% of patients with endocervical adenocarcinomas showed normal cytology and 80% of patients without grossly identifiable lesions had negative cytologic examinations.[34] Data such as these argue strongly for an expanded role for cytologic screening in the detection of asymptomatic endocervical lesions. A need exists for greater use of the new collection devices that better sample the higher areas of the endocervical canal where these glandular lesions arise. These devices, which were developed to provide adequate transformation zone sampling, have also enhanced the sensitivity for the detection of endocervical lesions. However, because the use of these newer sampling devices causes changes in the overall presentation of the smears, cytologists must continue to refine diagnostic criteria in order to better identify glandular lesions in routine cervical smears.

Endocervical AIS was initially described in 1953 by Friedell and McKay.[35] AIS is a lesion that consists of endocervical glands with marked architectural and cytologic abnormalities, but without evidence of stromal invasion. It has been postulated to be a precursor lesion to invasive endocervical adenocarcinoma and is often found adjacent to invasive adenocarcinoma of the cervix. There are no studies currently available that address the relative risk of the development of invasive cancer when AIS is identified. Further studies to define progression rates and the time course of progression are also needed. Similar to invasive endocervical adenocarcinoma, AIS appears to be increasing in incidence, possibly as a result of increased exogenous hormone use, as well as heightened clinical awareness and improved detection methodologies. As with the invasive lesions of the endocervical canal, colposcopic examination does not detect many cases of AIS. Therefore, cytologic identification assumes a premier role in the early detection and management of this lesion.

THE HISTOLOGY OF INVASIVE AND IN SITU ENDOCERVICAL ADENOCARCINOMA

Invasive endocervical adenocarcinoma may show a variety of histologic patterns. The most common (70% of all cases) is the so-called endocervical type. This form is so named because it recapitulates the typical columnar mucus-producing appearance of normal endocervical epithelium (Figs. 7-11 and 7-12). The histology of this tumor can range from well-differentiated to poorly differentiated. An association with squamous neoplasia is seen in up to 50% of cases.[36] One variant of endocervical adenocarcinoma is the minimal deviation adenocarcinoma (adenoma malignum), which accounts for approximately 10% of cases. This form of the tumor is very well differentiated, with deceptively benign nuclear features. Abnormally branched glands are noted to extend into the cervical muscular wall to a level below that normally noted for endocervical gland depth. Stromal reac-

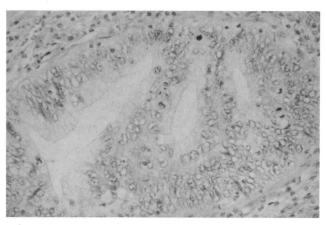

FIG. 7-12. Example of endocervical adenocarcinoma of the "endocervical" type. Note the recapitulation of normal endocervical-type tall columnar, mucous-producing epithelium. Often the glands may show prominent cribriforming as is shown in this case (hematoxylin and eosin).

tion may be present, and vascular invasion can sometimes be seen (Fig. 7-13). Endometrioid and serous papillary carcinomas are relatively uncommon as primary tumors in the cervix, but when present, closely mimic histologically their counterparts in the endometrium and ovary. Villoglandular papillary adenocarcinoma is a distinct variant that occurs in a younger population of patients and has a generally better prognosis than the other variants of invasive cancer.[37] This type of cancer shows prominent surface papillae of stratified columnar cells that demonstrate relatively mild nuclear atypia (Fig. 7-14).

Endocervical AIS has an appearance similar to that of invasive adenocarcinoma, but without evidence of stromal invasion (absence of invasive glands, stromal reac-

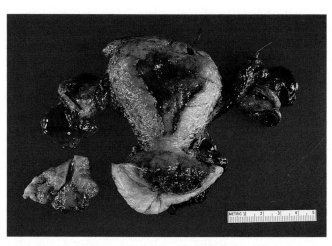

FIG. 7-11. Gross illustration of endocervical adenocarcinoma involving the area of the transformation zone. Note the exophytic nature of this tumor with obliteration and distortion of the normal endocervical canal and endocervical os.

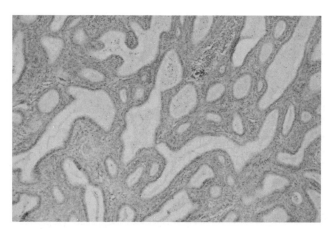

FIG. 7-13. Example of very well differentiated endocervical adenocarcinoma (adenoma malignum). In this form of cancer, the endocervical-type glands are very uniform, crowded, and extend to a depth greater than the normal extent of the endocervical crypts. The nuclei are very bland with only minimal cytologic abnormalities (hematoxylin and eosin).

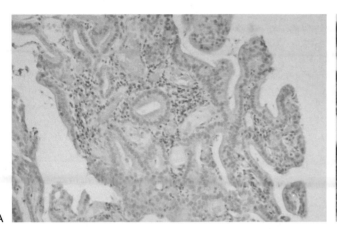 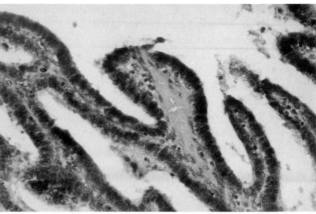

A   B

FIG. 7-14. Two examples of villoglandular endocervical adenocarcinoma are shown. (**A**) shows a low-magnification illustration of the well-differentiated nature of the tumor, with small, well-delineated glands and cribriform structures in the deeper portions of the tumor, and well-formed villous papillary structures extending from the surface. (**B**) shows a higher magnification of the surface villous papillary structures, which are lined by low columnar and cuboidal epithelial cells (hematoxylin and eosin).

tion, or glands below the normal depth). The neoplastic epithelium grows within the endocervical glands, replacing normal epithelium, generally with an abrupt transformation from benign to neoplastic (Fig. 7-15). The epithelium of AIS shows a pseudostratified architecture with nuclei extending to the surface of the columnar epithelium. Nuclear enlargement, irregularity, and hyperchromasia are present. Mitotic figures are commonly identified, along with nuclear breakdown granules[38] (apoptotic bodies; Fig. 7-16).

THE CYTOLOGY OF INVASIVE AND IN SITU ENDOCERVICAL ADENOCARCINOMA

In the spectrum of endocervical neoplasia, cell nuclei show progressive changes. Enlarging nuclei, hyperchro-

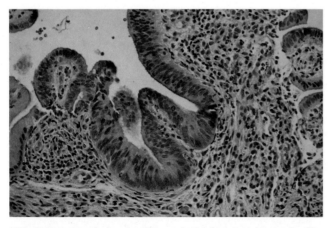

FIG. 7-15. Example of endocervical adenocarcinoma in situ. Note the abrupt transformation between normal endocervical mucosa (left) to the neoplastic epithelium, which shows loss of mucous-production and pseudostratification of nuclei throughout the height of the epithelium (hematoxylin and eosin).

masia, chromatin abnormality (increase in granular size and chromatin clearing), higher nuclear-to-cytoplasmic ratio, and increasing size of nucleoli are observed. Macronucleoli formation is an important differential diagnostic feature, because most invasive cancers show large nucleolar size, as well as the presence of multiple nucleoli. Throughout the advancing process, the cytoplasm retains its endocervical character, having a finely granular or vacuolated amphophilic to cyanophilic quality.

A number of investigators have studied the cytologic manifestations of endocervical AIS and have found some consistent features.[21,39–45] The cells of AIS are typically arranged in two-dimensional groups exhibiting nuclear crowding and overlap, with maintenance of palisading or polarity of the nuclear arrangements. The nuclear-to-cytoplasmic ratio is increased. The nuclei are oval to elongated and slightly larger (mean 75 μm^2) than normal endocervical cell nuclei. The nuclei show a highly distinctive, evenly dispersed but coarsely granular chromatin pattern. Mild degrees of nuclear pleomorphism of size and shape are noted within individual groups. Micronucleoli are present in most cells. Macronucleoli can be seen in some cells, but are not a consistent feature of in situ endocervical lesions. Proper attention to architectural features noted in groups of abnormal endocervical cells is crucial in distinguishing this type of neoplastic process from benign and reactive conditions, and from squamous neoplastic lesions (see later). The cell groups of AIS appear as cell strips with retention of columnar cytoplasmic features, nuclear stratification, and pseudostratification. Groups showing an acinar or "rosette" formation are common. Another characteristic architectural finding is the presence of nuclear "feathering" of the group edges (nuclear protrusions at the edges of the groups, compared with the usual

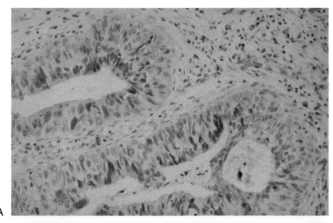
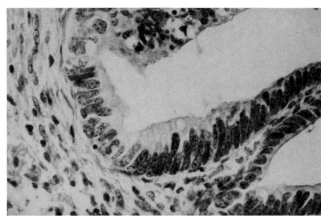
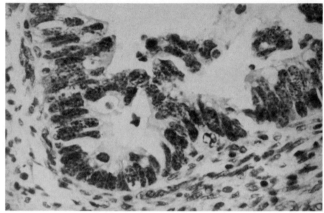

FIG. 7-16. Examples of endocervical adenocarcinoma in situ. **(A)** shows the complexity of the malignant glands with cribriformed pattern. **(B)** shows pseudostratified nuclei that are enlarged, hyperchromatic, and have a distinctive coarsely granular chromatin pattern. **(C)** shows similar nuclear features with prominent apoptotic bodies (nuclear breakdown fragments) indicative of increased cellular turnover (hematoxylin and eosin).

smooth borders). Examples of the individual cellular and architectural features of AIS are illustrated in Figure 7-17. These architectural features must be carefully sought in cases of suspected AIS. Such features are rarely seen together as a composite in nonneoplastic or nonendocervical lesions. The cytoplasm retains a typical endocervical granular amphophilic to cyanophilic character. Smear backgrounds are generally clean, although a variable number may show inflammatory or bloody patterns. As would be expected in this noninvasive lesion, a necrotic tumor diathesis is generally absent.

In contrast to noninvasive lesions, the smear background in cases of invasive endocervical adenocarcinoma commonly shows a tumor diathesis, with necrotic cellular breakdown material and blood. Cells from these lesions are abundant in routine smears when endocervical sampling devices are used, and most often show architectural and cytoplasmic features indicative of a columnar origin, particularly in the better-differentiated variants. Dyscohesion is increased, with more isolated tumor cells noted in smears from invasive cancer than in those from AIS. In addition, cell groupings derived from invasive cancer show an overall looser two-dimensional arrangement of the cells. Most of the architectural features of in situ lesions are retained in the invasive lesions. Two-dimensional sheets of cells with elongated nuclei are arranged in a side-by-side, fence-like orientation, of-

ten with retention of a rosette formation within the groups. Three-dimensional cell "clusters" are uncommon, and should suggest the possibility of a nonendocervical origin. (Table 7-3) Nuclei are generally larger than those of in situ lesions, ranging from approximately 75 μm^2 in the well-differentiated lesions to greater than 150 μm^2 in the more poorly differentiated examples. The nuclear-to-cytoplasmic ratio increases proportionately with decreasing differentiation, and the overall nuclear features of malignancy progressively worsen. Nuclei show increasing pleomorphism of size and shape. Chromatin patterns become progressively more abnormal, with increasing coarseness to the granular chromatin, areas of chromatin clearing, and the development of prominent macronucleoli, which are often multiple[9,21,46] (Fig. 7-18).

The villoglandular variant of endocervical adenocarcinoma, in addition to the malignant features noted earlier for typical endocervical adenocarcinoma, may show some degree of papillary grouping of cells in the cytologic pattern (Fig. 7-19). Such changes may give a more three-dimensional appearance to the tumor, which may make it somewhat difficult to distinguish from poorly differentiated endometrial adenocarcinoma. Generally, the large size of the cancer cells and the numerous cell groupings allows for a distinction between lesions of endometrial and endocervical origin. Because the villoglandular

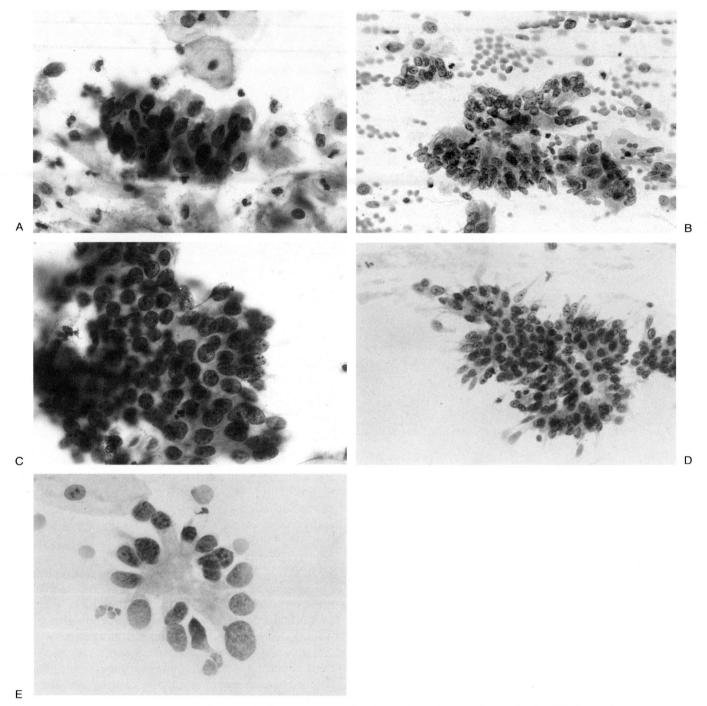

FIG. 7-17. Examples of the cytologic appearance of endocervical adenocarcinoma in situ. (**A**) shows the architectural pattern of pseudostratified strips of endocervical cells with loss of normal mucous production. (**B**) shows larger groups of pseudostratified cells with many smaller groups and isolated cells in the vicinity, indicative of decreased cellular cohesion. Note the clean background of the slide with no evidence of tumor diathesis in this noninvasive lesion. (**C**) shows a dense group of cells maintaining an architectural pattern highly reminiscent of the honeycombing of normal endocervical cell groups. However, nuclei are enlarged, hyperchromatic, and have a distinctly abnormal coarse chromatin pattern. Micronucleoli are present in many of the cell nuclei. (**D**) illustrates the prominent nuclear protrusion that can be seen at the margins of the groups of endocervical adenocarcinoma in situ. This phenomenon has been termed nuclear "feathering." (**E**) shows a glandular arrangement that has been markedly accentuated in this case by air-drying in the smear. Such features are termed "rosettes," and are commonly seen in cases of endocervical adenocarcinoma in situ (Papanicolaou stain).

TABLE 7-3. *Cytologic differential features between endocervical and endometrial carcinoma in cervical smears*

Feature	Endocervical	Endometrial
Cellularity	+++	+
Diathesis	Tumor	Watery
Cellular and nuclear size	Larger	Smaller
Cytoplasm	Amphophilic	Cyanophilic
Cytoplasm amount	+++	+
Nucleoli	+++	+
Multiple nucleoli	++	+
Cell configuration	Columnar	Round-oval
Group arrangement	Two-dimensional	Three-dimensional

+ = low/small; ++ = moderate; +++ = high/large.

variant is an invasive adenocarcinoma, a necrotic tumor diathesis is generally noted in the slide background.

In distinguishing poorly differentiated endocervical lesions from squamous carcinoma, nuclear features may be most helpful. Typically, squamous cancer nuclei have a more dense or opaque chromatin pattern, with no discernible macronucleoli. One of the more difficult tasks in evaluating glandular malignancies in cervical smears is differentiating between endocervical and endometrial adenocarcinomas. Further discussion of this differential diagnostic problem is presented after the section on the cytology of endometrial neoplasia.

THE PROBLEM OF ENDOCERVICAL ATYPIA

To this point, the discussion has involved the ends of the spectrum of endocervical cytology that are well studied and accepted, and for which morphologic criteria for diagnosis are well established. The cytologist should be able to render an accurate assessment at both ends of this continuum in the presence of the described cytologic features. The remainder of this review deals with those areas of endocervical cytology in which precise diagnoses are not yet routine or, in some cases, are not yet possible.

The use of the newer sampling devices mentioned previously has greatly improved the yield of endocervical cells present on cervical cytology specimens. These devices have also provided access to areas of the endocervical canal that subsequently have been found to show patterns and lesions with which cytologic observers may not yet be fully familiar. When compared with the traditional cervical swab specimens, the use of these new devices has been successful, in that the rate of unsatisfactory specimens attributable to lack of evidence of transformation zone sampling has diminished substantially.[1–7] With this increase in quantitative and topographic endocervical cellular sampling has come a broader presentation of the cytomorphologic appearance of the variety of normal endocervical cells, particularly endocervical cells derived from conditions in which the epithelium has been stimulated by traumatic or in-

flammatory processes, or in which the earliest manifestations of intraepithelial neoplasia (dysplasia) are occurring. Such samples can be very difficult to interpret, and may occasionally prompt overinterpretation or underinterpretation, even by the most experienced of observers. A wide variety of conditions may lead to a diagnosis of "atypical endocervical cells of undetermined significance," and many of the most common of these potential circumstances are listed in Table 7-4.

In some cases, merely the presence of abundant normal endocervical cells may prompt concern that an endocervical abnormality exists. This circumstance is often the case when an observer is new to the abundant endocervical sampling that may take place with the new canal-sampling devices. In such cases, the samples are very cellular, with numerous groups of endocervical cells present, along with large numbers of single, but normal, endocervical cells. Because the endocervical epithelium has been abundantly sampled by the bristles or cutting edges of the sampling device, groups are thick, with piled-up layers of overlapping cells, making the aggregates appear as if the cellular density is higher than would be expected. Such arrangements can give a false impression of an elevated nuclear-to-cytoplasmic ratio of the individual cells, loss of the normal honeycomb or columnar architectural pattern, and nuclear hyperchromasia (Fig. 7-20). In addition, the mild anisonucleosis that can be present in completely normal endocervical cells (see Fig. 7-8) may provide additional cause for concern in these large groups of densely packed endocervical cells. When such features are present in samples obtained with the canal-sampling instruments, the observer should look for additional specific features of endocervical neoplasia, as described earlier. The composite of the architectural and cellular features of diagnosable endocervical neoplasia is rarely seen in nonneoplastic conditions, even though the individual cytologic features seen in endocervical neoplasia occasionally may be present in such examples. Important differential diagnostic features to consider in nonneoplastic conditions are nuclear size and chromatin pattern, both of which are similar to those seen in normal endocervical cells. Examples of clearly normal cells on the same slide should be sought for comparison with the "atypical" cells in question.

A wide variety of benign reactive processes can involve the epithelium of the endocervical canal. Reparative changes in endocervical cells (Fig. 7-21) have distinctive cytologic features. Cells remain cohesive and, hence, are found in cell groupings, with isolated cells being present only at the edges of groupings of similar cells. The groups have a typical appearance that also suggests normal cohesion in that strands of cytoplasm from each cell remain attached to portions of neighboring cells despite the high shearing forces that are applied in the making of the smear. We have termed this feature *cells hanging on for dear life.* Individual cells generally show retention of a

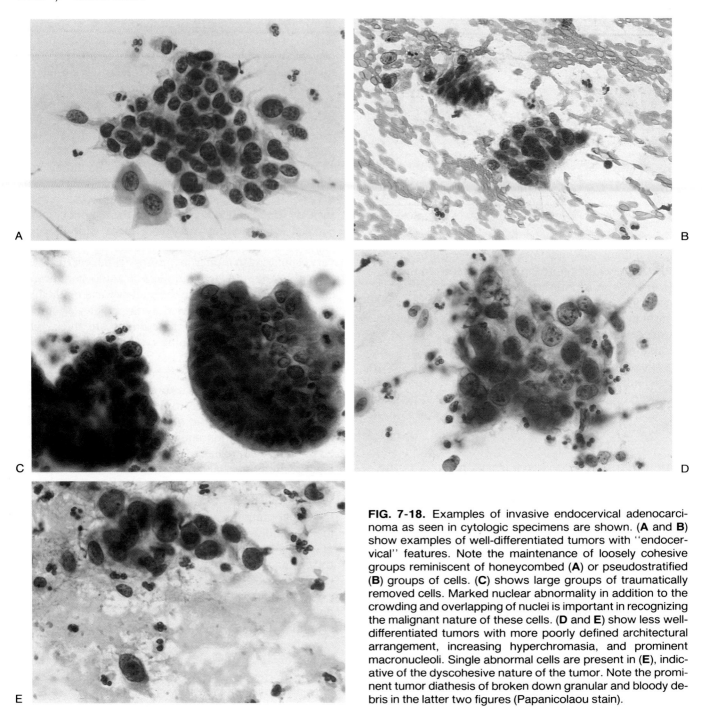

FIG. 7-18. Examples of invasive endocervical adenocarcinoma as seen in cytologic specimens are shown. (**A** and **B**) show examples of well-differentiated tumors with "endocervical" features. Note the maintenance of loosely cohesive groups reminiscent of honeycombed (**A**) or pseudostratified (**B**) groups of cells. (**C**) shows large groups of traumatically removed cells. Marked nuclear abnormality in addition to the crowding and overlapping of nuclei is important in recognizing the malignant nature of these cells. (**D** and **E**) show less well-differentiated tumors with more poorly defined architectural arrangement, increasing hyperchromasia, and prominent macronucleoli. Single abnormal cells are present in (**E**), indicative of the dyscohesive nature of the tumor. Note the prominent tumor diathesis of broken down granular and bloody debris in the latter two figures (Papanicolaou stain).

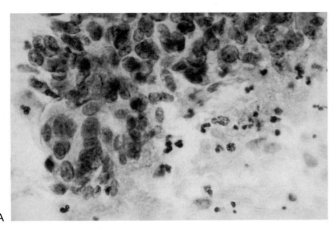
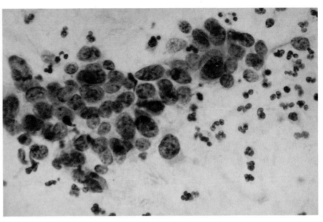

A

B

FIG. 7-19. Examples of villoglandular endocervical adenocarcinoma are illustrated. **(A)** shows a predominantly two-dimensional grouping of cells with a portion of the group (lower left) showing more three-dimensional (ball-like) configuration. **(B)** shows an arrangement more reminiscent of typical endocervical adenocarcinoma with honeycombed configuration, nuclear enlargement, and prominent macronucleoli (Papanicolaou stain).

normal to slightly increased nuclear-to-cytoplasmic ratio and slight nuclear enlargement, but without significant pleomorphism of size and shape. Prominent macronucleoli are present in most cells, but the chromatin remains generally finely granular and evenly dispersed.[47]

The presence of an intrauterine device causes significant changes in the endocervical mucosa, most likely secondary to irritation from the string that extends from the uterine fundus to the external os. The type of cells most commonly seen in association with an intrauterine device effect appear to be derived from the upper portions of the endocervical canal because of their strong resemblance to the cells of this area and to the cells of the lower uterine segment. These cells appear to be spontaneously exfoliated, because they are arranged most commonly in three-dimensional clusters. They have prominent cytoplasmic vacuolization, which may be secondary to degenerative phenomena. Their nuclei are small, with bland chromatin and little pleomorphism of size and shape[48] (Fig. 7-22).

Trauma from conization[49] and radiation[50] have been reported to produce reactive changes in endocervical

TABLE 7-4. *Nonneoplastic causes of endocervical glandular "atypia"*

Abundant normal endocervical cells in groups—"brush artifact"
Reparative or inflammatory processes
  After cone biopsy or other trauma
  Intrauterine device
  Chronic follicular cervicitis (*Chlamydia*)
  Radiation
Tubal metaplasia (ciliated cell metaplasia)
Endometrial cells from lower uterine segment or endometriosis of cervix
Colonic cells in rectovaginal fistula
Microglandular hyperplasia of the endocervical mucosa

cells that may also be difficult to differentiate from a neoplastic endocervical process. Endocervical cells, when reactive, may also be multinucleate. This appearance may lead to an erroneous diagnosis of herpetic infection.[51] The presence of endometrial cells sampled from the lower uterine segment or from areas of endometriosis in the endocervical canal is another potential pitfall in the differential diagnosis of "endocervical atypia." With vigorous use of the endocervical brush, endometrial cells can be traumatically removed from the uterine corpus and deposited on the cervical slide. In this circumstance, the endometrial cells are not spontaneously exfoliated and, hence, do not always take on their characteristic three-dimensional group appearance. This criterion of group conformation is one that cytologists have traditionally utilized to distinguish endometrial cells from their typically two-dimensional groups of neighboring endocervical cells. Hence, erroneous interpretations can be made, based on the tightly packed, but more two-dimensional, groups of densely chromatic cells that may be present on the cervical smear. Particular attention to the size of the endometrial cell nucleus, which is substantially smaller ($35 \mu m^2$) than the endocervical cell nucleus, generally allows for a correct interpretation of normal endometrial cells. In our laboratory, we have seen several cases of rectovaginal fistula in which goblet-type colonic cells presented in the cervical smear, prompting an erroneous diagnosis of atypical endocervical cells. Close attention to the cytologic features of the goblet columnar cells (Fig. 7-23), as well as to the clinical history, allows the observer to avoid an incorrect diagnosis in such cases.

This group of benign endocervical processes may present the observer with significant alterations in the cytologic appearance of endocervical cells. Recognition of the clinical history and the cytologic features in such

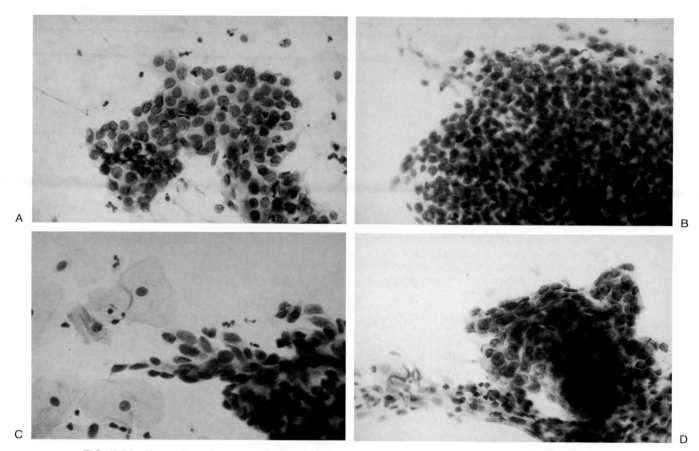

FIG. 7-20. Examples of normal or reactive endocervical cells that may be overinterpreted as derived from a preneoplastic or neoplastic process. **(A)** shows normal endocervical cells in a dense two-dimensional aggregate with minor degrees of nuclear overlap and irregularity. **(B)** shows a dense three-dimensional grouping of normal endocervical cells. Note the small size and regularity of the nuclei at the margins of the group. **(C** and **D)** show examples of normal/reactive endocervical cells that may be more difficult to interpret. Increasing nuclear pleomorphism, hyperchromasia, and possible nuclear feathering are present in these groups. Review of the entire slide in such cases is necessary to determine if the composite of diagnostic features is present in order to make a definitive diagnosis of neoplasia. In these two examples, no such composite of features was present and no positive follow-up was subsequently obtained (Papanicolaou stain).

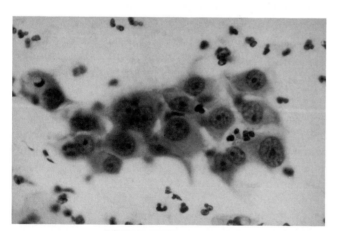

FIG. 7-21. Endocervical repair is shown in this slide. Note the overall cohesive nature of the grouping with the maintenance of tight attachments, as if the cells are "hanging on for dear life." Prominent macronucleoli are present in every cell and the nuclear chromatin pattern is uniform (Papanicolaou stain).

cases is imperative in order to avoid overinterpretation of cells derived from these processes as being neoplastic.

TUBAL METAPLASIA OF THE ENDOCERVICAL CANAL

The most common benign process that can lead to a diagnosis of atypical endocervical cells mimicking an endocervical neoplastic process is benign tubal, or ciliated cell, metaplasia. In this process, cells similar to those that normally line the uterine tubes replace portions of the normal endocervical canal and gland lining. Three cell types are typically seen: the ciliated columnar cell, the nonciliated mucin-producing cell, and the nonsecretory intercalated or "peg" cell (Fig. 7-24). This type of process has been well documented to involve the endometrial tissue, and has been suggested to be stimulated by estrogenic compounds.[52] The process has also been well de-

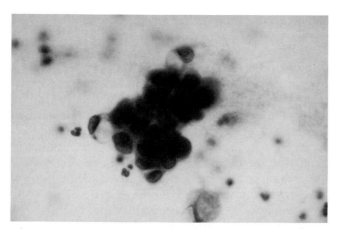

FIG. 7-22. Endocervical cells in the presence of an intrauterine contraceptive device are shown. Note the tight three-dimensional cluster of cells resembling cells derived from the upper reaches of the endocervical canal. These cells often show prominent intracytoplasmic vacuolizations, which are most likely degenerative effects caused by chronic irritation. Due to the cohesive and overlapping nature of these groupings, diagnoses of "atypical" can often be entertained. Such findings ought to prompt requests for additional clinical history regarding the presence of an intrauterine device (Papanicolaou stain).

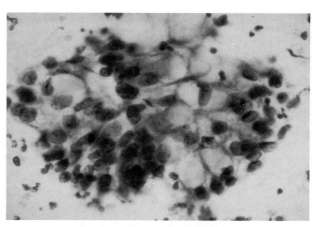

FIG. 7-23. This slide shows cells in a routine cervical smear that are of colonic origin. Follow-up of the patient revealed that she had a rectovaginal fistula. The presence of glandular cell groups showing complete goblet cell differentiation, and the absence of dyscohesion and nuclear atypia should prompt a consideration of normal colonic cells (Papanicolaou stain).

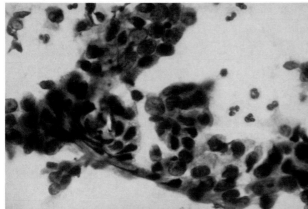

A

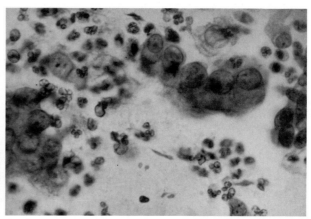

B

C

FIG. 7-24. Examples of tubal (ciliated cell) metaplasia are shown. (**A**) shows a group of endocervical cells with a partial maintenance of the honeycombed architectural pattern. Increasing nuclear overlap and nuclear size and hyperchromasia are noted. In the midportion of the group, cells with prominent cilia and terminal bars are noted. (**B**) shows endocervical nuclei with enlargement and mildly disrupted architecture also exhibiting cilia. (**C**) shows a group of densely packed endocervical cells with goblet cell metaplasia, and slender spindled cells consistent with origin from the intercalated metaplastic cells. When viewed together on the same slide, the three features of ciliated, goblet, and intercalated cells are consistent with the presence of tubal metaplasia (Papanicolaou stain).

scribed in the endocervical canal, where one group found tubal metaplasia in 31% of a retrospective series of cervical cone biopsy samples and hysterectomy specimens.[53] In a prospective series of 25 consecutive hysterectomy specimens removed for noncervical disease in our own laboratory, tubal metaplasia was identified in 100% of cases.[8] Most studies have shown that tubal metaplasia is increasingly more common in women older than 35 years of age. The changes of tubal metaplasia are most commonly seen in the upper portions of the endocervical canal, and can involve the surface epithelium, superficial portions of the endocervical glands, and deep portions of the endocervical glands.[8,53] In the study from our laboratory, the upper reaches of the endocervical canal showed, in addition to classic tubal metaplasia, columnar epithelial cells of both ciliated and nonciliated type, which lost the normal mucus-producing, basilar nuclear appearance and demonstrated increasing levels of pseudostratification, nuclear enlargement, and anisonucleosis. We have termed these changes *glandular crowding* (see Fig. 7-4). Such cellular changes are commonly found at the outlets of the endocervical glands. The new sampling devices undoubtedly obtain cells from areas involved by these normal processes far more commonly than did the previously utilized cervical cotton swab. Such changes, when seen on cytology, have often been termed *brush*

artifact and can mimic the tightly packed cellular groups of endocervical neoplasia.

A number of reports have appeared in the recent past detailing problem cases in which tubal metaplasia was overinterpreted on cytologic examination as endocervical atypia, glandular dysplasia, or endocervical AIS.[54–57] These studies all point to several common features that are useful in differentiating such processes from endocervical neoplasia (Table 7-5). Tubal metaplasia maintains many features that are suggestive of endocervical neoplasia, including the presence of large, crowded groups of cells arranged in two-dimensional sheets; rare architectural changes, including occasional rosettes; and frequent single cells. Nuclei may vary in size, tending to be larger than those of normal, nonneoplastic endocervical cells, and may show some irregularity and mild hyperchromasia.[54,57] In the study from our own laboratory mentioned previously, we examined the cellular changes that were present on high endocervical brushing samples from histologically proven nonneoplastic cervices.[8] Two experienced cytotechnologists were given smears made from lower, middle, and upper portions of the endocervical canal. They were blinded as to which portion of the canal was represented on each slide. The cytotechnologists were instructed to identify and mark endocervical groups they found to be "troublesome" because of their

TABLE 7-5. *Differential diagnostic features distinguishing endocervical adenocarcinoma in situ, adenocarcinoma, and tubal metaplasia*

Feature	Adenocarcinoma in situ	Adenocarcinoma	Tubal metaplasia
Cellularity	Moderate to high	High	Low to high
Crowded sheets	Numerous	Numerous	Few to numerous
Honeycombed sheets	Few	Few	Few to numerous
Feathered edges	Frequent	Frequent	Infrequent and focal
Isolated strips	Few to numerous	Numerous	Absent to few
Rosettes	Few to numerous	Numerous	Rare
Single cells	Few	Few to numerous	Few to numerous
Terminal bars/cilia	Absent	Absent	May be present
Cell shapes	Columnar and cuboidal, uniform in rosettes	Columnar and cuboidal, more variable than adenocarcinoma in situ	Columnar
Cytoplasm	Granular, uniform	Granular or vacuolated	Uniform, dense, cyanophilic
Nuclei	Enlarged, crowded	Enlarged, crowded	Enlarged, may be crowded
Shape	Variable, elongated	Less elongation than adenocarcinoma in situ	Oval and broad
Arrangement	Stratified, palisading	Stratified, palisading	Evenly spaced, polarized to base
Anisonucleosis	Moderate	Moderate to marked	Slight to moderate
Chromatin	Moderate to coarse, dense, even	Moderate to coarse, uneven	Fine to moderate, even, less dense than adenocarcinoma in situ
Nucleoli	Inconspicuous, micronucleoli	Macronucleoli	Inconspicuous, micronucleoli
Mitoses	Few to numerous	Numerous	Rare
Background	Clean	Diathesis	Clean

Adapted from Novotny DB, Maygarden SJ, Johnson DE, et al. Tubal metaplasia of the uterine cervix: a prevalence study in patients with gynecologic pathology findings. Int J Gynecol Pathol 1992;11:89.

TABLE 7-6. *Cytologic features of the normal endocervical canal*

Cytologic finding	A (lower)	B (middle)	C (upper)
Endocervical cellularity	+	+++	++
"Troublesome" groups	37	50	118

+ = low; ++ = moderate; +++ = high

potential for representing (or mimicking) endocervical neoplasia. Table 7-6 shows a compilation of the findings of the study. It can be clearly noted that as samples were obtained from the higher regions of the endocervical canal, the number of troublesome groups increased. Arrangements that the cytotechnologists identified as challenging in these known benign smears were many of the features characteristic of endocervical neoplasia, including rosettes, crowded groups with nuclear overlap, nuclear feathering, and anisonucleosis with chromatin irregularity. As can be seen by comparing Table 7-6 with the histologic results noted in Table 7-1, this increase in troublesome groups corresponds directly with the increased presence of tubal metaplasia and glandular crowding in the upper reaches of the canal. Therefore, we have postulated that many of the cytologic changes seen in atypical but benign smears are manifestations of the sampling of this region of the endocervical epithelium.

However, in our own experience and that of the previously cited groups, the overall appearance of the smears should generally allow the observer to avoid an overdiagnosis. In cases of tubal metaplasia, cellular groups tend to show cohesion, with regular nuclear spacing and preservation of normal columnar configuration. Cases containing only tubal metaplasia show a relative lack of the full range of the typical architectural features of AIS. Strips of pseudostratified cells, well-developed rosettes, and nuclear protrusion at group margins (nuclear feathering) can be seen as individual features in some cases, but the composite of all these cytologic changes is rare in tubal metaplasia. Metaplastic endocervical nuclei can be enlarged, but the nuclei of AIS are consistently enlarged above 75 μm^2 and, more importantly, have a highly distinctive, evenly distributed but coarsely granular chromatin pattern with hyperchromasia (see Fig. 7-17). This chromatin pattern would be very unusual in cases of benign metaplastic endocervical epithelium, which typically have a bland chromatin pattern that is finely granular and evenly distributed, sometimes appearing washed-out. In addition, we have observed that cases of tubal metaplasia often show groups containing several markedly enlarged individual nuclei that are out of proportion to the other uniformly smaller nuclei in the group (Fig. 7-25). In summary, cases of typical tubal metaplasia may occasionally show individual features seen in AIS, but rarely show a composite of the architectural and nuclear features of AIS. Overall, these cytologic characteristics make the correct diagnosis of benign metaplasia less difficult if the cases are studied carefully.

Most cases of tubal metaplasia show ciliated cells; however, cilia are often fragile structures and can be partially or completely lost during the sampling, preparation, and fixation process. Often, only the presence of prominent eosinophilic terminal bars, or the cytoplasmic granular eosinophilic remnants of the terminal bars, may be present. Therefore, the lack of ciliated cells should not deter the cytologist from entertaining a diagnosis of tubal metaplasia when the overall features of the case do not indicate a definitive diagnosis of endocervical neoplasia.

It is also imperative that the cytologist remember that neoplastic processes can often coexist in smears with the more ubiquitous tubal metaplasia. Novotny and associates found that ciliated cell metaplasia was present in association with squamous dysplasia in nearly 40% of the

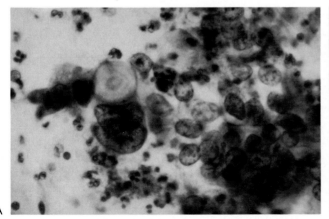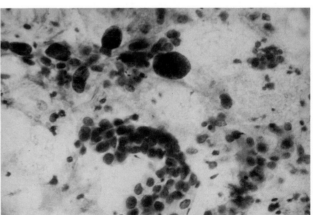

FIG. 7-25. Examples of tubal metaplasia in which anisonucleosis was a particularly prominent feature are shown. The presence of nuclei that appear to be outside the normal continuum of size for the remainder of endocervical cells on the slide are commonly seen in cases of tubal metaplasia. **(A)** The goblet cell is the cell that is affected. **(B)** Several gigantic stripped nuclei are noted above the group of relatively normal endocervical cells (Papanicolaou stain).

cases in their series.[54] Its presence in 100% of cases in our "normal" study would argue that such changes would also be suspected to be present on cervical smears in many cases with definitive pathology. The observer should always keep in mind that the presence of unequivocal "normal" ciliated cell metaplasia on a cervical smear does not preclude a careful examination for associated disease.

In our laboratory, we have recently observed several very difficult cytologic smears from women who were typically in their late 30s and early 40s and had no prior history of cervical disease. Endocervical broom specimens presented with groups of crowded cells showing marked crowding and nuclear overlap, nuclear hyperchromasia, marked anisonucleosis, and mitotic figures. However, none of the classic architectural features of endocervical neoplastic disease were well developed in these cases. After a careful search, some of the "abnormal" groups showed cells with terminal bars or cilia (Fig. 7-26). Because of the atypical cytologic features in these cases, a concurrent dysplastic process could not be excluded and the patients were referred for further evaluation. In each case, the biopsy showed tubal metaplasia in the endocervical canal epithelium. However, the epithelium showed marked pseudostratification with significant nuclear enlargement, hyperchromasia, and anisonucleosis (Fig. 7-27). The significance of these findings is unknown, but such cases have raised concern that these changes may be manifestations of a form of ciliated "endocervical dysplasia," as was suggested in one case in the study by Novotny and associates.[54] It is well known that ciliated cells can exist in malignancies arising in other areas of the female genital tract, such as in well-differentiated cases of papillary serous carcinoma of the ovary. Further study of cases such as these to determine their HPV nucleic acid status and clinical follow-up is needed to understand fully the significance of these described cellular changes.

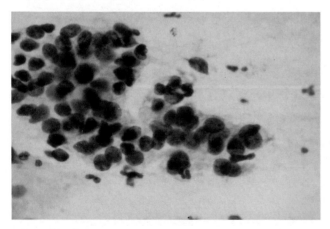

FIG. 7-26. Example of case called "atypical endocervical cells" in which cilia were identified in this abnormal group. Follow-up biopsy specimen slide is shown in figure 7-27 (Papanicolaou stain).

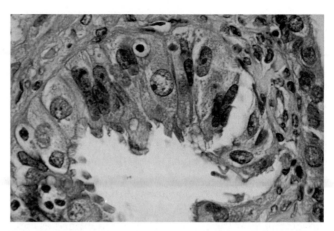

FIG. 7-27. Specimen from cervical biopsy performed in follow-up of cells depicted in figure 7-26 is shown. The biopsy specimen showed tubal metaplasia with cilia and marked anisonucleosis. The significance of these findings is unknown; however, some authors have suggested that such cases may represent a form of ciliated endocervical dysplasia[54] (hematoxylin and eosin).

ENDOCERVICAL GLANDULAR DYSPLASIA

The transformation from normal to malignant in most epithelia progresses through a series of morphologic stages in which there is a proportionately increased risk for the subsequent development of invasive cancer. This transformation has been clearly documented in squamous lesions of the cervix, with excellent studies showing the relative risk of progression or association of malignancy with the various precursor stages.[58] The concept of advancing degrees of dysplasia prior to the full development of in situ carcinoma has also been postulated for the endocervical epithelium. This hypothesis regarding endocervical glandular dysplasia has not yet been well studied in terms of criteria for diagnosis, natural history of the disease, and relative risk of subsequent development of AIS and invasive cancer.

Evidence to support the concept of endocervical preinvasive neoplasia (dysplasia) exists. Bousfield and colleagues, in a large series of cases of this putative endocervical neoplastic spectrum, showed a definitive age progression with increasing lesion severity similar to that noted for squamous lesions[39] (Table 7-7). Lesions described as endocervical glandular dysplasia have been reported to be found in association with classic lesions of AIS and invasive endocervical adenocarcinoma. This concept is similar to the presence of dysplasia adjacent to defined malignancy in other body sites, including the squamous epithelium of the cervix and the glandular epithelium of Barrett's esophagus.[59] In addition, a small number of studies have shown the presence of HPV nucleic acid in some lesions described as endocervical glandular dysplasia,[28,30,31] in a situation analogous to the

TABLE 7-7. *Mean age for the presentation of the various endocervical lesions*

Lesion	Age (y)	Range (y)
Dysplasia	36	33–38
In situ	37	22–70
Microinvasive	41	28–66
Invasive	49	26–85

presence of HPV in the definitive neoplastic lesions of the endocervix.

Various authors have defined endocervical glandular dysplasia in different ways. Bousfield and colleagues defined it as a lesion that shows a combination of architectural abnormalities of the columnar epithelium of the uterine cervix similar to, but less marked than, those described in AIS.[39] Brown and Wells subdivided endocervical atypia into two classifications: low-grade and high-grade. They described cases of high-grade atypia as those that show nuclear enlargement, with pleomorphism, hyperchromasia, and an increased nuclear-to-cytoplasmic ratio. Occasional mitoses, pseudostratification of nuclei in the lower two thirds of the epithelium, and glandular architectural changes such as irregular budding, tufting, and low papillae were also noted to be present. They described cases of low-grade atypia as those that exhibit fewer changes than in high-grade atypia but are different than the normal epithelium.[60]

Betsill and Clark studied cases across a spectrum of endocervical neoplasia ranging from atypia or dysplasia to invasive carcinoma.[44] They found that in dysplasia, cells demonstrate little variation in the size and shape of nuclei within clusters, with nuclear hyperchromasia, increased chromatin granule size with even distribution, and micronucleoli. In a follow-up morphometric study,[45] they found that dysplastic endocervical cells had a relative nuclear area almost twice as large as that of normal endocervical cells, but less than that of AIS or invasive adenocarcinoma.

Jaworski, in a review article on the subject, comments that because no well-accepted definition of endocervical glandular dysplasia currently exists, all lesions regarded as less than AIS should be placed in this category without subdivision into grades.[21] He points out key morphologic differences between endocervical glandular dysplasia and AIS, which are summarized in Table 7-8. This author supports this definition until adequate studies can be performed to define the natural history of this spectrum and reproducible criteria can be set forth for its diagnosis. In our own practice, on histologic biopsy samples, the following changes are accepted as indicative of endocervical glandular dysplasia. Nuclei are enlarged and variable in size and shape. Mitotic figures and apoptotic bodies are present (indicative of cell turnover), and the epithelium shows some degree of nuclear stratification that does not involve the full thickness. Architectural gland abnormalities, including irregular gland branching, epithelial tufting, and papillae, may be present, but are not necessary for the diagnosis. Examples of histologic changes this author would accept as endocervical glandular dysplasia are illustrated in Figure 7-28. Unfortunately, our ability to diagnose endocervical glandular dysplasia on cytologic specimens is more limited. Reproducible criteria for the diagnosis of endocervical glandular dysplasia, as are now available for the cytologic diagnosis of AIS, are not currently well accepted. There is significant overlap in the cytologic features of normal, reactive, metaplastic, and neoplastic endocervical epithelia. It is our current policy to place all cases of "atypical" endocervical cells that cannot be attributed directly to a normal, reactive, or reparative process, or to AIS, into the category of AGCUS using the Bethesda System guidelines.[61] Further work to define the criteria for a workable classification of endocervical glandular dysplasia is currently under way. Additional studies using markers of neoplastic transformation, HPV infection, or morphometry may be necessary to distinguish biologic disease from morphologic mimickers. With increased

TABLE 7-8. *Differential diagnostic features of endocervical glandular dysplasia and endocervical adenocarcinoma in situ*

Feature	Endocervical glandular dysplasia	Adenocarcinoma in situ
NUCLEAR		
Enlargement	Present	Present (greater)
Chromatin granularity	Fine to moderate	Moderate to coarse
Nucleoli	Inconspicuous	Micronucleoli
Shape	Oval	Oval to irregular
Pseudostratification	Minimal	Moderate to marked
Apoptosis	Present	Present (greater)
Mitoses	Occasional	Frequent
ARCHITECTURAL		
Glandular budding	May be present	May be present
Papillary processes	May be present	May be present
Cribriform glands	Absent	May be present

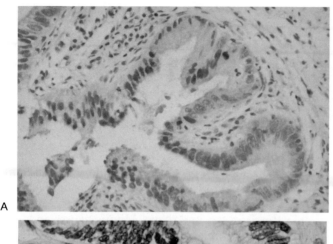

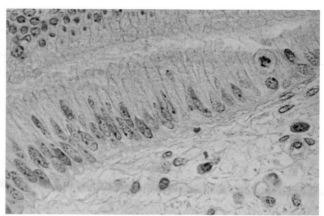

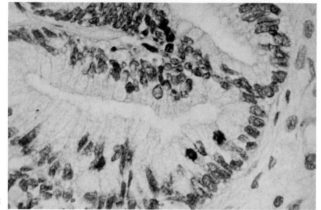

FIG. 7-28. (A, B, C) Examples of potential cases of endocervical dysplasia are shown. In these cases, the biopsy specimens shown were from areas adjacent to definitive endocervical neoplastic lesions. In these examples note the lack of full-thickness nuclear pseudostratification, mild degrees of nuclear enlargement, and the presence of mitotic figures. Changes such as these are not marked enough for a diagnosis of adenocarcinoma in situ and are thus postulated to represent an earlier stage in the neoplastic progression of noninvasive endocervical neoplasia (hematoxylin and eosin). (Figure **B** courtesy of Jagmohan Sidhu, MD, United Health Services, Binghamton, NY.)

awareness and experience in this area, helpful criteria will undoubtedly evolve in the future.

SQUAMOUS NEOPLASIA PRESENTING AS ATYPICAL ENDOCERVICAL CELLS

The use of the new endocervical sampling devices has allowed for an increased ability to sample not only endocervical processes, but also squamous lesions that may be present in the upper reaches of the transformation zone and may extend into the endocervical gland necks and crypts. Cells derived from squamous neoplasia may show different morphologic appearances when sampled from these areas as compared with the classic cytologic features of squamous dysplasia from the lower regions and surfaces of the transformation zone. Squamous lesions involving endocervical glands may show architectural arrangements that resemble those of endocervical cells and groups. They may also acquire some of the nuclear and cytoplasmic features that are more characteristic of cells of glandular origin. Such cellular features

may cause the observer to question the origin of the cells, and potentially to misclassify the abnormal squamous cells as atypical endocervical cells. These patterns are not completely new. In our laboratory, we have for many years utilized the following phrase: *Atypical cells of endocervical origin are present; squamous carcinoma in situ cannot be excluded.* This diagnosis was utilized in instances where many of the cytologic features were indicative of endocervical differentiation but some features suggestive of squamous differentiation were also present. Pacey also noted this differential diagnostic difficulty and has particularly related the phenomenon to endocervical brush specimens.[46] Since the introduction of a variety of endocervical sampling devices into routine clinical practice, this diagnostic problem has dramatically increased.

In such specimens, the cytologist observes large groups of densely packed cells with an endocervical-type architecture. This includes columnar configuration of the cells, with palisading and maintenance of cell polarity and granular, amphophilic cytoplasm (Fig. 7-29). These architectural features are accentuated at the margins of the groups, giving an overall appearance of columnar

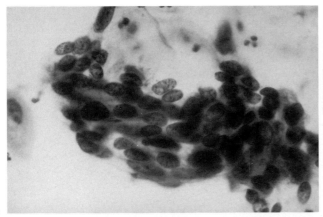

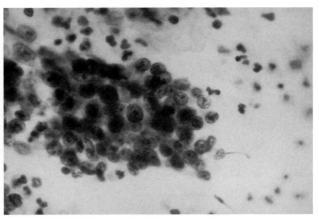

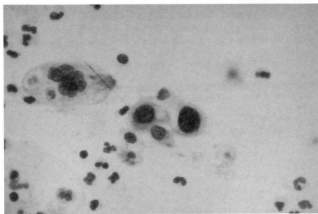

FIG. 7-29. (A) An example of high-grade squamous dysplasia presenting in the cervical smear as "atypical endocervical cells." Note the prominent streaming or palisading of cells in this group, which gives it a columnar, nonsyncytial appearance. An important clue to the proper diagnosis is the presence of markedly hyperchromatic, opaque nuclear features. (B) Another grouping of "glandular" appearing cells that show prominent macronucleoli. Macronucleoli are generally not considered to be a feature of the cells of squamous dysplasia, however, in squamous lesions sampled from endocervical glands, nucleoli may often be found in the cells. (C) Isolated dysplastic cells, which must be searched for diligently in such cases. Their presence will be an important key in correctly identifying the lesion as of squamous origin (Papanicolaou stain).

differentiation. Cell groupings do not have the classic "syncytial" patterns described in squamous carcinoma in situ, in which polarity and visible cell boundaries are lost. In contrast to classic descriptions of squamous dysplasia, these cells may also have very prominent macronucleoli. It is important to review the slide carefully for the presence of isolated cells showing classic features of squamous dysplasia. If such cells are found, it has been this author's experience that there is unlikely to be a glandular lesion present. The presence of occasional cells showing dense, eosinophilic cytoplasm and opaque, hyperchromatic nuclei also aids in the suspicion or definite classification of a squamous lesion. The lack of distinct architectural features characteristic of AIS, such as rosettes, pseudostratified strips of cells, and nuclear feathering, should also guide the observer away from this diagnosis. Follow-up surgical biopsies confirm that the features noted on cytology are also noted on the squamous lesions present in the endocervical glands (Fig.

7-30). Of course, squamous and endocervical lesions may coexist, but as can be seen in the follow-up data presented later, it is far more common for a squamous lesion to represent the ultimate outcome from a case containing atypical endocervical cells that are not specifically diagnostic of AIS.

A number of studies addressing this problem have resulted in conclusions similar to those arrived at in our practice. Covell and Frierson described seven cases of high-grade squamous lesions that were present in endocervical glands sampled by the endocervical brush.[62] They noted cellular changes that they interpreted as suggestive of microinvasion. The cells showed prominent macronucleoli and an irregular chromatin pattern. When these features are associated with palisading cells in some of the groups, a glandular origin may be suggested. Selvaggi studied 25 cases of squamous carcinoma in situ and found two distinctive cytologic patterns that appeared to correlate with endocervical glandular

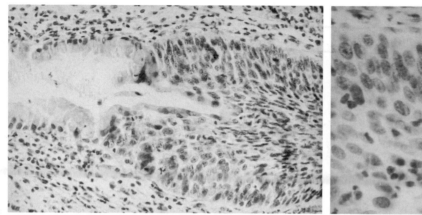
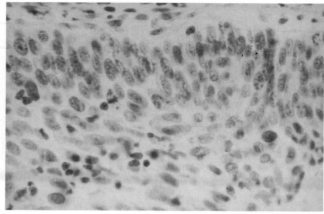

FIG. 7-30. These figures show the findings upon followup of the cells illustrated in figure 7-29. **(A)** High-grade squamous dysplasia was identified in the midportion of the endocervical canal, and extended into the endocervical gland crypts. **(B)** The prominent macronucleoli present in many of the cells, recapitulating the findings in the cytologic sample (hematoxylin and eosin).

involvement.[63] One pattern showed cells in three-dimensional clusters having smooth external cell borders and internal spindle-shaped or whorled arrangements. The other pattern consisted of sheets of columnar cells with peripheral palisading and nuclear pseudostratification. Selvaggi concluded that these features may be erroneously classified as AIS. However, no cases in her study showed histologic evidence of a glandular lesion. It is expected that with increased experience and recognition of this "new" pattern of squamous intraepithelial neoplasia, increased accuracy in diagnosis will ensue.

FOLLOW-UP OF ATYPICAL ENDOCERVICAL CELLS

Several studies have reported the incidence and follow-up of cases diagnosed as showing atypical endocervical cells. A comparison of the results of three of these studies is presented in Table 7-9. Goff and colleagues reported 100 examples of endocervical atypia, which represented 0.46% of the cases in their practice from 1988 and 1989.[64] They utilized a category of "endocervical atypia of indeterminate significance," which they defined as a minor loss of cohesion, overlapping of nuclei in groups, an increased nuclear-to-cytoplasmic ratio, nuclear hyperchromasia, and minor nuclear pleomorphism of size and shape. Thirty-seven patients (37%) had no documented follow-up. Of the 63 patients who had follow-up studies, 20 patients (20%) had benign diagnoses and 2 patients (2%) had endometrial hyperplasia without cytologic atypia. The largest group, with 22 patients (22%), had squamous lesions ranging from mild dysplasia to squamous carcinoma in situ. Only 7 patients (7%) were found to have true neoplastic lesions of the endocervical epithelium (5 patients with AIS and 2 with invasive endocervical adenocarcinoma). In this study,

when squamous atypia was present along with the endocervical changes, data showed that the outcome was never an endocervical lesion. Such cases were more likely to display the lower grades of squamous dysplasia. Neoplastic lesions that were found as the outcome when only glandular atypia was present were more likely to be true endocervical lesions or squamous carcinoma in situ. This finding is in keeping with the previously discussed similarities in the cytologic presentations of the last two entities, particularly when squamous carcinoma in situ involves the endocervical glands.

In another study of 44 cases diagnosed as showing "abnormal endocervical cells of uncertain significance," Bose and colleagues found 9 cases (20%) to represent benign reactive conditions and 35 cases (80%) to represent squamous intraepithelial lesions. No cases in their study were found to have an associated endocervical neoplastic process.[65]

In this author's laboratory, we have recently com-

TABLE 7-9. Three studies on the follow-up of "atypical" endocervical cells

Follow-up	Goff et al.[64]	Bose et al.[65]	Wilbur et al.[66]
No follow-up	37%		15%
Benign	20%	20%	35%
EM HP	2%		
ASCUS			5%
LSIL	8%	37%	11%
HSIL	14%	41%	27%
SCC			3%
EC neoplasia	7%	0%	4%
Total number of cases	100	44	265
Incidence	0.46%	NS	0.15%

EM HP, endometrial hyperplasia; *ASCUS,* atypical squamous cells of undetermined significance; *LSIL,* low-grade squamous intraepithelial lesion; *HSIL,* high-grade squamous intraepithelial lesion; *SCC,* squamous cell carcinoma; *EC,* endocervical.

pleted a review of our own experience with cases diagnosed as showing "atypical endocervical cells."[66] Cases from 1989 through 1991 were studied. Cases in which reparative or reactive atypia was suspected based on cytologic features were excluded. In addition, all cases were excluded in which an outright diagnosis of in situ or invasive endocervical adenocarcinoma was rendered. During this time period, 265 cases were diagnosed, representing 0.15% of the total gynecologic cytology volume. The results are remarkably similar to those of the two studies noted earlier.[64,65] No follow-up was available for 40 patients (15%). Among patients with adequate follow-up, benign results were found in 92 cases (35%). The largest category of abnormal follow-up was squamous lesions. One hundred twenty-two patients (46%) had squamous lesions, ranging from atypical squamous cells of undetermined significance to squamous cell carcinoma. True endocervical neoplasia (AIS or invasive endocervical adenocarcinoma) was seen in only 11 cases (4%).

Three additional studies have recently reported similar findings in series of AGCUS. Squamous lesions were most commonly identified in the follow-up of this diagnosis, with true glandular lesions of the cervix representing only a minor component of the findings.[67–69]

Data from these studies show that both benign and reactive processes, and the various degrees of squamous neoplasia, account for most of the follow-up in cases originally diagnosed as showing atypical endocervical cells. The presence of squamous dysplasia in endocervical glands and the improved sampling of these portions of the lesions clearly account for most of the cases in which the original interpretations were of lesions of endocervical origin. Of interest is the observation that continued study and experience with such cases substantially improves the ability to discriminate between lesions of squamous and endocervical origin. In the series from this author's laboratory, three experienced observers reviewed all 265 cases, blinded to the original diagnosis and the follow-up information. Fifty-four percent of the benign cases and 83% of the squamous lesions were correctly classified upon review. In addition, 64% of the true endocervical neoplastic lesions were diagnosed outright on blinded review as opposed to being termed "atypical." Further experience with these cases, careful documentation and study of follow-up cases, and definition of specific criteria will improve the observer's ability to be more specific in the accurate classification of benign and neoplastic processes occurring in the endocervical canal.

MANAGEMENT OF ENDOCERVICAL NEOPLASIA AND ATYPICAL ENDOCERVICAL CELLS

The entertainment of a diagnosis of atypical endocervical cells on a cervical smear should prompt the cyto-logic observer to run through a mental differential diagnosis of benign reactive processes, squamous neoplasia, and true endocervical dysplasia and carcinoma. The cytologist should make every possible attempt to classify each case correctly in order to avoid unnecessary work-up and significant undue worry to the patient where possible, and to ensure prompt and definitive treatment where indicated. It must be emphasized that well-prepared cell studies with excellent cell preservation, fixation, and staining are imperative in order to recognize many of the cytologic features discussed earlier and to make the fine distinctions between the various benign, reactive, and neoplastic categories encountered.

The current recommendations utilized in this author's laboratory for the management of a case suspected of showing an endocervical abnormality are outlined in Table 7-10. For a case in which an identifiable and completely benign process is suspected, no specific recommendation is made except for routine cytologic screening. For a case suspected of having an inflammatory or reparative etiology, repeated cytologic evaluation at slightly decreased follow-up intervals (6 to 12 months) is recommended because of the slight increase in the rate of subsequent lesion identification in the presence of presumed repair. In a case of atypical endocervical cells whose significance cannot be explained as benign, reactive, or definitively neoplastic (the AGCUS category), a short-term repeated cytologic examination (3 months) is recommended, with a colposcopic examination accompanied by endocervical curettage or cone biopsy if the abnormal cells are found to persist. In a case that is suspicious for endocervical neoplasia, immediate colposcopy is warranted, with either endocervical curettage or cone biopsy at the discretion of the clinician. An argument can be made for immediate performance of a cone biopsy, because the taking of an initial endocervical curettage may significantly disrupt the endocervical mucosa, making a definitive diagnosis difficult on subsequent procedures. If a lesion cannot be identified on the initial diagnostic biopsies, and these procedures are felt to have yielded adequate representations of the endocer-

TABLE 7-10. *Management of "atypical" endocervical cells*

Atypical endocervical cells of probable reparative or inflammatory origin
    Repeat cytologic examination in 6–12 mo.
Atypical endocervical cells of undetermined significance (AGUS)
    Repeat cytologic examination in 3 months with colposocopy and endocervical curettage for persistence.
Atypical endocervical cells suspicious for endocervical neoplasia
    Colposcopic examination with endocervical curettage. If a lesion is not identified, cytologic slides are rereviewed. If suspicion of neoplasia is confirmed, cone biopsy is recommended for definitive assessment.

vical canal, the cytologic sample is rereviewed. If a benign process in the biopsy specimen can be correlated with the cytologic changes, then further follow-up cytologic screening is recommended. If the cytologic changes cannot be explained on the basis of the biopsy material, then further action must be initiated by the clinician, the nature of which depends on the circumstances in each individual case.

These recommendations for follow-up must be individually tailored to the clinical circumstances, and may be modified by interaction between the cytologist and the clinician, with a full view of the particular needs of each patient.

ENDOMETRIAL NEOPLASIA

General Concepts

As a result of the success of cervical screening programs in diminishing the rate of cervical cancer and the increased use of unopposed estrogen therapy in an aging population, endometrial cancer has surpassed cervical cancer as the most common malignant tumor of the female genital tract in the United States. The cervical smear examination is far less sensitive for the detection of endometrial neoplasia than for the detection of lesions of cervical origin. In addition, abnormal endometrial cells, when present, are more difficult to detect than their cervical counterparts because of their relatively small size and the subtlety of the cytologic changes that typify an abnormal condition, particularly in the preinvasive stages of disease. Although many strategies and devices for directly sampling the endometrium have been proposed and have shown higher rates of lesion detection, no effective screening program is currently available for the detection of endometrial cancer and its precursor lesions. High costs and the inherent difficulties in the cytologic interpretation of such specimens have been the major roadblocks to date.

The great bulk of endometrial cancer arises in postmenopausal women. In addition to the increased risk attributed to estrogen use, other risk factors include obesity, hypertension, diabetes, nulliparity, and high socioeconomic status. The association with estrogen use is further strengthened by studies demonstrating a subsequent drop in endometrial cancer rates coinciding with a decrease in the amount of estrogen sales in this country.[70] In addition, women diagnosed with tumors of other sites that are known to produce estrogenic substances, such as granulosa cell tumors of the ovary, are at higher risk for the development of endometrial neoplasia.

Cytologic Detection

Because standard cervical cytologic techniques do not directly sample the endometrial cavity, the cytologist must rely on spontaneously exfoliated endometrial cells, related cells, and smear patterns for evaluation of endometrial pathology. Endometrial cells travel down the endocervical canal, where they may be picked up on the sampling device. Unfortunately, reliance on spontaneously exfoliated cells often means that the cellular sample available in cases of endometrial pathology is scant and poorly preserved. In addition, endometrial cells and groups take on configurations reminiscent of fluid suspensions rather than traumatically removed samples. This situation leads to a marked discordance between cytologic and histologic morphology.

In the correct clinical context, normal-appearing endometrial cells, or cells with only minimal cytologic changes, may be clinically significant (see later). Therefore, an adequate clinical history (including age, menopausal status, hormonal therapy, and the presence of clinical symptoms such as postmenopausal bleeding) must be obtained for accurate interpretation of smears that are suspicious for endometrial pathology.

HISTOLOGY OF THE NORMAL ENDOMETRIUM

The lining of the uterine fundus is composed of endometrial epithelial cell groupings that are surrounded by endometrial stromal cells. The appearance of the normal endometrium is dependent on a number of factors, including the age and menstrual status of the patient and the hormonal environment on the day the sample was taken. In a patient with a normal cycle, the endometrial lining is at minimal thickness during the early proliferative phase, which follows active menstrual shedding. Throughout the proliferative phase, the main task of the endometrial glands and stroma is to increase parenchymal bulk through active cellular replication. The typical proliferative endometrium shows epithelial cells arranged in simple columnar pseudostratified glands. As the proliferative phase progresses, the glands become larger and more elongated, and glandular mitoses increase (Fig. 7-31). The endometrial stromal cells also participate in the proliferative process, becoming plumper and showing numerous mitotic figures.

At the time of normal ovulation, the endometrial lining is approaching maximal thickness, which is reached during the early to middle secretory phase. At this point, the normal function of the endometrial glands and stroma changes from that of increasing cell number to providing a lining that is receptive to the fertilized ovum. In this regard, the epithelial component reverts to a simple non-pseudostratified columnar epithelium that demonstrates vacuolization, followed by the apical secretion of mucus (Figs. 7-32 and 7-33). In the late phases of the secretory process, the glands become markedly crowded and tortuous in configuration, with a prominent serrated appearance (Fig. 7-34), prior to undergoing sloughing

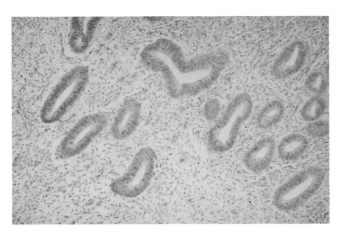

FIG. 7-31. Normal proliferative endometrium is shown. Note the regularity of the glands, and the pseudostratified configuration of this simple epithelium (hematoxylin and eosin).

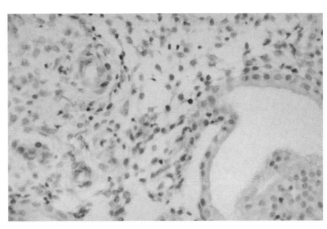

FIG. 7-34. Normal secretory endometrium at day 24 (postovulatory day 10) is shown. The glands have become dormant with no evidence of secretion and a simple low columnar to cuboidal appearance. The stroma has begun the process of pseudodecidualization (hematoxylin and eosin).

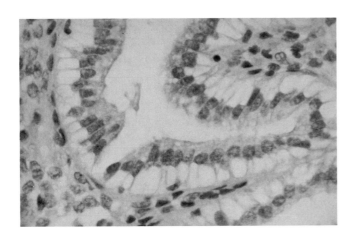

FIG. 7-32. Normal secretory endometrium at day 17 (postovulatory day 3) is shown. Note the prominent subnuclear vacuoles and the change from a pseudostratified to a simple unstratified epithelium (hematoxylin and eosin).

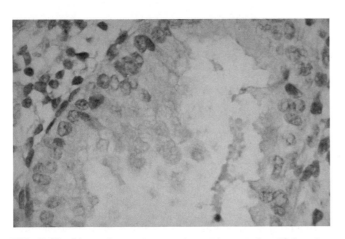

FIG. 7-33. Normal secretory endometrium at day 19 (postovulatory day 5) is shown. Note the prominence of apical secretion within the glands (hematoxylin and eosin).

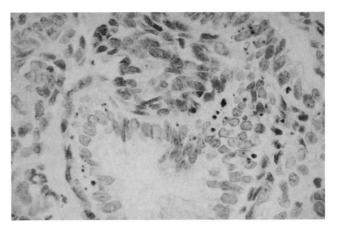

FIG. 7-35. Normal menstrual endometrium is shown. Note the prominent enlargement and reactive atypia present in the endometrial glandular cells. These types of changes can make endometrial cells appear atypical in menstrual smears. The endometrial stroma is also undergoing dissolution during this phase. Stromal cells may be prominently displayed as cohesive groups of small hyperchromatic cells in the cervical smear during menses, making their recognition very important in the differential diagnosis of glandular lesions (hematoxylin and eosin).

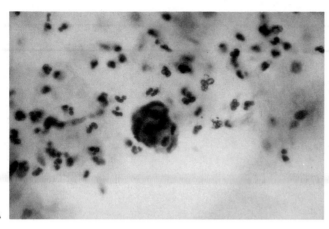
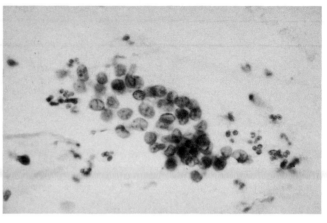

A   B

FIG. 7-36. Two examples of normal endometrial cells are shown. **(A)** shows a three-dimensional cluster of cells with a high nucleus to cytoplasmic ratio, and a scant amount of cytoplasm. **(B)** shows a more two-dimensional arrangement of endometrial epithelial cells, which has more likely been directly sampled. Note the scant amount of cytoplasm, the uniformity of the nuclei, and the presence of small chromocenters (Papanicolaou stain).

during the menstrual phase (Fig. 7-35). During the secretory phase, the endometrial stroma also undergoes characteristic changes consisting of prominent edema, followed by a pseudodecidual reaction, infiltration by inflammatory cells, and, finally, dissolution during the menstrual phase.

CYTOLOGY OF THE NORMAL ENDOMETRIUM

Spontaneously exfoliated endometrial cells show a morphology reminiscent of cells that have been suspended in a fluid medium. As described in the histology section, the endometrial lining is a simple columnar epithelium. When directly sampled, it shows cytologic features that recapitulate this morphology, consisting of individual columnar cells and two-dimensional groupings. Exfoliated endometrial cells, which travel down the endocervical canal within the endocervical mucus, appear as they do in fluid suspensions, with rounding up of individual cells and three-dimensional clusters as cell groupings. Normal endometrial cells are small, only slightly larger than mature lymphocytes or segmented neutrophils. Isolated cells show a generally round to oval configuration. The cytoplasm is scant, poorly defined, and sometimes vacuolated or finely granular, and generally has a cyanophilous staining reaction. The nuclei measure 35 to 40 μm^2 in area (similar to intermediate squamous cell nuclei). The nuclei are round to oval and often eccentrically placed within the cytoplasm. The chromatin is finely granular and evenly distributed, and small chromocenters are present (Fig. 7-36). Because of frequent degeneration in cervical specimens, endometrial cells occasionally have opaque, contracted, and pyknotic nuclei. When present as groupings, endometrial cells typically form densely packed three-dimensional

clusters, contrasting with the more two-dimensional groupings noted for endocervical cells. Endometrial cytoplasm within the groups is typically arranged in a round to oval configuration and is densely cyanophilic, with subtle granularity.

Endometrial stromal cells may also be exfoliated and can appear in cervical smear preparations. They are often difficult to distinguish from endometrial glandular cells, but are generally larger with more pleomorphic or reniform nuclei, and may resemble small histiocytes. Such cells may appear spindle-shaped, with more abundant granular cyanophilic cytoplasm. They are generally isolated, but often appear in loosely cohesive groupings

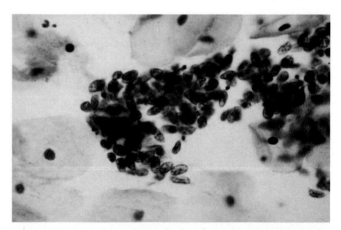

FIG. 7-37. An example of endometrial stroma cells is shown. These cells are commonly seen on smears taken during the menstrual period. Although these cells are of mesenchymal origin, they often appear as cohesive groups of cells with prominent ovoid to spindled configuration. They typically have more abundant granular cyanophilic cytoplasm when compared with endometrial epithelial cells. Because of their more two-dimensional configuration, endometrial stromal cells may also enter into the differential diagnosis of "atypical endocervical cells" (Papanicolaou stain).

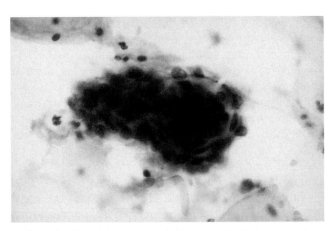

FIG. 7-38. This figure shows a characteristic pattern of endometrial epithelial and stromal cells in the typical "exodus" pattern seen between days 6 and 10 of the menstrual cycle. In this arrangement, endometrial epithelial cells are present on the periphery of the group, whereas the central area is composed of degenerating endometrial stroma. (Papanicolaou stain).

(Fig. 7-37). Stromal cells are commonly noted in the menstrual smear and also can be seen in the day 6 to 10 smear, where they exhibit the so-called *exodus* pattern of three-dimensional stromal balls surrounded by endometrial glandular cells (Fig. 7-38).

Endometrial cells of both types are normally present in cyclic women during the proliferative phase of the menstrual cycle. During the menstrual period (days 1 to 5), endometrial cells are abundant and may show significant reactive atypia (enlargement, nuclear pleomorphism of size and shape), which is secondary to degeneration. Such changes should not be interpreted as indicative of a neoplastic process, making the date of the last menstrual period and the patient's menopausal status imperative portions of the clinical information when evaluating endometrial cells in a cervical smear.

ENDOMETRIAL HYPERPLASIA AND CARCINOMA

General Features

Cytologically, as one progresses through the spectrum of endometrial neoplasia, several general features hold true. With increasing severity of the lesion, the number of cells spontaneously exfoliated increases. The cells become larger, as do the nuclei. Nuclear chromatin shows an increasingly more "malignant" pattern, with irregular distribution and more coarse granulation. The percentage of cells showing first micronucleoli and then macronucleoli increases. The dividing line between hyperplasia and carcinoma is cytologically difficult to discern; however, the presence of nuclei measuring 60 μm^2 or greater, micronucleoli in more than 70% of the abnormal cells, and a change from even to irregularly distributed chro-

matin would appear to represent a useful cytologic dividing line.[71] As the grade of the endometrial carcinoma increases, the diagnosis of malignancy becomes less difficult because cells acquire clearly abnormal features, including macronucleoli with irregularity, very large nuclei, a high nuclear-to-cytoplasmic ratio, and marked chromatin irregularity. The presence of single abnormal cells in addition to three-dimensional clusters, indicating decreased cohesion, is also a useful differential diagnostic feature.

Histopathology

Endometrial hyperplasia is a condition wherein there is an increase in the amount of endometrial tissue due to an abnormal proliferation of endometrial glands and stroma. Hyperplasia develops in situations where there is relative hyperestrogenism or unopposed estrogen effect. The process is considered to be a precursor lesion to endometrial adenocarcinoma, particularly in its more severe forms.

Endometrial hyperplasia is classified into three histologic types: simple, complex (adenomatous), and atypical. Although in the past, some authors have recognized endometrial carcinoma in situ as a separate entity, at the present time, most pathologists do not distinguish between atypical hyperplasia and carcinoma in situ.

The histologic types of endometrial hyperplasia are distinguished from each other by the degree of complexity of the glandular proliferation and the presence or absence of cellular (nuclear) atypia. Simple hyperplasia is characterized by an excess of relatively simple glands, many of which may be cystically dilated (Fig. 7-39). Complex hyperplasia consists of endometrial glands that typically demonstrate increased density and complex

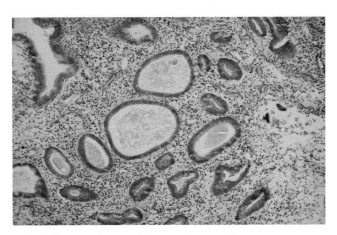

FIG. 7-39. An example of endometrium from a postmenopausal woman involved by simple hyperplasia is shown in this slide. Note the increased glands to stroma ratio, with only round to oval glands being present. The epithelium is pseudostratified, with mitotic activity, but shows no evidence of cytologic atypia (hematoxylin and eosin).

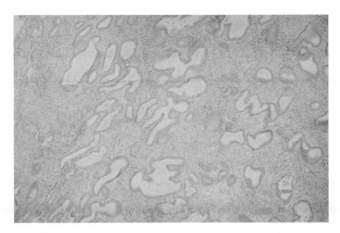

FIG. 7-40. An example of complex hyperplasia is shown. The epithelial lining is similar to that described for simple hyperplasia, however, the glandular configurations have become more complex with irregular outpouchings and configurations. As in simple hyperplasia, no cytologic atypia is present within the epithelial cells (hematoxylin and eosin).

outpouchings and infoldings produced by the excessive proliferation of the epithelium (Fig. 7-40). Atypical hyperplasia is characterized by atypical cytologic features, including enlarged nuclei that tend to be rounded rather than oval, epithelial stratification, the presence of conspicuous nucleoli, and an increased mitotic rate (Fig. 7-41). Atypia may be associated with either a simple or complex glandular pattern, but is more common with the latter.

The variants of endometrial hyperplasia differ considerably in their apparent rates of progression to adenocarcinoma. Simple hyperplasia, according to most studies, has a progression rate to adenocarcinoma of less than 5%. Complex hyperplasia has been shown to progress to adenocarcinoma in 25% of cases or less, and atypical hyperplasia in 50% of cases or more.[72-74] However, in a more recent study, Kurman and associates report much lower progression rates.[75] In this study, the progression rates from simple and complex hyperplasia to adenocarcinoma were 1% and 3%, respectively, and the progression rate from atypical hyperplasia to adenocarcinoma was 23%. Most cases of progression were found in the group in which atypical changes were observed together with the complex architectural pattern. It is apparent from these studies that the degree of cytologic atypia that is present in association with the architectural hyperplastic pattern plays a pivotal role in determining the relative risk of progression for each patient.

Cytopathology

The cytologic detection of endometrial hyperplasia is difficult and cannot be accomplished with the degree of accuracy with which abnormalities of the epithelium of the cervix can be detected. As mentioned previously, cytologic detection is dependent on the identification of spontaneously exfoliated endometrial cells, which, unfortunately, are not shed in any regular pattern from endometrial lesions. In addition, the cytologic changes associated with hyperplasia are much more subtle than those associated with the precursors of cervical carcinoma. Procedures that produce direct endometrial samples have been more successful than routine cytologic techniques in the detection of hyperplasia, but are generally not applicable to routine screening programs because of the complexity of their performance and interpretation, and their high cost.

The degree of cytologic abnormality noted corresponds with the degree of severity of the hyperplastic process. Cells derived from simple and complex hyperplasia closely resemble normal endometrial cells, whereas cells derived from atypical hyperplasia are often difficult to distinguish from low-grade adenocarcinoma. The most detailed studies of cells derived from endometrial hyperplasia and adenocarcinoma have been published by Reagan and Ng.[76] A summary of their findings is presented in Table 7-11. Cells identified as only slightly larger than normal cells may well originate from a hyperplastic endometrium (Fig. 7-42). However, at this lower end of the disease spectrum, other nonneoplastic conditions may produce slight enlargement of endometrial cells and nuclei, creating situations where potential false-positive diagnoses may occur. Such conditions include endometrial polyp and anovulatory cycling with endometrial breakdown and cellular degeneration. As the hyperplastic process becomes more severe, cells progressively show greater degrees of nuclear enlargement, nuclear chromatin abnormalities, and the presence of nucleoli (Fig. 7-43). In such cases, after careful review

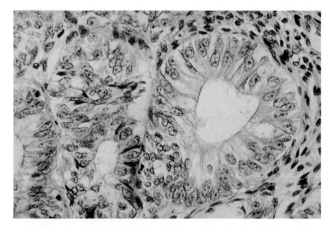

FIG. 7-41. A high-magnification of atypical endometrial hyperplasia is shown. Atypical hyperplasia may show architectural patterns that are either simple or complex. This form of hyperplasia must have significant cytologic atypia consisting of nuclear enlargement, hyperchromasia, and pleomorphism. Atypical hyperplasia has a risk of progression to adenocarcinoma of about 25%, which is much higher than either of the two nonatypical forms of endometrial hyperplasia (hematoxylin and eosin).

TABLE 7-11. *Cytologic criteria for the distinction of the endometrial hyperplasias from adenocarcinoma*

Feature	Hyperplasia			Cancer
	Simple	Complex	Atypical	
Number of cells per slide	107	142	245	538
Cell area (μm²)	89	98	116	149
Nuclear area (μm²)	42	49	53	68
Relative nuclear area (%)	47	50	46	46
Irregular chromatin (%)	4	10	21	97
Nucleoli (%)	2	6	17	88

Adapted from Regan JW, Ng ABP. The cells of uterine adenocarcinoma, 2nd ed. Basel: S Karger, 1973:121.

of the clinical situation, it may be possible to suggest a diagnosis of endometrial hyperplasia. However, because of the subtlety of such findings, particularly in the lower grades, a diagnosis of "AGCUS—endometrial type" would be most appropriate. This diagnosis should prompt further investigation on the part of the clinician, generally in the form of direct endometrial sampling, to establish a firm histologic diagnosis.

HISTOPATHOLOGY OF ENDOMETRIAL ADENOCARCINOMA

Endometrial adenocarcinoma is characterized by several different morphologic patterns. The current histologic classification scheme reflects these histologic variants (Table 7-12).

The typical histologic pattern of endometrial adenocarcinoma is made up of a complex proliferation of neoplastic endometrial glands whose overall conformation resembles that of the normal endometrium. The malignant glands are characterized by pseudostratification of the lining epithelial cells and a back-to-back arrange-

ment of the glands with little or no intervening stroma (Fig. 7-44). Often, the glandular proliferation may take on a cribriform growth pattern. The back-to-back arrangement and cribriform growth pattern are the most characteristic morphologic features that correspond to stromal invasion. In addition, there are individual cellular changes evident that reflect further progression of the cytologic abnormalities noted in the spectrum of hyperplasia. These include an increase in nuclear size and nuclear-to-cytoplasmic ratio, and prominent nucleoli (Fig. 7-45). Mitoses are identifiable, but vary from relatively few to many. In some cases of low-grade endometrial carcinoma, the degree of cytologic abnormality may be relatively minor and the diagnosis based principally on the architectural features mentioned earlier. The carcinoma may be limited to small areas of the endometrium or may involve the entire endometrial cavity. Low-grade lesions are often entirely confined to the endometrium, whereas high-grade lesions are often associated with more extensive invasion. Exceptions occur in both situations, however, and low-grade lesions that are deeply invasive and high-grade lesions that are superficial may be encountered.

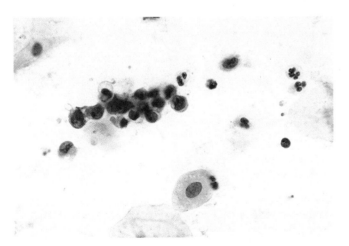

FIG. 7-42. An example of cells identified in the cervical smear from women shown to have nonatypical endometrial hyperplasia. The changes found in these endometrial cells are very subtle and consist only of increased numbers of endometrial cells, some with slightly enlarged nuclei (Papanicolaou stain).

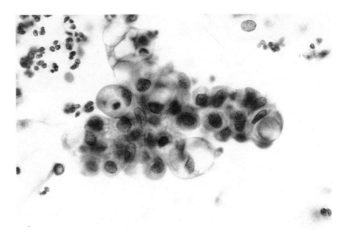

FIG. 7-43. In patients with atypical hyperplasias, the cytologic changes increase in severity, with further degrees of nuclear enlargement and irregularity, as well as hyperchromasia, and nucleoli formation, as are noted in this example (Papanicolaou stain).

TABLE 7-12. *Morphologic variants of endometrial adenocarcinoma*

Endometrioid ("typical") adenocarcinoma
  Secretory
  Ciliated cell
  Adenocarcinoma with squamous differentiation
    Adenoacanthoma (benign squamous metaplasia)
    Adenosquamous carcinoma
Papillary serous adenocarcinoma
Clear cell adenocarcinoma
Mucinous adenocarcinoma
Squamous carcinoma
Undifferentiated carcinoma

Endometrial adenocarcinoma is graded on the basis of its architectural features. Tumors that contain less than 5% solid (nonsquamous) component are classified as grade I. Tumors that show between 5% and 50% solid component are classified as grade II, and those that show greater than 50% solid pattern are classified as grade III.

Occasional endometrial adenocarcinomas may show prominent cytoplasmic secretory activity recapitulating secretory endometrium. When this type of differentiation is predominant in the tumor, the term *secretory adenocarcinoma* may be utilized. Such tumors are typically well differentiated and demonstrate minimal cytologic atypia.

Adenoacanthoma and *adenosquamous carcinoma* are terms that have been applied to endometrial adenocarcinomas that contain areas of squamous differentiation. *Adenoacanthoma* (Fig. 7-46) refers to adenocarcinomas that contain a histologically benign squamous component, and *adenosquamous carcinoma* refers to those tumors that have a malignant-appearing squamous component. However, it is now more common to refer to endometrial carcinomas with areas of squamous differentiation as simply *endometrial adenocarcinomas with partial squamous differentiation*. The previous division resulted largely from the work of Ng and associates, who showed that adenoacanthomas, which are usually well-differentiated tumors, had a prognosis similar to that of pure adenocarcinomas of the same grade, whereas mixed adenosquamous tumors tended to have a very poor prognosis.[77] Although the studies of some others have supported this concept, others have refuted it. In a study performed in our laboratory, for example, no difference in prognosis for mixed adenosquamous carcinomas was noted when compared with pure adenocarcinomas of the same histologic grade.[78] The concept remains controversial, but it is clear that endometrial carcinomas that contain a benign-appearing squamous component are generally low-grade neoplasms and those that contain a malignant-appearing squamous component generally also contain a high-grade glandular component.

Some adenocarcinomas of the endometrium show

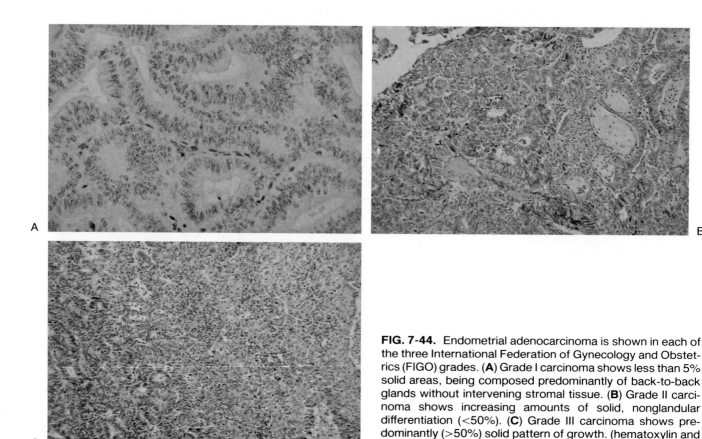

FIG. 7-44. Endometrial adenocarcinoma is shown in each of the three International Federation of Gynecology and Obstetrics (FIGO) grades. **(A)** Grade I carcinoma shows less than 5% solid areas, being composed predominantly of back-to-back glands without intervening stromal tissue. **(B)** Grade II carcinoma shows increasing amounts of solid, nonglandular differentiation (<50%). **(C)** Grade III carcinoma shows predominantly (>50%) solid pattern of growth. (hematoxylin and eosin).

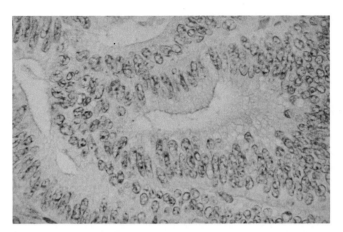

FIG. 7-45. In this high-magnification slide, the histologic appearance of endometrial adenocarcinoma is displayed. Endometrial carcinoma cells show increased size, pleomorphism, and hyperchromasia, when compared with normal endometrium. Macronucleoli become more prominent as the degree of differentiation diminishes (hematoxylin and eosin).

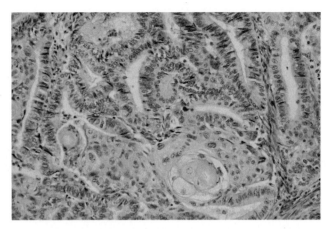

FIG. 7-46. An example of adenoacanthoma is shown. This designation refers to an otherwise typical endometrial adenocarcinoma in which prominent benign squamous metaplasia is present. Note the keratinizing morules of squamous epithelium in this example. This pattern in endometrial adenocarcinoma carries no difference in prognosis from adenocarcinomas of the same grade without the squamous differentiation (hematoxylin and eosin).

differentiation that is identical to other carcinomas of müllerian type. These include clear-cell, papillary serous, and mucinous adenocarcinomas. The clear-cell type of endometrial adenocarcinoma is histologically identical to the clear-cell carcinomas that occur elsewhere in the female genital tract. These tumors may have a papillary, glandular, solid, or tubulocystic pattern. This variant of endometrial carcinoma represents a high-grade neoplasm characterized by markedly atypical nuclear features. The cells are large, with eosinophilic or clear cytoplasm. The so-called *hobnail-type cell* is a feature of the papillary and tubulocystic areas of these tumors (Fig. 7-47). The differential diagnosis usually includes papillary serous and secretory carcinomas. The marked nuclear abnormalities of the clear-cell tumors as compared with the less atypical appearance of the nuclei of the other neoplasms is a helpful differential feature.

Papillary serous carcinoma is a primary endometrial

cancer that is histologically similar to the primary serous tumors of the ovary. It must be distinguished from the other two endometrial papillary neoplasms, clear-cell carcinoma and the papillary variant of the typical endometrial adenocarcinoma. The serous lesions are characterized by arborizing, thin, fibrous stalks that are lined by cuboidal or polygonal cells, without evidence of a prominent clear-cell pattern. The nuclear abnormalities are usually intermediate in severity. Deep myometrial invasion and lymphatic space involvement are typical with this tumor type, which characteristically shows an ovarian carcinoma–like spread pattern when present in the abdominal cavity. This tumor variant has a prognosis that is consistently poorer than that of the typical form of endometrial adenocarcinoma (Fig. 7-48).

Mucinous adenocarcinoma of the endometrium is his-

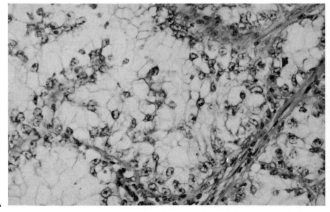
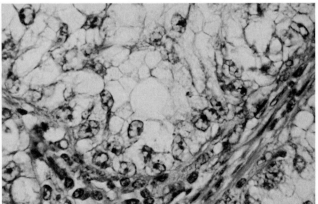

A   B

FIG. 7-47. An example of clear cell carcinoma of the endometrium is shown at low- and high-magnification. Note the prominent clear cytoplasm and the marked nuclear atypism present in these lesions (hematoxylin and eosin).

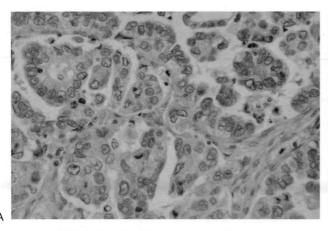

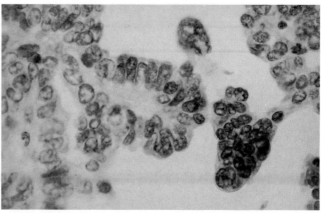

FIG. 7-48. Papillary serous carcinoma of the endometrium is shown in the two figures. Papillary serous carcinoma is identical in appearance to the tumor of the same name arising in the ovaries and pelvic peritoneum. It consists of papillary tufts lined by highly atypical cells showing marked degrees of nuclear enlargement and pleomorphism and a high mitotic rate. The prognosis is significantly poorer than endometrial carcinomas of the usual histologic type, when compared on a stage-for-stage basis (hematoxylin and eosin).

tologically identical to the common pattern of endocervical adenocarcinoma. Focal mucin production is not unusual in typical endometrial adenocarcinoma, but tumors classified as mucinous adenocarcinoma show a predominance of this form of differentiation (Fig. 7-49). Malignant tumors of this type should be distinguished from benign mucinous metaplasia of the endometrium. Ross and colleagues emphasize architectural complexity, epithelial stratification, loss of polarity, and nuclear atypia as important differential diagnostic features.[79] There is no reliable histologic method of differentiating endocervical primary mucinous tumors from those arising in the endometrium,[80] but differences in the appearance of the associated stroma and normal epithelium, or the presence of in situ disease components sometimes help in suggesting the primary site of origin. Localization by examination and differential curettage is usually necessary to make a definitive distinction. There is no apparent difference in the biologic behavior of this type of endometrial carcinoma and that of the typical variant.

CYTOPATHOLOGY OF ENDOMETRIAL ADENOCARCINOMA

Cells derived from endometrial adenocarcinoma are shed irregularly and may appear in cervical cytologic samples taken by the usual techniques. Most commonly, these abnormal cells are identified in material derived from the endocervical canal, because they are often entrapped in endocervical mucus. The most detailed studies of the cells of adenocarcinoma have been published by Reagan and Ng.[76]

The cytologic manifestations of carcinoma of the endometrium are related to the tumor's histologic type, degree of differentiation, and extent in the uterus. As mentioned earlier, the most common endometrial adenocarcinoma demonstrates the typical endometrioid pattern, and most cytologic studies of endometrial adenocarcinoma refer to cells derived from this type of neoplasm. The cytologic features of significance are the size of the cells, the size of the nuclei, the arrangement of the cells on the slide, the chromatin pattern, and the presence and size of nucleoli. Cells derived from endometrial adenocarcinoma are generally relatively sparse on routinely obtained samples, particularly in low-grade lesions. In higher-grade lesions, the number of abnormal cells present in the cell study increases progressively through the spectrum of disease. The cells are generally

FIG. 7-49. An example of mucinous carcinoma of the endometrium is illustrated. Mucinous carcinomas show a predominance of mucous-producing columnar cells recapitulating the appearance of tumors arising in the endocervix. Often, large amounts of extracellular mucous are also present (hematoxylin and eosin).

round to oval, with cyanophilic, often vacuolated cytoplasm (Fig. 7-50). Intracytoplasmic neutrophils are often present within individual tumor cell cytoplasm and may displace the nucleus to the margin of the cell in a "signet-ring" fashion (Fig. 7-51). The nuclei are enlarged (generally greater than 60 μm^2), with finely granular, often irregularly distributed chromatin. Nucleoli are evident and prominent nucleoli may be encountered in high-grade tumors. Like the number of abnormal cells, the size of the cells, the size of the nuclei, and the number and size of the nucleoli all are related directly to the differentiation of the tumor.

Endometrial adenocarcinoma does not generally exhibit a necrotic tumor diathesis background pattern. A more typical pattern is the presence of a blue-tinged, finely granular background throughout the slide. This pattern has been referred to as a *watery* diathesis (Fig. 7-52).

In cases of endometrial carcinoma that show partial squamous differentiation, a malignant-appearing squamous component may be recognized along with the malignant endometrial cells on the cervical smear. In such cases, it may not be possible to differentiate a primary endometrial lesion from a mixed adenosquamous carcinoma of the cervix on a cytologic basis alone.

Cells derived from clear-cell carcinoma of the endometrium are cytologically identical to cells derived from its counterpart in the vagina or cervix. The cells may be single or arranged in clusters or sheets. The cytoplasm is ill defined and may appear clear or vacuolated. In alcohol-fixed material, however, the cytoplasm may have a pale amphophilic to eosinophilic, finely granular appearance. The nuclei are large and round or oval, with irregular clumped chromatin and prominent nucleoli, which may be multiple[81-83] (Fig. 7-53).

Mucinous carcinoma of the endometrium resembles typical endocervical adenocarcinoma histologically and sheds cells that are also similar to those of endocervical adenocarcinoma. There are usually fewer cells present than are encountered in the case of an endocervical primary lesion because the tumor is not sampled directly. The morphologic characteristics of the cells themselves,

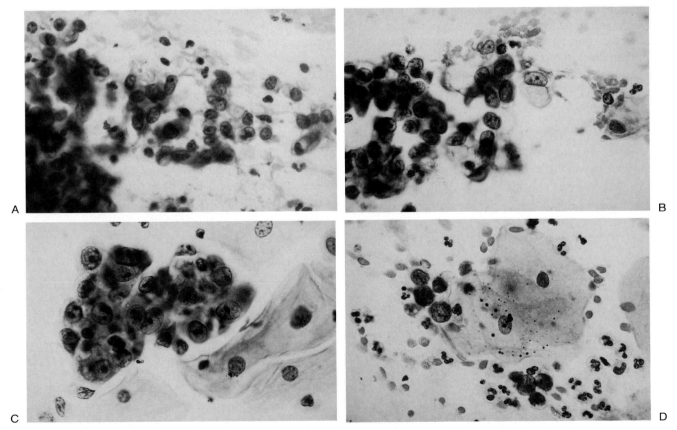

FIG. 7-50. Examples of endometrial adenocarcinoma obtained in cervical cytologic samples are shown. In the spectrum of increasing tumor grade, a continuum of cytologic changes shows progression of nuclear size, pleomorphism, formation of macronucleoli, and dyscohesion. **(A)** Cells derived from grade I adenocarcinoma. **(B)** Cells derived from grade II adenocarcinoma. **(C and D)** Cells derived from grade III adenocarcinoma. Note the very prominent macronucleoli and the presence of numerous single tumor cells in the grade III lesion (Papanicolaou stain).

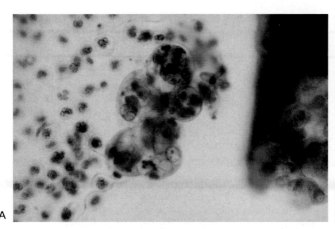
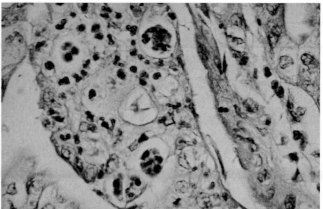

A   B

FIG. 7-51. Cells of endometrial adenocarcinoma often exfoliate cells with intracytoplasmic vacuolizations containing neutrophils. (**A**) These types of cells in the cytologic sample. (**B**) Similar cells present in the endometrial biopsy specimen from the same patient (**A,** Papanicolaou stain; **B,** hematoxylin and eosin).

however, usually do not permit distinction between an endocervical and an endometrial primary lesion in tumors of this type.

The morphologic appearance of serous carcinoma of the endometrium reflects the papillary nature of this neoplasm and its similarity to the common ovarian neoplasms of serous type. Characteristically, the cells are larger than those of typical endometrial adenocarcinoma and are often found arranged in tightly cohesive, three-dimensional papillary groups. The nuclei are hyperchromatic and often contain irregular and sometimes multiple macronucleoli (Fig. 7-54). In some cases, psammoma bodies may be identified. Kuebler and associates, in a study comparing the cytologic features of this variant of adenocarcinoma with the typical endometrial adeno-

carcinoma, noted several other potentially helpful differential cytologic features.[84] Included among these is the presence of a necrotic tumor diathesis in the slide background with serous carcinoma and the relatively rare identification of neutrophilic phagocytosis by tumor cells. The latter finding is a common feature of endometrial adenocarcinoma of the typical type.

Distinguishing papillary serous tumors arising in the endometrium from their counterparts in the ovary may not always be possible. The presence of numerous tumor cells or of a background diathesis pattern (watery or necrotic) on the slide, however, should prompt strong consideration of the possibility of an endometrial primary tumor. Generally, cells of ovarian carcinoma that appear in the cervical smear travel through the uterine tubes and uterine fundus, and are not associated with the necrotic patterns of directly invasive tumors. This feature is the most reliable, but not absolute, criterion allowing distinction between primary sites for tumors of the papillary serous type.

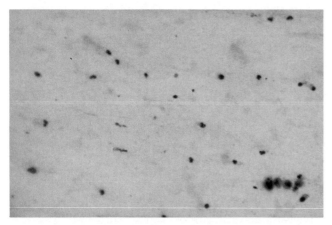

FIG. 7-52. The typical "watery," or granular, diathesis pattern noted on cytologic preparations from patients with endometrial adenocarcinoma is shown. The background contains finely granular cyanophilic material with very little coarse necrotic material, inflammation, or blood (Papanicolaou stain).

CYTOLOGIC DIFFERENTIAL DIAGNOSIS OF ENDOMETRIAL ADENOCARCINOMA

Cells derived from a number of benign and malignant processes may mimic the cytologic appearance of adenocarcinoma of the endometrium.

Several types of normal cells of the uterus may be mistaken for endometrial carcinoma cells. Perhaps the most common problem is mistaking normal endometrial cells for cancer cells. As has been mentioned previously, the features distinguishing low-grade adenocarcinoma from normal endometrial cells may be subtle. The difficulties may be magnified if cellular preservation, specimen fixation, and staining are less than optimal. This is espe-

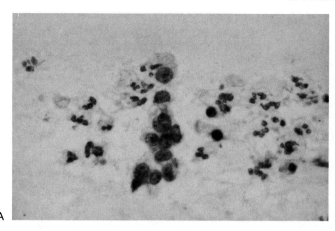
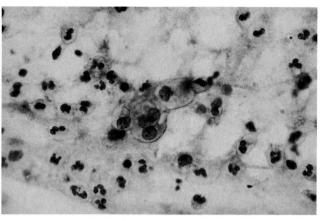

FIG. 7-53. Cells derived from clear cell adenocarcinoma of the endometrium are illustrated (**A** and **B**). Note the abundant clear cytoplasm and the prominent macronucleoli present in most cells. A prominent tumor diathesis pattern is noted in the background (Papanicolaou stain).

cially true if the cells have undergone minor degenerative changes. Accurate clinical information always helps to avoid problems in this regard, and obtaining such information is absolutely necessary if accurate interpretation is to be rendered regarding potential endometrial lesions.

Aggregates of other cell types may also cause differential diagnostic difficulties. Groups of small histiocytes or granulocytes may superficially mimic groups of endometrial adenocarcinoma. In postmenopausal women in particular, aggregates of atrophic endocervical cells or

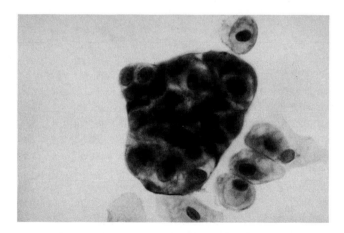

FIG. 7-54. A three-dimensional cluster of malignant cells from a case of papillary serous carcinoma of the endometrium is shown in this thin-layer preparation. Cells from this process typically form such clusters, similar to the papillary structures that are seen in the histologic preparations (see figure 7-48). The nuclei are large and contain prominent macronucleoli. Overall, their appearance is very similar to that of ovarian serous carcinomas present in body cavity fluid specimens. In making the differential diagnosis between an endometrial and ovarian origin for this tumor, the presence of tumor diathesis will often be helpful, as primary ovarian tumors most often present with a clean background (Papanicolaou smear—ThinPrep).

bare endocervical nuclei may resemble the cell groupings of endometrial carcinoma. Accurate interpretation in these instances depends on familiarity not only with the cytologic features of normal and abnormal endometrium, but also with the variations in the cytologic characteristics of other normal cells.

Reactive and inflammatory processes that are associated with cellular changes may also be confused with adenocarcinoma of the endometrium. These include endometrial polyp, chronic endometritis, and, less commonly, acute and chronic endocervicitis. With endometrial polyp and chronic inflammation of the endometrium, cells are shed irregularly. Superficial endometrial cells shed in this fashion may be atypical in their appearance, with nuclear enlargement and prominent nucleoli secondary to the increased metabolic activity resulting from proliferation, inflammation, and degeneration. Although less commonly confused with cells of endometrial origin, reactive endocervical cells, particularly those derived from inflamed endocervical polyps, may cause cytologic difficulty.

The differentiation of adenocarcinomas of endocervical origin from those of endometrial origin is an important clinical consideration when tumor cells are identified in the cervical smear. Reagan and Ng suggested the use of the following differential cytologic features[76]:

Endocervical carcinomas shed significantly more cells than do endometrial adenocarcinomas.

Endocervical carcinoma cells and nuclei are larger.

The cytoplasm of endocervical carcinomas typically is less cyanophilic than that of endometrial carcinomas.

Nucleoli are more common and larger in endocervical carcinomas.

Endometrial carcinomas are typically arranged in three-dimensional clusters, whereas endocervical carcinomas are present in side-by-side, two-dimensional sheet arrangements.

Endometrial carcinomas show a watery background, whereas endocervical carcinomas show a necrotic tumor diathesis.

Obviously, as endometrial carcinomas of higher grade are encountered, such differential features become less helpful in making definitive distinctions.

NORMAL ENDOMETRIAL CELLS AT ABNORMAL TIMES

Endometrial cells are rarely present in the secretory phase of women with normal cycles. In most cases, such shedding cannot be traced to a specific abnormality. However, among women younger than 40 years of age, such shedding is unlikely to be caused by a malignant process. Identifiable causes of such shedding include dysfunctional uterine bleeding, hormonal therapy, and the presence of an intrauterine device. Among women older than 40 years of age, however, there is an increasing probability that the shedding of cytologically normal endometrial cells is associated with endometrial hyperplasia or carcinoma. Ng and associates reported that 37% of women older than 40 years of age with endometrial cells seen in the second half of the cycle had endometrial hyperplasia, and 20% had endometrial cancer.[85] In addition, they noted that the incidence of cancer increased with advancing age. A more recent study by Cherkis and colleagues identified a 36% rate of endometrial pathology, with 11% being cancer, in a follow-up of normal endometrial cells present in the second half of the cycle or in postmenopausal women. Again, the authors noted an increase in the association of cancer with advancing age.[86]

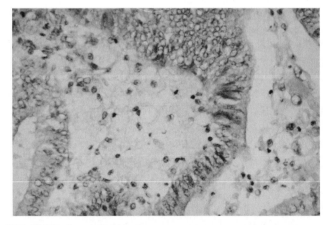

FIG. 7-55. Large lipid-laden macrophages may be commonly seen in the stroma of endometrial adenocarcinomas as shown here (hematoxylin and eosin).

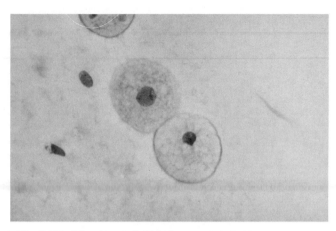

FIG. 7-56. The large lipid-laden macrophages, as shown here and in figure 7-55, may be seen in cervical cytologic smears from patients harboring endometrial neoplasia. When significant numbers of such "lipophages" are identified in patients at risk for the development of endometrial neoplasia, further clinical follow-up is routinely recommended (Papanicolaou stain).

ENDOMETRIAL STROMAL HISTIOCYTES (FOAM CELLS, LIPOPHAGES)

In tissue sections of endometrial adenocarcinoma and hyperplasia, it is not uncommon to find large, vacuolated histiocytes within the endometrial stroma between neoplastic glands (Fig. 7-55). A number of studies have identified a link between the presence of such cells in cervical cytologic samples and endometrial neoplasia. Ng and colleagues reported a 4% association between the presence of such cells and endometrial neoplasia.[85] Patten and Patten reported a 17% incidence of endometrial cancer when large, vacuolated histiocytes containing lipid (lipophages; Fig. 7-56) are present in the cytologic sample within the background of an inappropriately elevated estrogenic effect.[87] Recently, in this author's laboratory, Dressel and associates showed a 12% association between the presence of large numbers of histiocytes in the cervical smear and endometrial neoplasia (10%) or extrauterine carcinoma (2%) on subsequent follow-up studies.[88] It is important to identify these large, vacuolated histiocytic cells in patients who are clinically at risk for the development of endometrial neoplasia (ie, those who are postmenopausal, have postmenopausal bleeding, are taking hormonal therapy, or show an inappropriate estrogen effect), and to recommend close clinical follow-up or endometrial biopsy.

REFERENCES

1. Taylor PT, Andersen WA, Barber SR, et al. The screening Papanicolaou smear: contribution of the endocervical brush. Obstet Gynecol 1987;70:734.

2. Schumann JL, O'Connor DM, Covell JL, et al. Pap smear collection devices: technical, clinical, diagnostic, and legal considerations associated with their use. Diagn Cytopathol 1992;8:492.

3. Hutchinson M, Fertitta L, Goldbaum B, et al. Cervex-Brush and Cytobrush. Comparison of their ability to sample abnormal cells for cervical smears. J Reprod Med 1991;36:581.

4. Kawaguchi K, Nogi M, Ohya M, et al. The value of the Cytobrush for obtaining cells from the uterine cervix. Diagn Cytopathol 1987; 3:262.

5. Boon ME, Alons-van-Kordelaar JJM, Rietveld-Scheffers PEM. Consequences of the introduction of combined spatula and Cytobrush sampling for cervical cytology: improvements in smear quality and detection rates. Acta Cytol 1986;30:264.

6. Trimbos JB, Arentz NPW. The efficacy of the Cytobrush versus the cotton swab in the collection of endocervical cells in cervical smears. Acta Cytol 1986;30:261.

7. Buntinx F, Boon ME, Beck S, et al. Comparison of Cytobrush sampling, spatula sampling and combined Cytobrush-spatula sampling of the uterine cervix. Acta Cytol 1991;35:64.

8. Babkowski RC, Rutkowski MA, Facik MJ, et al. Endocervical cytologic atypia: the effects of endocervical canal topography and high endocervical sampling on the cytologic presentation of normal endocervical cells. Am J Clin Pathol 1994;101:376.

9. Reagan JW, Ng ABP. Cellular detection of glandular neoplasms of the uterine cervix. In Wied GL (ed). Compendium on diagnostic cytology, 6th ed. Chicago: Tutorials of Clinical Cytology, 1988: 146.

10. Vesterinen E, Forss M, Nieminen U. Increase of cervical adenocarcinoma: a report of 520 cases of cervical carcinomas including 112 tumors with glandular elements. Gynecol Oncol 1989;33:49.

11. Goodman HM, Buttlar CA, Niloff JM, et al. Adenocarcinoma of the uterine cervix: prognostic factors and patterns of recurrence. Gynecol Oncol 1989;33:241.

12. Davis JR, Moon LB. Increased incidence of adenocarcinoma of the uterine cervix. Obstet Gynecol 1975;45:79.

13. Greer BE, Figge DC, Tamimi HK, et al. Stage 1B adenocarcinoma of the cervix treated by radical hysterectomy and pelvic lymph node dissection. Am J Obstet Gynecol 1989;160:1509.

14. Valente PT, Hanjani P. Endocervical neoplasia in long-term users of oral contraceptives: clinical and pathologic observations. Obstet Gynecol 1986;67:695.

15. Dallenbach-Hellweg G. On the origin and histologic structure of adenocarcinoma of the endocervix in women under 50 years of age. Pathol Res Pract 1984;179:38.

16. Deligdisch L, Escay-Martinez E, Cohen CJ. Endocervical carcinoma: a study of 23 patients with clinicopathological correlation. Gynecol Oncol 1984;18:321.

17. Jones MW, Silverberg SG. Cervical adenocarcinoma in young women: possible relationship to microglandular hyperplasia and use of oral contraceptives. Obstet Gynecol 1989;73:984.

18. Horowitz IR, Jacobsen LP, Zucker PK, et al. Epidemiology of adenocarcinoma of the cervix. Gynecol Oncol 1988;31:25.

19. Brinton LA, Tashima KT, Lehman HF, et al. Epidemiology of cervical cancer by cell type. Cancer Res 1987;47:1706.

20. Parazzini F, LaVechchia C, Negri E, et al. Risk factors for adenocarcinoma of the cervix: a case control study. Br J Cancer 1988;57: 201.

21. Jaworski RC. Endocervical glandular dysplasia, adenocarcinoma in situ, and early invasive (microinvasive) adenocarcinoma of the uterine cervix. Semin Diagn Pathol 1990;7:190.

22. Griffin NR, Dockey D, Lewis FA, et al. Demonstration of low frequency of human papillomavirus DNA in cervical adenocarcinoma and adenocarcinoma in situ by the polymerase chain reaction and in situ hybridization. Int J Gynecol Pathol 1991;10:36.

23. Tase T, Okagaki T, Clark BA, et al. Human papillomavirus DNA in adenocarcinoma in situ, microinvasive adenocarcinoma of the uterine cervix, and coexisting cervical squamous intraepithelial neoplasias. Int J Gynecol Pathol 1989;8:8.

24. Smotkin D, Berek JS, Fu YS, et al. Human papillomavirus deoxyribonucleic acid in adenocarcinoma and adenosquamous carcinoma of the uterine cervix. Obstet Gynecol 1986;68:241.

25. Gordon AN, Bornstein J, Kaufman RH, et al. Human papillomavirus associated with adenocarcinoma and adenosquamous carcinoma of the cervix: analysis by in situ hybridization. Gynecol Oncol 1989;35:345.

26. Wilczynski SP, Walker J, Liao SY, et al. Adenocarcinoma of the cervix associated with human papillomavirus. Cancer 1988;62: 1331.

27. Duggan MA, Benoit JL, McGregor SE, et al. The human papillomavirus status of 114 endocervical adenocarcinoma cases by dot blot hybridization. Hum Pathol 1993;24:121.

28. Farnsworth A, Laverty C, Stoler MH. Human papillomavirus messenger RNA expression in adenocarcinoma in situ of the uterine cervix. Int J Gynecol Pathol 1989;8:321.

29. Duggan MA, Benoit JL, McGregor SE, et al. Adenocarcinoma in situ of the endocervix: human papillomavirus determination by dot blot hybridization and polymerase chain reaction amplification. Int J Gynecol Pathol 1994;13:143.

30. Leary J, Jaworski R, Houghton R. In-situ hybridization using biotinylated DNA probes to human papillomavirus in adenocarcinoma-in-situ and endocervical glandular dysplasia of the uterine cervix. Pathol 1991;23:85.

31. Tase T, Okagaki T, Clark BA, et al. Human papillomavirus DNA in glandular dysplasia and microglandular hyperplasia: presumed precursors of adenocarcinoma of the uterine cervix. Obstet Gynecol 1989;73:1005.

32. Korhonen MO. Adenocarcinoma of the uterine cervix. An evaluation of the available diagnostic methods. Acta Pathologia et Microbiologia Scandinavia (A) 1978;(Suppl 264:1).

33. Young RH, Scully RE. Invasive adenocarcinoma and related tumors of the uterine cervix. Semin Diagn Pathol 1990;7:205.

34. Hurt WG, Silverberg SG, Frable WJ, et al. Adenocarcinoma of the cervix: histopathologic and clinical features. Am J Obstet Gynecol 1977;129:304.

35. Friedell GH, McKay DG. Adenocarcinoma in situ of the endocervix. Cancer 1953;6:887.

36. Oster AG, Pagano R, Davoren RAM, et al. Adenocarcinoma in situ of cervix. Int J Gynecol Pathol 1984;3:179.

37. Young RH, Scully RE. Villoglandular papillary adenocarcinoma of the uterine cervix. A clinicopathological analysis of 13 cases. Cancer 1989;63:1773.

38. Jaworski RC, Pacey NF, Greenberg ML, et al. The histologic diagnosis of adenocarcinoma in situ and related lesions of the cervix uteri. Cancer 1988;61:1171.

39. Bousfield L, Pacey F, Young Q, et al. Expanded cytologic criteria for the diagnosis of adenocarcinoma in situ of the cervix and related lesions. Acta Cytol 1980;24:284.

40. Ayer B, Pacey F, Greenberg M, et al. The cytologic diagnosis of adenocarcinoma in situ of the cervix uteri and related lesions. I. Adenocarcinoma in situ. Acta Cytol 1987;31:397.

41. Lee KR, Manna EA, Jones MA. Comparative cytologic features of adenocarcinoma in situ of the uterine cervix. Acta Cytol 1991;35: 117.

42. Pacey F, Ayer B, Greenberg M. The cytologic diagnosis of adenocarcinoma in situ of the cervix uteri and related lesions. III. Pitfalls in diagnosis. Acta Cytol 1988;32:325.

43. Kudo R, Sagae S, Hayakawa O, et al. Morphology of adenocarcinoma in situ and microinvasive adenocarcinoma of the uterine cervix. A cytologic and ultrastructural study. Acta Cytol 1991;35: 109.

44. Betsill WL, Clark AH. Early endocervical glandular neoplasia I. Histomorphology and cytomorphology. Acta Cytol 1986;30:115.

45. Clark AH, Betsill WL. Early endocervical glandular neoplasia II. Morphometric analysis of the cells. Acta Cytol 1986;30:127.

46. Pacey NF. Glandular neoplasms of the uterine cervix. In Bibbo M (ed). Comprehensive cytopathology. Philadelphia: WB Saunders, 1991:231.

47. Flenker H. Tissue repair in the cervix. In Wied GL (ed). Compendium on diagnostic cytology, 7th ed. Chicago: Tutorials of Clinical Cytology, 1992:75.

48. Bibbo M, Weid GL. Inflammation. In Keebler C, Somrak T (eds) The manual of cytotechnology, 7th ed. Chicago: ASCP Press, 1993:90.

49. Lee KR. Atypical glandular cells in cervical smears from women who have undergone cone biopsy. A potential diagnostic pitfall. Acta Cytol 1993;37:705.

50. Frierson HF, Covell JL, Andersen WA. Radiation changes in endocervical cells in brush specimens. Diagn Cytopathol 1990;6:243.

51. Stowell SB, Wiley CM, Powers CN. Herpesvirus mimics: a potential pitfall in endocervical brush specimens. Acta Cytol 1994;38:43.

52. Hendrickson MR, Kempson RL. Endometrial epithelial metaplasias: proliferations frequently misdiagnosed as adenocarcinoma. Report of 89 cases and proposed classification. Am J Surg Pathol 1980;4:525.

53. Jonasson JG, Wang HH, Antonioli DA, et al. Tubal metaplasia of the uterine cervix: a prevalence study in patients with gynecologic pathology findings. Int J Gynecol Pathol 1992;11:89.

54. Novotny DB, Maygarden SJ, Johnson DE, et al. Tubal metaplasia. A frequent potential pitfall in the cytologic diagnosis of endocervical glandular dysplasia on cervical smears. Acta Cytol 1992;36:1.

55. Van Le L, Novotny D, Dotters DJ. Distinguishing tubal metaplasia from endocervical dysplasia on cervical Papanicolaou smears. Obstet Gynecol 1991;78:974.

56. Suh KS, Silverberg SG. Tubal metaplasia of the uterine cervix. Int J Gynecol Pathol 1990;9:122.

57. Ducatman BS, Wang HH, Jonasson JG, et al. Tubal metaplasia: a cytologic study with comparison to other neoplastic and non-neoplastic conditions of the endocervix. Diagn Cytopathol 1993;9:98.

58. Patten SF. Diagnostic cytopathology of the uterine cervix. Basel: S Karger, 1978:138.

59. Hamilton SR, Smith RRL. The relationship between columnar epithelial dysplasia and invasive adenocarcinoma arising in Barrett's esophagus. Am J Clin Pathol 1987;87:301.

60. Brown LJR, Wells M. Cervical glandular atypia associated with squamous intraepithelial neoplasia: a premalignant lesion? J Clin Pathol 1986;39:22.

61. Kurman RJ, Solomon D. The Bethesda system for reporting cervical/vaginal cytologic diagnoses. New York: Springer-Verlag, 1994:62.

62. Covell JL, Frierson HF. Intraepithelial neoplasia mimicking microinvasive squamous-cell carcinoma in endocervical brushings. Diagn Cytopathol 1992;8:18.

63. Selvaggi SM. Cytologic features of squamous cell carcinoma in situ involving endocervical glands in endocervical brush specimens. Acta Cytol 1994;38:687.

64. Goff BA, Atanasoff P, Brown E, et al. Endocervical glandular atypia in Papanicolaou smears. Obstet Gynecol 1992;79:101.

65. Bose S, Kannan V, Kline TS. Abnormal endocervical cells. Really abnormal? Really endocervical? Am J Clin Pathol 1994;101:708.

66. Wilbur DC, Mulford DM, Sickel JZ, et al. The problem of endocervical atypia: new cytologic presentations of normal endocervical cells and squamous neoplasia. Acta Cytol 1994;38:808.

67. Pisharodi LR, Ramirez N, Gudlangsson E, et al. The spectrum and significance of atypical glandular cells of undetermined significance (AGUS) on Papanicolaou smears. Acta Cytol 1994;38:794.

68. Currie MM, Casm Z, Balign M, et al. The significance of atypical glandular cells on Papanicolaou smears: an eight-year follow-up study. Acta Cytol 1994;38:810.

69. Lee KR, Manna EA, St John T. Diagnostic accuracy of cervical smears with atypical glandular cells. Mod Pathol 1995;8:42A.

70. Walker AM, Jick H. Declining rates of endometrial cancer. Obstet Gynecol 1980;56:733.

71. Reagan JW, Ng ABP. The cells of the uterine cervix, 2nd ed, p 45. Basel: S Karger, 1973.

72. Huang SJ, Amparo EG, Fu YS. Endometrial hyperplasia: histologic classification and behavior. Surg Pathol 1988;1:215.

73. Sherman AI, Brown S. The precursors of endometrial carcinoma. Am J Obstet Gynecol 1979;135:947.

74. Fox H, Buckley CH. The endometrial hyperplasias and their relationship to endometrial neoplasias. Histopathology 1982;6:493.

75. Kurman RJ, Kaminski PF, Norris HJ. The behavior of endometrial hyperplasia. A long term study of "untreated" hyperplasia in 170 patients. Cancer 1985;56:403.

76. Reagan JW, Ng ABP. The cells of uterine adenocarcinoma, 2nd ed. Basel: S Karger, 1973:121.

77. Ng ABP, Reagan JW, Storaasli JP, et al. Mixed adenosquamous carcinoma of the endometrium. Am J Clin Pathol 1973;59:765.

78. Salazar OM, DePapp EW, Bonfiglio TA, et al. Adenosquamous carcinoma of the endometrium: an entity with an inherent poor prognosis? Cancer 1977;40:119.

79. Ross J, Eifel PH, Cox RS, et al. Primary mucinous adenocarcinoma of the endometrium. A clinicopathologic and histochemical study. Am J Surg Pathol 1983;7:715.

80. Czernobilsky B, Katz Z, Lancet M, et al. Endocervical-type epithelium in endometrial carcinoma. A report of 10 cases with emphasis on histochemical methods for differential diagnosis. Am J Surg Pathol 1980;4:481.

81. Taft PD, Robboy SJ, Herbst AL, et al. Cytology of clear cell adenocarcinoma of the genital tract in young females. Review of 95 cases from the registry. Acta Cytol 1974;18:279.

82. Young QA, Pacey NF. The cytologic diagnosis of clear cell adenocarcinoma of the cervix uteri. Acta Cytol 1978;22:3.

83. Vooijs PG, Ng ABP, Wentz WB. The detection of vaginal adenosis and clear cell carcinoma. Acta Cytol 1973;17:59.

84. Kuebler DL, Nikrui N, Bell DA. Cytologic features of endometrial papillary serous carcinoma. Acta Cytol 1989;33:120.

85. Ng ABP, Reagan JW, Hawliezak S, et al. Significance of endometrial cells in the detection of endometrial adenocarcinoma and its precursors. Acta Cytol 1974;18:356.

86. Cherkis RC, Patten SF, Andrews TJ, et al. Significance of normal endometrial cells detected by cervical cytology. Obstet Gynecol 1988;71:242.

87. Patten SF, Patten FW. Cellular detection of endometrial stromal lipophages: an incidental observation or marker for endometrial adenocarcinoma and its precursors (unpublished data). In Syllabus for differential diagnostic cytopathology of adenocarcinomas of the female genital tract. 39th Annual Meeting, American Society of Cytology, Los Angeles, California, November 1991.

88. Dressel DM, Dressel IJ, Wilbur DC. Stromal histiocytes in routine Papanicolaou smears: histopathologic and clinical significance. Acta Cytol 1992;36:629.

Gynecologic Cytopathology. Edited by
Thomas A. Bonfiglio and Yener S. Erozan.
Lippincott–Raven Publishers, Philadelphia, © 1997.

CHAPTER 8

Uncommon Tumors of the Cervix, Vagina, and Uterine Corpus

Thomas A. Bonfiglio

Although the common glandular and squamous epithelial neoplasms make up the vast majority of tumors that involve the female genital tract, there are a large number of other neoplasms that occur here. Although these are uncommon, they are of significant importance clinically and must be recognized by the pathologist in both cytologic and tissue samples. Many of these lesions are very well described in the cytopathology literature, whereas a few are seen so rarely that their cytologic manifestations have not yet been extensively detailed. Nevertheless, most of these tumors can be detected and accurately diagnosed in cytologic samples.

SMALL-CELL CARCINOMA (NEUROENDOCRINE CARCINOMA)

Small-cell carcinoma accounts for about 5% of cervical carcinomas and rarely occurs at other sites in the female genital tract. It was formerly classified as a subtype of squamous carcinoma. It is now recognized, however, that this is a poorly differentiated variant of neuroendocrine carcinoma akin to small-cell carcinoma of the lung. Unlike its pulmonary counterpart, cervical small-cell neuroendocrine carcinoma is strongly associated with human papillomavirus type 18.[1] This highly aggressive neoplasm is composed of diffusely infiltrating aggregates of small, polygonal to irregular cells with little visible cytoplasm and small, rounded to irregularly shaped nuclei that are hyperchromatic and contain small nucleoli. Mitoses are common and necrosis is frequently evident (Figs. 8-1 and 8-2). Electron microscopy or immunocy-

tochemical staining demonstrates the presence of neurosecretory cytoplasmic granules. This neoplasm should be distinguished from nonkeratinizing squamous cell carcinoma composed of relatively small cells, especially because small-cell neuroendocrine carcinoma has a worse prognosis and usually is treated with a different therapeutic approach, often utilizing chemotherapeutic agents.

In cytologic samples, the abnormal cells from this tumor usually exist in a dirty background caused by the destructive process of the invading neoplasm. The cells are small and relatively uniform, with a mean area of approximately 170 μm^2. They are either isolated or in loose syncytial arrangements. The cytoplasm is quite scant and cyanophilic. The nuclei, which average 65 μm^2, are round to oval with hyperchromatic, coarsely granular chromatin. Nuclear angulation and molding may be evident and nucleoli are common but not prominent[2] (Figs. 8-3 through 8-7).

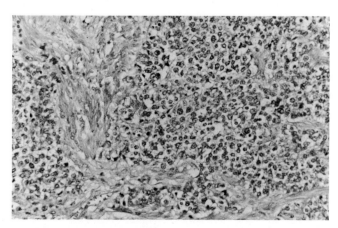

FIG. 8-1. Small-cell carcinoma, cervix. Tissue, hematoxylin and eosin, medium power.

T. A. Bonfiglio: Department of Pathology and Laboratory Medicine, University of Rochester Medical Center, Rochester, New York 14642.

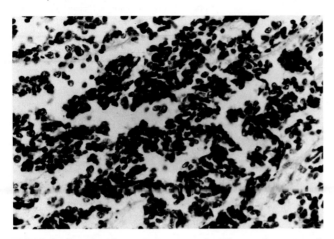

FIG. 8-2. Small-cell carcinoma, cervix. Tissue, hematoxylin and eosin, medium power.

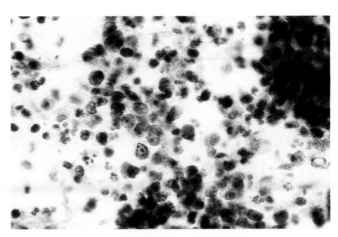

FIG. 8-5. Small-cell carcinoma. Dischohesive tumor cells and tight aggregates. Note opaque nuclear forms in degenerated cells and irregular angulated nuclei in other cells.

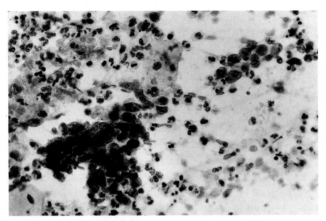

FIG. 8-3. Small-cell carcinoma. The tumor cells are arranged in tight syncytial aggregates.

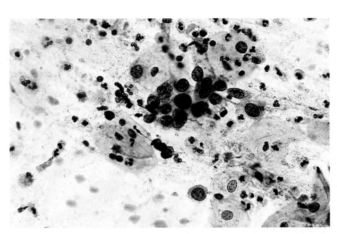

FIG. 8-6. Small-cell carcinoma. Syncytial aggregate of tumor cells. Scant cytoplasm is evident.

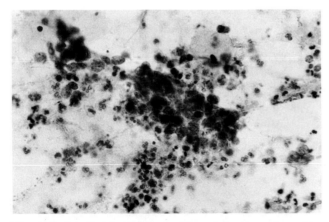

FIG. 8-4. Small-cell carcinoma. Syncytial aggregates of tumor cells with necrotic cellular debris in the background.

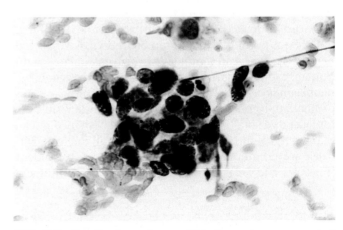

FIG. 8-7. Small-cell carcinoma. This tumor is composed of somewhat larger cells but retains neuroendocrine features.

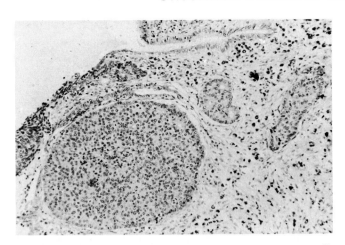

FIG. 8-8. Carcinoid tumor. Low-power view, hematoxylin and eosin stain.

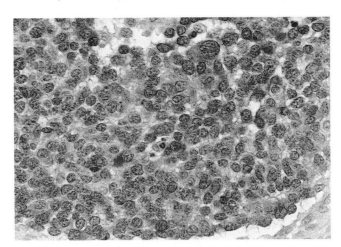

FIG. 8-10. Carcinoid tumor, medium power. Positive immunocytochemical stain for neuron-specific enolase.

CARCINOID TUMORS

Carcinoid tumors of the uterine cervix are rare but well recognized.[3-6] They are histologically similar to carcinoid tumors at other body sites and consist of small, relatively uniform cells growing in an insular or trabecular pattern with or without rosette formation (Figs. 8-8 and 8-9). The presence of argyrophilic cytoplasmic granules is confirmatory evidence for this diagnosis. Neurosecretory granules can also be demonstrated by electron microscopy, and immunocytochemical techniques can be used to demonstrate neuroendocrine markers such as neuron-specific enolase, chromogranin, or synaptophysin (Fig. 8-10). The relationship between this neuroendocrine tumor and the human papillomavirus is unknown.

Although there are some reports in the literature,[7] the cytologic findings in these well-differentiated neuroendocrine lesions of the cervix are not well established. The tumors often coexist with typical squamous carcinomas or adenocarcinomas, producing a complex cytologic pattern. In the cases seen by the author, the cells believed to be derived from the carcinoid component presented as single cells or small aggregates of cells that were relatively small and uniform with round to oval nuclei, granular chromatin, and inconspicuous nucleoli (Fig. 8-11).

ADENOID CYSTIC AND ADENOID BASAL CELL CARCINOMAS

Adenoid cystic and adenoid basal cell carcinomas are rare neoplasms of the cervix that only recently were clearly differentiated from each other.[8] Adenoid cystic tumors of the cervix resemble adenoid cystic carcinomas of the salivary gland in their histologic appearance and aggressive biologic behavior. They are composed of small basaloid cells arranged in sheets and nests, often

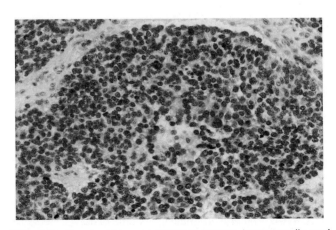

FIG. 8-9. Carcinoid tumor. Medium power, hematoxylin and eosin stain.

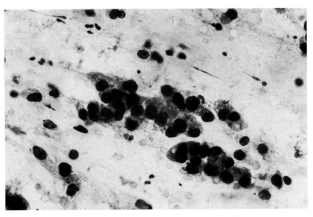

FIG. 8-11. Cells derived from cervical carcinoid tumor. Note relative uniformity of tumor cells and cuboidal to low columnar configuration.

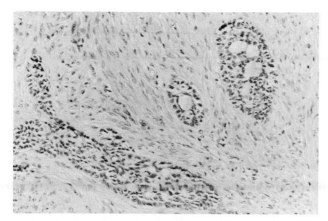

FIG. 8-12. Adenoid cystic carcinoma of cervix. Hematoxylin and eosin, medium power.

having a cribriform pattern or small cyst-like formations that contain a hyaline-like material. These tumors frequently coexist with squamous cell carcinomas (Fig. 8-12). Adenoid basal carcinomas are composed of small nests of basaloid cells that have a morphea-like pattern. In the center of some nests, miniature gland-like formations are identified. Hyaline material is not identified and a cribriform pattern is not seen. These tumors may also be associated with typical squamous cell carcinomas (Fig. 8-13). They tend to occur in older women, but are not as aggressive in their biologic behavior as are adenoid cystic tumors.

The cytologic features of these two neoplasms have not been well described. In a single case of adenoid basal cell carcinoma seen in our laboratory and described by Patten, the tumor cells resembled those derived from a small-cell type of squamous carcinoma in situ.[9] Because both adenoid cystic and adenoid basal cell carcinomas often coexist with intraepithelial and invasive squamous lesions, the cytologic distinction of these neoplasms may be difficult.

VERRUCOUS CARCINOMAS

Verrucous carcinomas are rare tumors that may occur in either the cervix or the vagina. They are characterized by a bulky exophytic growth of well-differentiated squamous epithelium that invades the underlying stroma as broad sheets of tumor cells with rounded, pushing borders. There are few reports of the cytologic manifestations of these neoplasms in the literature. Because of the well-differentiated nature of the tumors and the minimal cytologic abnormalities noted in the component cells, particularly at the surfaces of the lesions, they are unlikely to be diagnosed on the basis of a cytologic sample. Smears may show no abnormalities or contain only evidence of hyperkeratosis or parakeratosis. In a case described by Ramzy and colleagues,[10] "atypical" squamous cells were reported, whereas dyskaryotic cells, squamous pearls, and anucleate squames were described by DeTorres and Mora.[11]

LYMPHOMAS

Lymphomas rarely involve the uterus or cervix, but both primary and secondary involvement of these tissues has been reported with both large- and small-cell lymphomas of various types.[12,13] Hodgkin disease with cervical involvement has also been reported.[14] Cells diagnostic of either Hodgkin lymphoma or non-Hodgkin lymphoma can be detected in cervical cytologic samples. The cells appear singly and may be present in large numbers. The differential diagnosis includes chronic follicu-

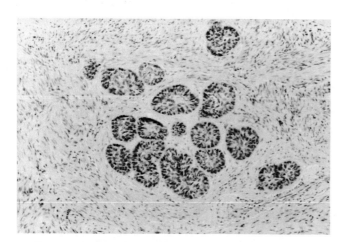

FIG. 8-13. Adenoid basal cell carcinoma of cervix. Hematoxylin and eosin, medium power.

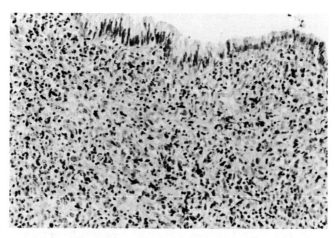

FIG. 8-14. Primary malignant lymphoma of cervix. Hematoxylin and eosin, low power.

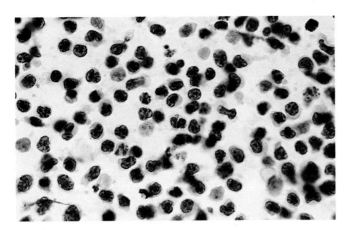

FIG. 8-15. Malignant lymphoma of cervix in cytologic sample.

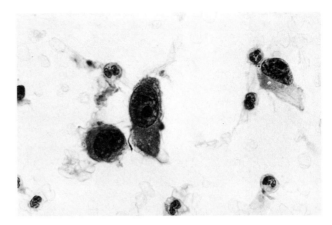

FIG. 8-17. Cytology of vaginal malignant melanoma. Note prominent macronucleoli.

lar (lymphocytic) cervicitis and pseudolymphomatous infiltrates[15] (Figs. 8-14 and 8-15).

MALIGNANT MELANOMAS

Malignant melanomas are also rare primary malignancies in the vagina or cervix (Fig. 8-16). The cytologic features of melanomas at other body sites are well described.[16-18] Because the tumors in the vagina or cervix are similar to those at other sites, the tumor cells are fairly easy to recognize. The cells often appear as single isolated cells rather than as cellular aggregates. They usually have a round to oval configuration, but may also be polygonal or spindle-shaped. Melanin granules are frequently identifiable within the cytoplasm. The nuclei are large and often eccentric, with prominent macronucleoli (Figs. 8-17 and 8-18). Multinucleate or bizarre forms may be present.

VAGINAL ADENOSIS AND CLEAR-CELL CARCINOMA

Glandular-type epithelium is not normally found in the vagina. Its occurrence is referred to as *vaginal adenosis*. Its presence in women other than those exposed to diethylstilbestrol appears to be unusual, but is well documented.[18] The change is most well known, however, for its association with diethylstilbestrol use during pregnancy by mothers of affected young women. In these cases, the reported incidence rate has ranged from 35% to 90%, although the most recent rates have been at the lower end of this spectrum.[19] The vaginal glandular epithelium, which is most commonly detected in young women, usually in their adolescence or early 20s, is gradually replaced by squamous epithelium through the process of squamous metaplasia (Figs. 8-19 and 8-20).

Adenosis is most common in the upper portion of the vagina and is reported to be more frequent on the ante-

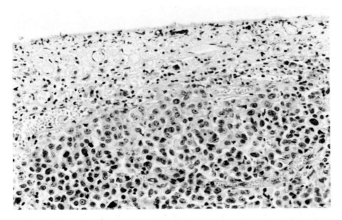

FIG. 8-16. Biopsy section of malignant melanoma of vagina. Hematoxylin and eosin, low power.

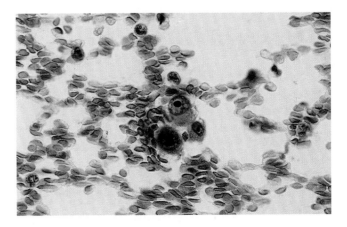

FIG. 8-18. Malignant melanoma.

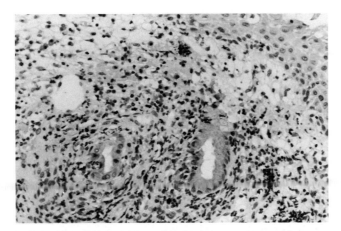

FIG. 8-19. Vaginal adenosis. Endocervical type glands are present within the vaginal stroma. The mucosal surface epithelium is of squamous metaplastic type.

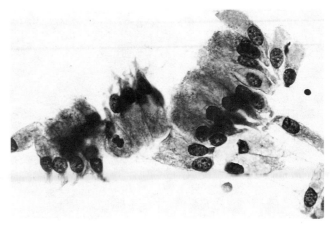

FIG. 8-21. Columnar endocervical mucinous epithelial cells in a vaginal wall scrape originating in adenosis.

rior wall.[20] In order to detect the abnormality on cytology, vaginal scrape specimens are the sample of choice, with care taken to avoid contaminating the specimen with cervical material either from the cervix itself or from the vaginal pool. The use of four-quadrant vaginal wall scrapes, each placed on a separately labeled slide, can aid in identifying the sites of involvement.

Adenosis in these samples is characterized by the presence of columnar glandular cells, similar to those of the cervix, or immature squamous metaplastic cells (Figs. 8-21 and 8-22). Atypia of the glandular epithelium has been described in some cases, but the significance of this finding remains undefined.

Primary clear-cell carcinoma is a very uncommon tumor of the cervix or vagina and is extremely rare in the absence of a history of diethylstilbestrol exposure in utero. In the 1970s, however, a relatively large number of cases of this tumor were reported in the daughters of

mothers who had taken this drug during pregnancy. Although the cases were numerous, the scope of the problem fortunately never reached the size that early data suggested.

This tumor, like the adenosis discussed earlier, primarily occurs in young women who were exposed to diethylstilbestrol in utero (mean age 19 years).[21] Histologically, its appearance is identical to clear-cell carcinoma as it occurs elsewhere in the female genital tract, and is characterized by a solid, tubulocystic, or papillary growth pattern (Fig. 8-23).

On cytology, the tumor cells appear singly or in sheets or clusters of variable size. Sometimes, three-dimensional papillary-like structures are present. The cytoplasm may be clear or finely granular with a pale amphophilic or eosinophilic staining reaction. Cytoplasmic vacuoles may be present. Nuclei are large, vary from round to pleomorphic with irregularly distributed chro-

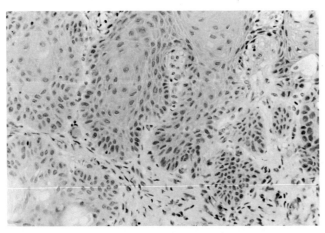

FIG. 8-20. Vaginal adenosis. The glandular type epithelium formerly covering this area of mucosa and extending into the stroma has been replaced by squamous metaplasia.

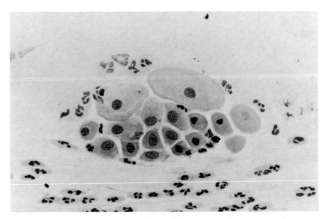

FIG. 8-22. Squamous metaplastic cells in a vaginal wall scrape from a young cyclic patient with adenosis. If contamination of the sample with cervical material can be excluded, this finding is consistent with adenosis.

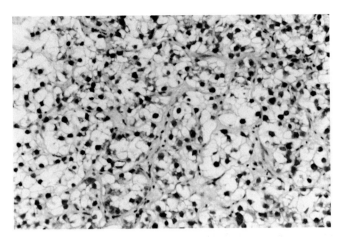

FIG. 8-23. Tissue biopsy specimen of clear cell carcinoma. In addition to this solid pattern, papillary or tubulocystic patterns are commonly seen.

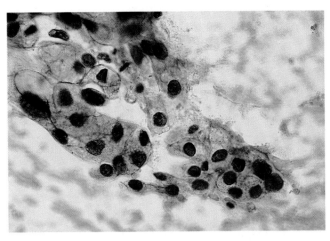

FIG. 8-25. Clear cell carcinoma. The granular eosinophilic cytoplasm is a common feature of clear cell carcinomas in cytologic specimens.

matin, and often have one or more prominent nucleoli[22] (Figs. 8-24 and 8-25).

METASTATIC TUMORS

Malignant tumor cells in samples obtained from the vaginal fornix or cervix are occasionally derived from neoplasms that do not originate in the uterus or vagina. These tumor cells may appear on a cervical or vaginal Papanicolaou smear when tumors that originate elsewhere directly invade the vagina or uterus, or, more commonly, when tumor cells that are shed into the peritoneal cavity are carried into the uterine tubes, through the uterus, and out through the cervical os. In some cases, the presence of these tumor cells on a routine Papanicolaou smear is the first sign of an intraabdominal malignancy. The most common primary site of malig-

nant tumor cells detected in this fashion is the ovary. Less frequently, cells derived from a gastrointestinal or tubal primary tumor are observed. Other primary sites have also been reported. Nearly all these tumors are adenocarcinomas. Their cytologic presentation is characterized by the appearance of tumor cells on a slide preparation with a clean background. The tumor diathesis that is characteristic of cervical primary tumors or the watery diathesis that is seen with endometrial primary adenocarcinomas is generally absent. The exception to this clean background occurs when there is direct invasion into the vagina or uterus. This produces a tumor diathesis similar to that seen in cervical primary neoplasms. The tumors most commonly associated with this pattern of involvement arise in the colon or rectum (Fig. 8-26).

Ovarian cancers make up the majority of the lesions that present as tumor cells on cytologic smears with clean backgrounds. In general, these cells tend to be larger than those associated with the most common types of either

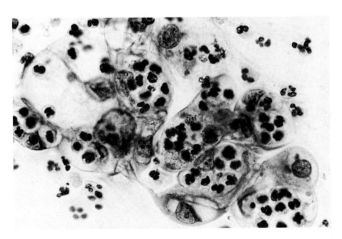

FIG. 8-24. Clear cell carcinoma. The large tumor cells have abundant cytoplasm with numerous intracytoplasmic neutrophils and pleomorphic nuclei.

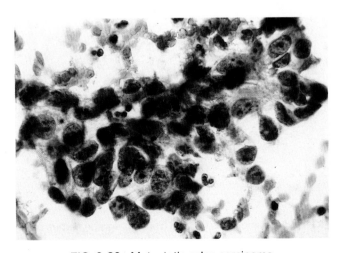

FIG. 8-26. Metastatic colon carcinoma.

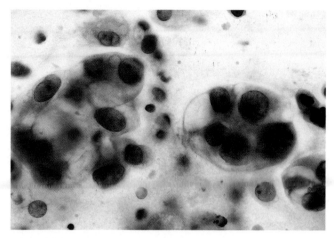

FIG. 8-27. Metastatic high-grade ovarian adenocarcinoma with clear cell features.

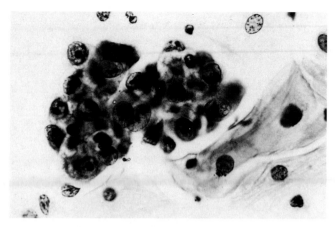

FIG. 8-29. Poorly differentiated ovarian adenocarcinoma cells. Clean slide background is typical with "metastatic" tumors.

endometrial or endocervical adenocarcinoma. They are found in tight, three-dimensional clusters or ball-like arrangements and generally have prominent and conspicuous macronucleoli. The number of tumor cells present is quite variable, and in some cases, only one or two clusters may be observed on an entire slide (Figs. 8-27 through 8-29). Psammoma bodies may be identified in association with papillary serous neoplasms. It should be noted, however, that the presence of psammoma bodies alone is not pathognomonic evidence of an ovarian neoplasm, either benign or malignant. Psammoma bodies are also associated with primary serous tumors of the uterus and with benign lesions such as mesothelial hyperplasia, benign papillary tumors of the ovary, and other benign conditions.[23–27]

Primary tubal neoplasms shed cells that are similar in appearance to cells of serous ovarian lesions (Fig. 8-30).

These types of neoplasms cannot be readily distinguished purely on a cytologic basis, but a tubal primary tumor should be considered when adenocarcinoma cells of this type are detected on a cervical or vaginal smear and there is no evidence of a neoplasm in the uterus or ovaries. One must also consider, however, that ovarian primary tumors can occur with normal-size ovaries, and that primary peritoneal papillary carcinomas do exist. These also have a similar cytologic appearance.

Transitional cell carcinomas of the bladder or urethra may secondarily involve the vagina, sometimes in a pagetoid manner, and present with malignant cells in a vaginal smear (Fig. 8-31). In this situation, confusion with the cytologic presentation of a squamous intraepithelial lesion or an invasive squamous carcinoma is possible. The possibility of pagetoid involvement of the vagina should be considered in any patient with a history of

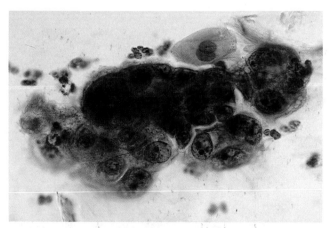

FIG. 8-28. Tumor cells derived from high-grade serous ovarian carcinoma in a cervical smear sample.

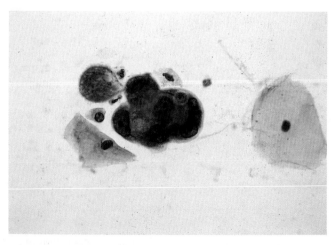

FIG. 8-30. Tumor cells derived from tubal adenocarcinoma.

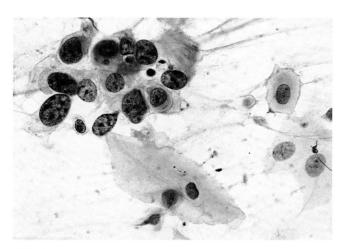

FIG. 8-31. Transitional cell carcinoma metastatic to vagina.

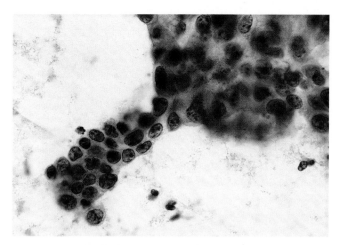

FIG. 8-32. Glandular tumor cells from malignant mixed Müllerian tumor of the uterus.

transitional cell carcinoma who has a positive Papanicolaou smear and no evident lesions by colposcopic examination.

MIXED MÜLLERIAN TUMORS AND SARCOMAS

Mixed müllerian tumors and pure sarcomas are rare as primary neoplasms of the cervix or vagina, but arise more commonly as primary tumors of the uterine corpus. Their primary diagnosis or detection by means of cytopathology is relatively uncommon, but these tumors do shed cells that may be found in routine cytologic samples from the cervix. There are a number of detailed discussions of the cytologic features of these neoplasms in the literature.[28–34]

Malignant mixed müllerian tumors are neoplasms that consist of a combination of malignant epithelial and mesenchymal elements. The epithelial component may be of glandular or squamous differentiation and can resemble that of any of the common neoplasms of müllerian epithelium. The mesenchymal component consists of sarcomatous elements homologous with tissue normally found in the uterus (ie, smooth muscle or stromal cells), or heterologous elements such as chondrosarcoma, osteogenic sarcoma, or some combination of these. These tumors, which typically occur in women beyond the sixth decade of life, are aggressive neoplasms with a poor prognosis.

Pure uterine sarcomas are usually either leiomyosarcomas or stromal sarcomas. Other patterns of differentiation are encountered, but are rare. Embryonal rhabdomyosarcoma, which is one of the more common examples, presents as a botryoid tumor (sarcoma botryoides) of the vagina in young girls. These tumors, which are classically described as grossly resembling a bunch

of grapes, are composed of small malignant tumor cells, typically aggregated in a layered arrangement below the epithelial surface overlying the neoplasm.

Malignant mixed müllerian tumors and pure uterine sarcomas both tend to present in routine cytologic samples as sparse populations of isolated tumor cells. This reflects the fact that the neoplasms most commonly arise within the fundus, and cytologic detection depends on spontaneous shedding rather than direct sampling of the tumors by cervical scrapers or brushes. Because the neoplasms are frequently large and partially necrotic, a tumor diathesis may be present. In the case of mixed müllerian tumors, the cytologic findings may reflect their biphasic nature, with both sarcomatous and epithelial elements being present (Figs. 8-32 and 8-33). The epithelial component of these tumors cytologically resembles the cells of pure epithelial tumors of the uterus. Cells derived from sarcomas or sarcomatous components of

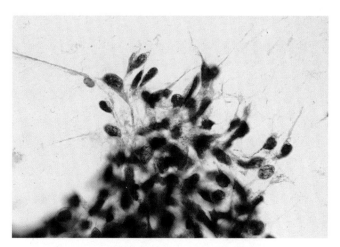

FIG. 8-33. Tumor cells with sarcomatous differentiation from malignant mixed Müllerian tumor of the uterus.

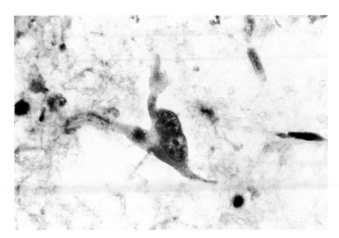

FIG. 8-34. Leiomysarcoma of uterus.

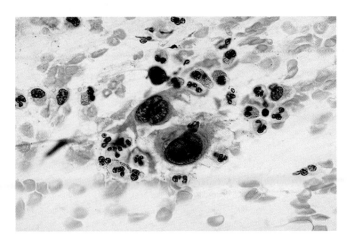

FIG. 8-36. Malignant fibrous histiocytoma, cervical primary.

uterine neoplasms vary in their appearance with the nature of the tumor. Because these neoplasms are often poorly differentiated, however, the two components may not be clearly distinguishable.

Leiomyosarcomas often present cytologically as spindle-shaped or elongated cells with pale, cyanophilic cytoplasm. The nuclei of these cells vary in appearance with the grades of the tumors (Fig. 8-34). Low-grade neoplasms may have relatively bland-appearing, oval to elongated nuclei with moderate hyperchromasia. In higher-grade neoplasms, the nuclei are more irregular in configuration, with marked hyperchromasia and coarse chromatin. Nucleoli are generally prominent, and irregular macronucleoli may be present.

Stromal sarcomas of low grade are characterized by relatively small cells with a high nuclear-to-cytoplasmic ratio and round to oval, hyperchromatic nuclei. Nucleoli are generally evident, but are not necessarily prominent. These single cells may be difficult to distinguish

from other small-cell neoplasms, including malignant lymphoma.

High-grade uterine sarcomas of any type are difficult to distinguish from one another in cytologic samples. Short of finding typical rhabdomyoblasts or cross-striations in tumor cells, the diagnosis of high-grade malignant neoplasm suggestive of uterine sarcoma may be as precise as one can be. High-grade sarcomas are often characterized by markedly pleomorphic cells with bizarre nuclei. Multinucleate tumor giant cells may also be present, and in cervical samples, their identification is strongly suggestive of a sarcomatous process (Figs. 8-35 and 8-36). The differential diagnosis of uterine sarcomas on a cytologic basis includes benign and malignant trophoblastic elements, markedly atypical reparative reactions, malignant melanoma, and some variants of squamous cell carcinoma.

The cells of embryonal rhabdomyosarcomas resemble other small, round-cell tumors seen in children. Their

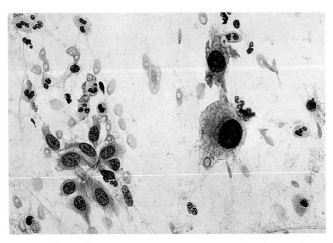

FIG. 8-35. Malignant fibrous histiocytoma, cervical primary.

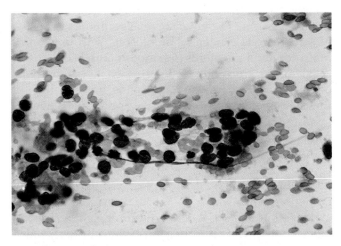

FIG. 8-37. Embryonal rhabdomyosarcoma. Note scant eosinophilic cytoplasm and small hyperchromatic nuclei.

characteristics have been more commonly described in other types of specimens, particularly fine-needle aspirates. They have small, hyperchromatic nuclei and relatively scant cytoplasm, which may be elongated and tapered. Nucleoli may be evident (Fig. 8-37).

GESTATIONAL TROPHOBLASTIC DISEASE

Gestational trophoblastic disease includes complete and partial hydatidiform mole, invasive mole, placental site trophoblastic tumor, and choriocarcinoma. All variants develop from an abnormal proliferation of trophoblastic cells. A detailed discussion of the histologic and clinical pathologic features of these neoplasms can be found in standard reference texts.[32,35] In brief, complete hydatidiform mole is an abnormal trophoblastic proliferation that is androgenic in origin, usually occurring when an empty egg is fertilized by a single sperm, which then divides. This results in a 46 XX phenotype. A partial mole is a result of trisomy, in which a single egg is fertilized by two sperm. Complete hydatidiform mole is characterized by molar changes involving all chorionic villi and trophoblastic hyperplasia of varying degrees. Partial moles show similar changes, but only a portion of the villi are involved. A small proportion of cases of complete hydatidiform mole are followed by the development of choriocarcinoma. However, partial moles seldom, if ever, evolve into malignancy.

Choriocarcinomas are characterized by a malignant proliferation of both syncytial trophoblastic and cytotrophoblastic elements, with myometrial invasion, hemorrhage, and necrosis as typical features of the tumors. They are distinguished from invasive moles by the absence of the villi that characterize the latter lesions.

Placental site trophoblastic tumor is an unusual neoplasm that appears to originate from the intermediate

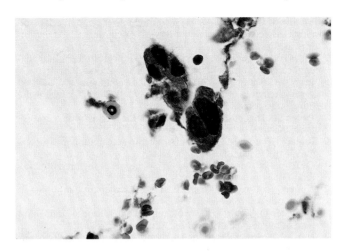

FIG. 8-39. Atypical trophoblastic cells from a patient with choriocarcinoma.

type of trophoblastic cell. It develops as a solid infiltrative neoplasm of polygonal cells without identifiable syncytial trophoblastic elements that invade between smooth muscle bundles of the uterine wall, resembling an exaggeration of the usual placental site reaction. This tumor, which was originally believed to be a benign proliferation, is now known to metastasize and behave aggressively in some patients.

Cytologic samples from patients with hydatidiform mole may contain syncytial trophoblasts, which can be impossible to distinguish from the similar cells sometimes encountered in smears from women with normal pregnancies. The nuclei, however, may be somewhat more hyperchromatic. Cytotrophoblastic cells may also be present (Fig. 8-38).

In cases of choriocarcinoma, atypical syncytial trophoblastic and cytotrophoblastic elements may be seen, along with evidence of necrosis and hemorrhage. Although some of the cells may be indistinguishable from the trophoblastic cells of normal pregnancy or hydatidiform mole, other bizarre-appearing tumor giant cells with marked pleomorphism and macronucleoli are typically present[36] (Fig. 8-39).

REFERENCES

1. Stoler MH, Mills SE, Gersell DJ, et al. Small-cell neuroendocrine carcinoma of the cervix. A human papillomavirus type 18-associated cancer. Am J Surg Pathol 1991;15:28.
2. Ng ABP, Reagan JW. The pathology and cytopathology of squamous cell carcinoma of the uterine cervix. In Wied GL, Keebler CM, Koss LG, et al (eds). Compendium on diagnostic cytology, 6th ed. Chicago: Tutorials of Cytology, 1988:123.
3. Alborees-Saavedra J, Rodriguez-Martinez HA, Larraza-Hernandez O. Carcinoid tumor of the cervix. Pathol Annu 1979;14:273.
4. Mackay B, Osborne BM, Wharton JT. Small cell tumor of the cervix with neuroendocrine features: ultra structural observation in two cases. Cancer 1979;43:1138.
5. Warner TF. Carcinoid tumor of the cervix. J Clin Pathol 1978;31:990.

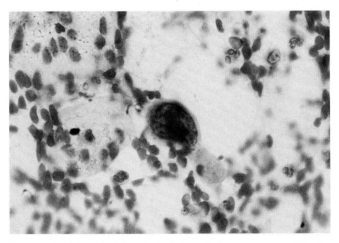

FIG. 8-38. Atypical trophobalstic cell from a case of hydatidiform mole. Note the hyperchromasia and coarse chromatin. (Courtesy of Dr. Yener Erozan).

6. Mullins JD, Hilliard GD. Cervical carcinoid (agyrophil cell carcinoma) associated with an endocervical carcinoma: a light and ultrastructural study. Cancer 1981;47:785.

7. Miles PA, Herrera GA, Mena H, et al. Cytologic findings in malignant carcinoid tumor of the cervix. Acta Cytol 1985;29:1003.

8. Ferry JA, Scully RE. "Adenoid cystic" carcinoma and adenoid basal carcinoma of the uterine cervix. A study of 28 cases. Am J Surg Pathol 1988;12:134.

9. Patten SF. Diagnostic cytopathology of the uterine cervix, 2nd ed. Basel: Karger, 1978:273.

10. Ramzy I, Smout MS, Collins JA. Verrucous carcinoma of the vagina. Am J Clin Pathol 1976;65:644.

11. DeTorres EF, Mora A. Verrucous carcinoma of the cervix uteri: a report of a case. Act Cytol 1981;25:307.

12. Komaki R, Cox JD, Hansen PM, et al. Malignant lymphoma of the uterine cervix. Cancer 1984;54:1699.

13. Whitaker D. The role of cytology in the detection of malignant lymphoma of the uterine cervix. Acta Cytol 1976;20:510.

14. Harris NL, Scully RE. Malignant lymphoma and granulocytic sarcoma of the uterus and vagina. Cancer 1984;53:2530.

15. Hajdu SI, Salvino A. Cytologic diagnosis of malignant melanoma. Acta Cytol 1973;17:320.

16 Masubichi S, Nagai I, Hirata M, et al. Cytologic studies of malignant melanoma of the vagina. Acta Cytol 1975;19:527.

17. Yu HC, Ketabchi M. Detection of malignant melanoma of the uterine cervix from Papanicolaou smears: a case report. Acta Cytol 1987;31:73.

18. Sandburg EC. The incidence and distribution of occult vaginal adenosis. Am J Obstet Gynecol 1968;101:322.

19. Reagan JW, Ng ABP. Vaginal and vulvar disease. In Wied GL, Keebler CM, Koss LG, et al (eds). Compendium on diagnostic cytology, 7th ed. Chicago: Tutorials of Cytology, 1992:167.

20. Ng ABP, Reagan JW, Nadji M, et al. Natural history of vaginal adenosis in women exposed to diethylstilbestrol in utero. J Reprod Med 1977;18:1.

21. Herbst AL, Noruses MJ, Rosenow PJ, et al. An analysis of 346 cases of clear cell carcinoma of the vagina and cervix with emphasis on recurrence and survival. Gynecol Oncol 1979;7:111.

22. Taft PD, Robboy SJ, Herbst AL, et al. Cytology of clear cell adenocarcinoma of the female genital tract in young females: review of 95 cases from the registry. Acta Cytol 1973;18:279.

23. Kirkland N, Hardy N. Psammoma bodies found in cervicovaginal smears. Acta Cytol 1979;23:131.

24. Picoff RC, Meeker CI. Psammoma bodies in the cervicovaginal smear in association with benign papillary structures of the ovary. Acta Cytol 1970;14:45.

25. Dance EF, Fullmer CD. Extrauterine carcinoma cells observed in cervicovaginal smears. Acta Cytol 1970;14:187.

26. Rubin DK, Frost JK. The cytologic detection of ovarian cancer. Acta Cytol 1963;7:191.

27. Ng ABP, Teeple D, Lindner EA, et al. The cellular manifestations of extrauterine cancer. Acta Cytol 1974;18:108.

28. Hajdu S, Hajdu EO. Cytopathology of sarcomas and other nonepithelial tumors. Philadelphia: WB Saunders, 1976:183.

29. Parker JE. Cytologic findings associated with previous uterine malignancies of mixed cell types (malignant mixed mullerian tumor). Acta Cytol 1964;8:316.

30. Massoni EA, Hajdu SI. Cytology of primary and metastatic uterine sarcomas. Acta Cytol 1984;28:93.

31. Becker SN, Wong JY. Detection of endometrial stromal sarcoma in cervicovaginal smears. Report of 3 cases. Acta Cytol 1980;25:272.

32. Mazur MT, Kurman RJ. Gestational trophoblastic disease. In Kurman RJ (ed). Blaustein's pathology of the female genital tract, 3rd ed. New York: Springer-Verlag, 1987:835.

33. Bonfiglio TA, Patten SF, Woodworth FE. Fibroxanthosarcoma of the uterine cervix: cytopathologic and histopathologic manifestations. Acta Cytol 1976;20:501.

34. Patten SF, Patten FW, Bonfiglio TA. Cytopathology of uterine sarcomas. In Wied GL, Keebler CM, Koss LG, et al (eds). Compendium on diagnostic cytology, 6th ed. Chicago: Tutorials of Cytology, 1988:228.

35. Scully R, Bonfiglio TA, Kurman RJ, et al. Histologic typing of female genital tract tumors. New York: Springer-Verlag, 1994:32.

36. Taki I, Kashimura Y. Cytology of hydatidiform mole, invasive mole and choriocarcinoma. In Wied GL, Keebler CM, Koss LG, et al (eds). Compendium on diagnostic cytology, 7th ed. Chicago: Tutorials of Cytology, 1992:155.

Gynecologic Cytopathology. Edited by
Thomas A. Bonfiglio and Yener S. Erozan.
Lippincott–Raven Publishers, Philadelphia, © 1997.

CHAPTER 9

Fine-Needle Aspiration Cytology of the Ovary

Mehrdad Nadji and Parvin Ganjei

Fine-needle aspiration cytology is now well established as a simple and reliable method for the diagnosis of human tumors detected by palpation or imaging techniques. Its use in gynecology, however, has been limited to the occasional diagnosis of pelvic masses.[1–12] Unlike most gynecologic tumors, which are accessible to direct biopsy, ovarian masses are located in the pelvis or abdomen and can be reached only by laparoscopy or laparotomy. It appears, therefore, that fine-needle aspiration may be an ideal alternative to those traditional invasive diagnostic procedures. In fact, as a primary diagnostic tool, aspiration cytology has been employed successfully in the evaluation of ovarian tumors because it can provide information regarding their benign or malignant nature, cell type, and, sometimes, degree of histologic differentiation.[2–11] On the other hand, most clinicians prefer to investigate pelvic masses by exploratory laparotomy, followed by direct biopsy or surgical excision. In such cases, there appears to be no reason for performing a preoperative needle aspiration, particularly if the tumor is cystic and one fears perforation and spillage of tumor cells by the needle. However, spread of an ovarian neoplasm as a result of fine-needle aspiration, as cautioned by some authors,[13] has not been documented clinically or pathologically.[1–6,10–12,14–16]

Because of its simplicity, accuracy, and relatively atraumatic nature, fine-needle aspiration cytology is an ideal diagnostic procedure in patients with nonneoplastic pelvic masses, especially functional cysts, endometriosis, and inflammatory processes.[6] Similarly, aspiration cytology is of a great value in the follow-up of patients with ovarian malignancies who have undergone surgery with or without irradiation and chemotherapy.[10,11] In this group of patients, it can be used as an alternative to the traditional "second-look" surgery, with its associated morbidity. In addition to cytomorphologic evaluation, aspirated material can be used for a variety of ancillary studies, including immunocytochemistry and molecular biologic procedures.[17]

TECHNICAL ASPECTS

Ovarian masses can be aspirated directly or indirectly. Direct aspiration of ovarian neoplasms is accomplished by sampling the mass during surgery or at the time of laparoscopy.[4] Indirect aspiration is performed by the transvaginal, transrectal, or transabdominal approach.[1–7] Transrectal and transvaginal aspiration are performed using a Franzen needle guide.[2,3,6,11,12] Prior sedation or mild anesthesia may be necessary. The aspiration is carried out using a syringe holder and 22-gauge needles of appropriate lengths. The use of back-and-forth and lateral movements of the needle while maintaining a negative pressure increases the cellular yield.[11,12]

The aspirated material is spread over several glass slides that are fixed immediately in alcohol or sprayed with a spray fixative. Cytocentrifugation is used when fluid is aspirated from cystic masses or ascites. We prefer the Papanicolaou staining method, a rapid version of which can be completed in less than 5 minutes. In addition to preserving cell morphology, rapid fixation preserves cellular substances for subsequent cytochemistry or immunocytochemistry in the event they are needed.[17]

CYTOLOGIC INTERPRETATION

The female pelvis is a complex multiorgan region that is often the seat of a diverse group of pathologic processes, including inflammation, endometriosis, cysts, and a number of benign and malignant neoplasms. The ovary itself may be the site of a variety of primary and

---

M. Nadji: University of Miami School of Medicine, Miami, Florida 33101.

P. Ganjei: University of Miami School of Medicine, Miami, Florida 33101.

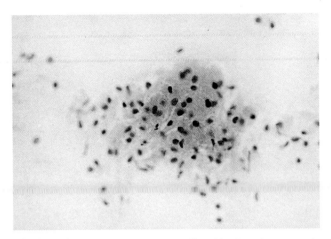

FIG. 9-1. Corpus luteum. Large cells with abundant granular eosinophilic cytoplasm and small nuclei. Papanicolaou, ×100.

secondary neoplasms, each further categorized by cell type and histologic grade. Accurate interpretation of fine-needle aspirates from the female pelvis, therefore, requires intimate familiarity with the histology and cytology of a wide range of pathologic processes. Furthermore, for correct evaluation of needle aspirates from the female pelvis, it is necessary to have an adequate cell sample, optimal fixation and staining, and, most importantly, pertinent clinical information. Knowledge of the patient's age, the laparoscopic and sonographic findings, the exact site of aspiration, and the patient's history of prior malignancy and treatment is essential. Therefore, close communication between the clinician and the pathologist is the basis for optimal utilization of aspiration cytology in the evaluation of ovarian lesions.[6,12]

In this chapter, we first examine the cytomorphology of the normal ovary and its nonneoplastic disorders, then review the aspiration cytology of common ovarian neoplasms. For a more detailed description of the cytomorphology of ovarian tumors, the reader is referred to several recent publications.[7–12,16,18,19]

NORMAL OVARY

Because of their relatively small size and compact nature, normal ovaries are rarely aspirated. On the route to adjacent pelvic masses, however, the needle may occasionally pass through an ovary and sample its normal cellular elements, which may be derived from stroma or epithelium. Aspirated ovarian stroma is usually composed of a few isolated cells with elongated nuclei containing dense chromatin. Cytoplasm, when present, is scant and pale-staining. Cells derived from ovarian surface epithelium are commonly arranged in small sheets with well-defined cytoplasmic borders and uniform oval

nuclei.[11,12] Binucleation and prominent nucleoli may be seen if the surface epithelium is irritated.

Cells from ovarian follicles are arranged in small groups and have round nuclei; scant, pale-staining cytoplasm; and indistinct cellular borders. Degenerated follicular cells of atretic follicles have pyknotic nuclei and vacuolated cytoplasm. Cells derived from corpora lutea have abundant granular eosinophilic cytoplasm; small, eccentrically located nuclei; and indistinct cell borders (Fig. 9-1).

In transvaginal and transrectal aspirates, nonovarian mesenchymal and epithelial elements are commonly present. Fibroadipose tissue, smooth and skeletal muscle, and segments of blood vessels may also be found. More commonly, epithelial elements of vaginal and colonic mucosa are sampled. Both mesothelial and urothelial cells may also appear in pelvic aspirates. An inexperienced observer may occasionally confuse the cytomorphology of normal and reactive transitional epithelium with a neoplastic process.[12]

NONNEOPLASTIC LESIONS

The most common nonneoplastic lesions of the ovary that may produce masses are cysts, inflammation, and endometriosis. Nonneoplastic cysts of the ovary include follicular and corpus luteum cysts, as well as various epithelial cysts arising from mesonephric or müllerian inclusions.[11,12]

Laparoscopically and ultrasonically guided aspiration cytology has assumed an important role in the management of nonneoplastic cysts of the ovary in recent years.[18–21] These lesions are usually discovered in women of reproductive age during pregnancy or the postpartum period,[15] at the time of infertility work-up, or, occasion-

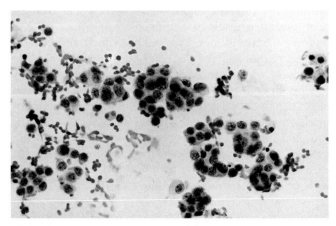

FIG. 9-2. Follicular cyst. Large number of cells, arranged in small groups, showing hyperchromatic nuclei with moderate pleomorphism. Papanicolaou, ×100.

ally, in the course of egg retrieval in patients undergoing in vitro fertilization.[22] Aspirates from follicular or luteinized follicular cysts contain proteinaceous fluid with or without red blood cells. In addition to isolated or small groups of cells resembling those aspirated from maturing follicles, they may contain abundant cells arranged in "cell balls" or small papillary clusters showing enlarged nuclei, prominent nucleoli, or chromocenters and indistinct cytoplasmic borders (Fig. 9-2). Mitotic figures may also be seen (Fig. 9-3). These morphologic features may be misinterpreted as evidence of malignancy and lead to unnecessary oophorectomy in a relatively young patient.[20,23,24] The combination of the clinical history, including the patient's age, and the benign appearance of the cyst on laparoscopy and sonography (small [less than 5 cm], unilocular, thin-walled, and lacking solid areas) should alert the pathologist to the nonneoplastic nature of the cyst.[23]

Aspirates from pelvic inflammatory disorders show a spectrum of inflammatory cells with or without necrosis. Causative organisms are rarely identified unless a portion of the aspirate is used for microbiologic studies. Endometriosis of the pelvic adnexa may also be mass-forming and, hence, subject to needle aspiration. The unequivocal diagnosis of endometriosis is made only when endometrial epithelial cells are identified in such aspirates (Fig. 9-4). These cells are often small, with scant cytoplasm and uniform, darkly stained, round nuclei.[8,11,12] They form loose aggregates with indistinguishable cell borders. Prior treatment with hormones changes the size and shape of endometrial cells. Endometrial stromal cells are less commonly found in needle aspirates of pelvic endometriosis. Fresh and lysed blood and hemosiderin-laden macrophages are commonly present in aspirates from endometriotic cysts.

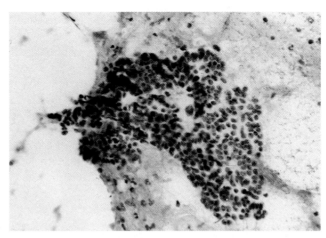

FIG. 9-4. Pelvic endometriosis. A loose cluster of endometrial epithelial cells with indistinguishable cytoplasmic borders on a background of fresh and lysed blood. Few hemosiderin-laden macrophages are also present. Papanicolaou, ×100.

NEOPLASMS OF THE OVARY

Ovarian neoplasms are a heterogeneous group of benign and malignant tumors of epithelial, stromal, and germ-cell origin. A number of secondary malignancies, such as metastatic carcinomas and malignant lymphomas, may also involve the ovaries. Because of this diversity, cytologic interpretation of needle aspirates from ovarian neoplasms is both interesting and challenging. The challenge resides not only in recognizing the ovarian neoplasm in the cytologic sample, but also in classifying it as benign or malignant and categorizing it further into a specific cell type.[11,12] It is evident, therefore, that only better-differentiated neoplasms lend themselves to cytologic subclassification. It is extremely difficult to subtype high-grade malignant neoplasms of the ovary accurately unless they are associated with better-differentiated components.[10,11]

Epithelial Neoplasms

Common epithelial tumors of the ovary include serous, mucinous, endometrioid, clear-cell, and Brenner types. Each cell type may form a benign (adenoma), borderline (low malignant potential), or malignant (carcinoma) neoplasm.

Fine-needle aspirates from *benign serous tumors* (serous cystadenomas and cystadenofibromas) may contain a few clusters of tightly packed, small cells forming sheets or simple papillary structures. Serous epithelial cells have a high nuclear-to-cytoplasmic ratio, hyperchromatic nuclei, and scant cytoplasm. There is usually a pale-staining eosinophilic and granular fluid in the slide background, containing a few histiocytes (Fig. 9-5). These cells probably represent previously desquamated

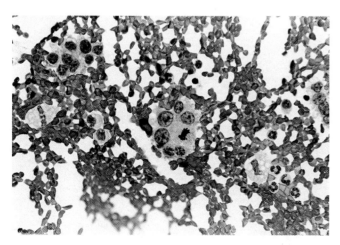

FIG. 9-3. Follicular cyst. Small groups of atypical follicular cells with a prominent mitotic figure. The smear also contains histiocytes, neutrophils, and numerous red blood cells. Papanicolaou, ×100.

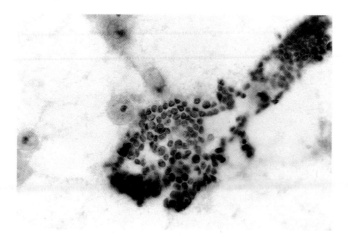

FIG. 9-5. Serous cystadenoma of the ovary. A sheet of tightly packed small cells with darkly stained nuclei and scanty cytoplasm. The histiocytic cells represent previously desquamated epithelial cells and may be the only elements found in the cyst fluid. Papanicolaou, ×100.

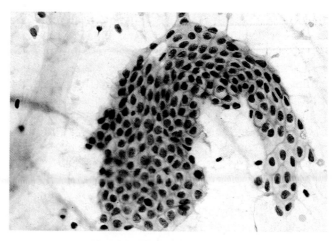

FIG. 9-7. Mucinous cystadenoma. Sheet of uniform cells with oval nuclei and abundant clear cytoplasms and well-defined cytoplasmic borders. Slide background contains mucin. Papanicolaou, ×100.

serous epithelial cells from the cyst lining and, at times, may be the only cellular elements found in the aspirates from benign serous cysts. In the aspirates from *serous tumors of low malignant potential,* the number of cells and the size of cellular aggregates increases. Papillary structures are also more complex and display frequent branching (Fig. 9-6). Although the nuclei may be larger and show slight pleomorphism, the overall morphology of the individual cells closely resembles that of benign serous tumors. In our experience, it is extremely difficult to separate epithelial tumors of low malignant potential from well-differentiated carcinomas.[10,11] Cells derived from *serous carcinomas* arrange themselves in large sheets and papillary groups with prominent branching. The cells are small, with scant cyanophilic cytoplasm and hyperchromatic nuclei with irregularly distributed,

coarsely granular chromatin. Nucleoli are not prominent. Nuclear size and pleomorphism increase with decreasing differentiation. Psammoma bodies may be found in serous tumors, but their presence is neither diagnostic of malignancy nor pathognomonic of serous neoplasms.[12]

Aspirates from mucinous tumors of the ovary contain variable amounts of mucin, which forms a film on the slide background and, depending on its thickness, stains anywhere from pale basophilic to eosinophilic with the Papanicolaou stain. *Mucinous cystadenomas* usually yield a limited number of uniform cells arranged in small sheets with a honeycomb appearance.[11,12] The cells have well-defined cytoplasmic borders, uniform round or oval nuclei, and abundant clear cytoplasm (Fig. 9-7). The chromatin is finely granular and micronucleoli may be

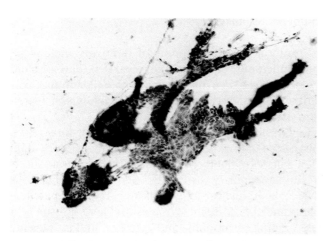

FIG. 9-6. Serous ovarian tumor of low malignant potential. Papillary group of tightly packed small cells with hyperchromatic nuclei and scanty cytoplasms. Papanicolaou, ×25.

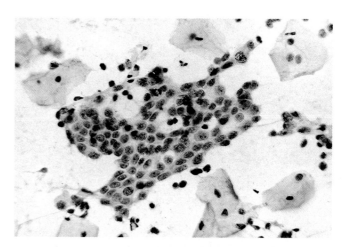

FIG. 9-8. Well-differentiated mucinous adenocarcinoma. In comparison to figure 9-7, the organized honeycomb arrangement of cells is lost. Mature squamous cells represent contamination in this transvaginal aspiration. Papanicolaou, ×100.

present. In well-differentiated *mucinous adenocarcinomas,* the nuclei are larger, have prominent nucleoli, and show frequent overlapping; hence, the organized honeycomb arrangement of the cells is lost (Fig. 9-8). As with serous tumors, the separation of well-differentiated mucinous carcinomas from tumors of low malignant potential is extremely difficult using cytology alone.

The overall morphology of cells derived from *endometrioid tumors* of the ovary is similar to that of mucinous neoplasms except for their cytoplasm, which is granular and eosinophilic (Fig. 9-9). Their abundant cytoplasm and nuclear characteristics distinguish endometrioid tumors from serous neoplasms. Endometrioid neoplasms may have squamous elements. In aspiration cytology, the glandular and squamous elements may appear in continuity with each other or in different areas of the slide.[12]

The cytomorphology of *clear-cell tumors* of the ovary is similar to that of their counterparts in the vagina and cervix. The cells are large and contain abundant, granular, pale-staining cytoplasm and pleomorphic nuclei with irregular folding of the nuclear membrane (Fig. 9-10). Peripheral protrusion of nuclei at the edges of cell groups gives the clusters a "hobnail" appearance.[11,12]

Brenner tumors of the ovary are seldom aspirated, which may be a consequence of their usually small size. If aspirated, the epithelial elements appear as small sheets of polygonal cells with a moderate amount of cytoplasm and uniformly oval nuclei. Stromal elements, if present, appear as isolated bare nuclei. Cytologic separation of *malignant Brenner tumors* of the ovary from transitional cell carcinomas of the urothelium is not possible without knowledge of the patient's clinical history.

Aspirates from *malignant mixed mesodermal tumors* of the ovary may contain epithelial and mesenchymal elements in variable proportions (Fig. 9-11). The epithe-

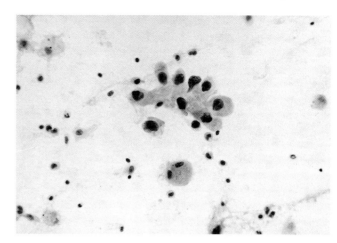

FIG. 9-10. Clear cell carcinoma of the ovary. Small group of epithelial cells with abundant cytoplasms and pleomorphic, darkly stained nuclei are arranged in a "hobnail-like" fashion. Papanicolaou, ×100.

lial elements are usually poorly differentiated carcinomas. The mesenchymal components cannot be specifically subtyped unless there is chondroid, smooth, or skeletal muscle differentiation. Sarcomatous cells are large and have pleomorphic nuclei and prominent nucleoli. They may occur singly or in tissue fragments with indistinct cytoplasmic borders.[11,12]

Sex Cord—Stromal Tumors

Fine-needle aspirates from *thecomas* of the ovary characteristically contain only a few isolated, dark-staining, spindle-shaped nuclei resembling those of normal ovarian stroma. Interlacing bundles of nuclei may be seen if small tissue fragments are aspirated.[11] The slide background often exhibits granular, eosinophilic mate-

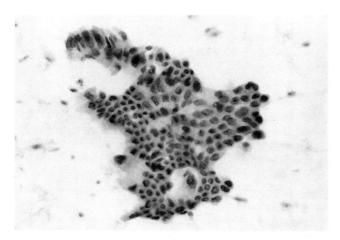

FIG. 9-9. Well-differentiated endometrioid adenocarcinoma. The overall morphology of the cells is similar to mucinous carcinoma except for the cytoplasm, which is granular and eosinophilic. Papanicolaou, ×100.

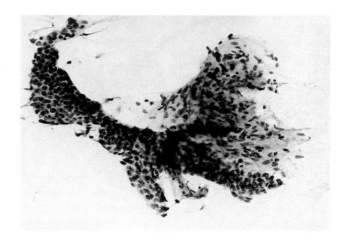

FIG. 9-11. Malignant mixed mesodermal tumor of the ovary. Group of moderately differentiated adenocarcinoma cells (left) and sarcomatous elements (upper right) are seen in continuity of each other. Papanicolaou, ×50.

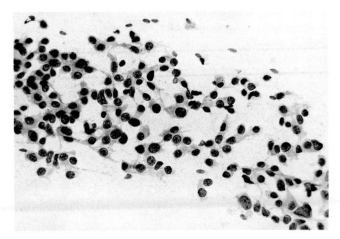

FIG. 9-12. Sertoli-Leydig cell tumor of the ovary. Isolated and small groups of cells with round, slightly pleomorphic nuclei and pale staining cytoplasms. Papanicolaou, ×100.

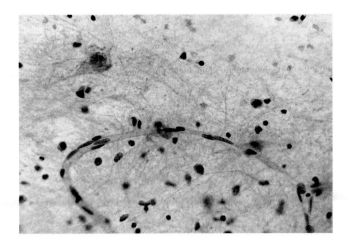

FIG. 9-14. Mature teratoma of the ovary. Glial tissue, a segment of capillary, and a single ganglion cell (upper left) are seen. Papanicolaou, ×100.

rial. Aspirates from luteinized thecomas may show groups of cells with ill-defined eosinophilic cytoplasm and oval nuclei.

Aspirates from *granulosa cell and Sertoli-Leydig cell tumors* of the ovary characteristically contain abundant cells arranged in small groups or isolated forms (Figs. 9-12 and 9-13). The nuclei are uniformly round to oval with finely granular chromatin and micronucleoli. Focal nuclear pleomorphism is occasionally seen (see Fig. 9-12). The cytoplasm is pale-staining and cell borders are usually ill-defined. Depending on the type and differentiation of the tumor, cellular arrangements such as cords, acini, or tubules may be seen. In well-differentiated granulosa cell tumors, cellular groupings suggestive of Call-Exner bodies may be present (see Fig. 9-13). On the basis of aspiration cytology, we are unable to differentiate granulosa cell and Sertoli-Leydig cell tumors.[10–12] The

cytology of ovarian carcinoids may resemble that of sex cord tumors. In carcinoids, however, the cytoplasmic borders are well defined. The nuclei are eccentrically located and contain the characteristic coarsely granular "salt and pepper" chromatin.

Germ-Cell Tumors

Aspirates from *mature cystic teratomas* of the ovary contain a large number of mature squamous cells, many of which are anucleate.[8,11,12] The background may exhibit amorphous amphophilic material suggestive of sebaceous gland secretions. Other types of epithelial cells, such as metaplastic squamous, ciliated columnar, and columnar mucin-producing, may also be present. Less commonly found are mesenchymal elements, including

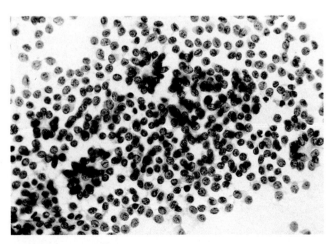

FIG. 9-13. Granulosa cell tumor. Abundant, loosely cohesive cells with round nuclei and indistinct cytoplasmic borders. Cell groupings suggestive of Call-Exner bodies are present. Papanicolaou, ×100.

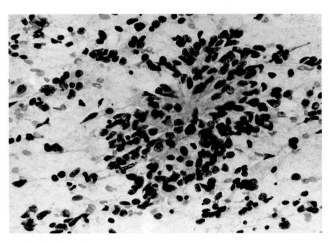

FIG. 9-15. Immature teratoma of the ovary. Primitive neuroepithelial elements are present in isolated forms and in a rosette-like cluster. Papanicolaou, ×100.

adipose tissue, smooth muscle, and glial elements (Fig. 9-14). It should be remembered that a few squamous cells of vaginal epithelial origin are always present in transvaginal pelvic aspirates. It is the presence of numerous isolated anucleate and superficial squamous cells that should raise the possibility of a mature cystic teratoma.[12]

Aspirates from *immature teratomas* may also contain a variety of epithelial cells, but usually in fewer numbers and smaller groups. The background displays granular eosinophilic material and many isolated, dark-staining, naked nuclei. Those cells that represent immature neuroepithelial elements often form loosely bound groups with occasional rosette-like formations (Fig. 9-15).

Dysgerminomas of the ovary frequently yield abundant cells in fine-needle aspirates. These cells occur both in isolation and in loosely cohesive groups. They contain large nuclei with prominent nucleoli and indistinct cytoplasmic borders (Fig. 9-16). Lymphocytes and histiocytes are usually admixed with tumor cells, but their absence does not exclude the diagnosis of a dysgerminoma.[11] Because these neoplasms often show focal necrosis, it is not uncommon for the background to contain necrotic material and inflammatory cells.

Embryonal carcinomas of the ovary are uncommon; aspirates often display a hemorrhagic and necrotic background. They are usually fairly cellular and contain highly abnormal and pleomorphic cells arranged in groups, with an overall pattern resembling that of poorly differentiated adenocarcinoma (Fig. 9-17). Nuclei are large and hyperchromatic, with irregularly distributed, coarsely granular chromatin and macronucleoli. Small nuclear fragments are often superimposed on cellular groups. Trophoblastic and yolk sac elements are difficult to distinguish in cytologic samples of embryonal carcinomas, unless immunocytochemistry is used. The de-

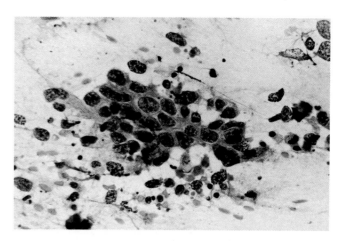

FIG. 9-17. Embryonal carcinoma of the ovary. Poorly differentiated carcinoma cells with large, hyperchromatic nuclei and marked pleomorphism. There is a hemorrhagic and necrotic background. Papanicolaou, ×100.

finitive diagnosis of embryonal carcinoma is difficult to establish on the basis of cytology alone. On the other hand, the combination of a poorly differentiated ovarian carcinoma in a young woman with elevated serum α-fetoprotein and chorionic gonadotropin levels is highly suggestive of an embryonal carcinoma.[12]

Monodermal teratomas of the ovary such as struma ovarii and carcinoid are uncommon tumors and, therefore, rarely encountered in aspirates. The cytomorphology of *ovarian carcinoid* resembles that of endocrine tumors of other organs. The aspirates usually contain abundant cells arranged in small groups or as isolated forms. The eccentric nuclei are uniformly round or oval and display the typical "salt and pepper" chromatin pattern. Cytoplasmic borders are well defined. The cytologic presentation of *strüma ovarii* resembles that of adenomatous goiter or colloid cyst of the thyroid (Fig. 9-18).

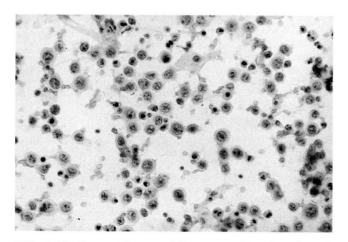

FIG. 9-16. Dysgerminoma of the ovary. Abundant, loosely cohesive cells with large nuclei and prominent nucleoli. Few lymphocytes and histiocytes are also present. Papanicolaou, ×100.

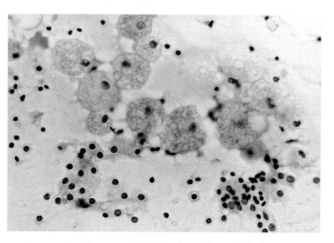

FIG. 9-18. Strüma ovarii. Follicular cells and histiocytes on a background of colloid. This morphology is identical to that seen in an aspirate from a colloid goiter. Papanicolaou, ×100.

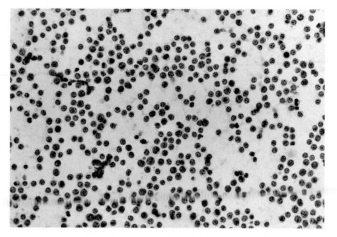

FIG. 9-19. Malignant lymphoma involving the ovary. Abundant, isolated, abnormal lymphocytes. Papanicolaou, ×100.

Finally, extragonadal germ-cell tumors may be found anywhere near the midline, including that of the pelvis and retroperitoneum. This possibility should be kept in mind when needle aspirates from sites other than the ovaries display the characteristic cytomorphology of a germ-cell tumor.[11,12]

Secondary Tumors

Most metastatic carcinomas in the ovary are of gastrointestinal or breast origin and, hence, represent adenocarcinomas of variable differentiation. Cytologic classification of these tumors as adenocarcinomas does not usually create a problem. Their identification as metastatic tumors, however, is extremely difficult in aspiration cytology.

Malignant lymphomas in the ovary are usually secondary tumors. The cytologic recognition of extranodal malignant lymphomas is important because it may be difficult to distinguish them from exuberant chronic inflammation or undifferentiated carcinomas. In contrast to inflammatory exudates, malignant lymphomas are composed of uniform populations of abnormal lymphocytes (Fig. 9-19). The isolated, noncohesive arrangement of the cells separates lymphomas from carcinomas and dysgerminomas. Aspirates from the latter may resemble large-cell lymphomas. Unlike lymphoma cells, however, germinoma cells are, at least focally, loosely cohesive.[12]

SUMMARY

Aspiration cytology is a safe, accurate, and cost-effective method of evaluating ovarian lesions. It is particularly helpful in establishing the benign nature of nonneoplastic adnexal cysts in young women. It also is a relatively atraumatic technique for the follow-up of patients with treated ovarian cancer. Cytologic assessment of aspirates from the female pelvis requires experience, and collaboration between the clinician and the pathologist is of utmost importance in the proper evaluation of gynecologic lesions.

REFERENCES

1. Mintz M, Dupre-Froment J, DeBrux J. Ponctions de 94 kystes para-uterins sous coelioscopie et etude cytologique des liquides. Gynaecologia 1967;163:61.
2. Kjellgren O, Angstrom T, Bergman F, et al. Fine needle aspiration biopsy in diagnosis and classification of ovarian carcinoma. Cancer 1971;28:967.
3. Angstrom T, Kjellgren O, Bergman F. The cytologic diagnosis of ovarian tumors by means of aspiration biopsy. Acta Cytol 1972; 16:336.
4. Kovacic J, Rainer S, Levicnik A, et al. Cytology of benign ovarian lesions in connection with laparoscopy. In Zajicek J (ed). Aspiration biopsy cytology, part 2. Cytology of infradiaphragmatic organs. Basel: S Karger, 1979:57.
5. Kjellgren O, Angstrom T. Transvaginal and transrectal aspiration biopsy in diagnosis and classification of ovarian tumors. In Zajicek J (ed). Aspiration biopsy cytology, part 2. Cytology of infradiaphragmatic organs. Basel: S Karger, 1979:80.
6. Sevin B-U, Greening SE, Nadji M, et al. Fine needle aspiration cytology in gynecologic oncology. I. Clinical aspects. Acta Cytol 1979;23:277.
7. Ramzy I, Delaney M. Fine needle aspiration of ovarian masses. I. Correlative cytologic and histologic study of celomic epithelial neoplasms. Acta Cytol 1979;23:97.
8. Nadji M, Greening SE, Sevin B-U, et al. Fine needle aspiration cytology in gynecologic oncology. II. Morphologic aspects. Acta Cytol 1979;23:380.
9. Ganjei P. Fine needle aspiration cytology of the ovary. Clin Lab Med 1995;15:705.
10. Ganjei P, Nadji M. Aspiration cytology of ovarian neoplasms. A review. Acta Cytol 1984;28:329.
11. Nadji M. Aspiration cytology in the diagnosis and assessment of ovarian neoplasms. In Roth LM, Czernobilsky B (eds). Tumors and tumorlike conditions of the ovary. New York: Churchill Livingstone, 1985:153.
12. Nadji M, Sevin BU. Pelvic fine needle aspiration cytology in gynecology. In Linsk JA, Franzen S (eds). Clinical aspiration cytology, 2nd ed. Philadelphia: JB Lippincott, 1989:261.
13. Hajdu SI, Melamed MR. Limitations of aspiration cytology in the diagnosis of primary neoplasms. Acta Cytol 1984;28:337.
14. Geier GR, Strecker JR. Aspiration cytology and E$_2$ content in ovarian tumors. Acta Cytol 1981;25:400.
15. Khaw KT, Walker WJ. Ultrasound guided fine needle aspiration of ovarian cysts: diagnosis and treatment in pregnant and nonpregnant women. Clin Radiol 1990;41:105.
16. Wojcik EM, Selvaggi SM. Fine-needle aspiration cytology of cystic ovarian lesions. Diagn Cytopathol 1994;11:9.
17. Nadji M, Ganjei P, Morales AR. Immunocytochemistry in contemporary cytology, the technique and its application. Lab Med 1994;25:502.
18. Selvaggi SM. Cytology of nonneoplastic cysts of the ovary. Diagn Cytopathol 1990;6:77.
19. Davila RM. Cytology of benign cystic uterine adnexal masses. Acta Cytol 1993;37:385.
20. Nunez C, Diaz JI. Ovarian follicular cysts: a potential source of false positive diagnoses in ovarian cytology. Diagn Cytopathol 1992;8:532.
21. Dordoni D, Zaglio S, Zucca S, et al. The role of sonographically guided aspiration in the clinical management of ovarian cysts. J Ultrasound Med 1993;12:27.
22. Greenebaum E, Mayer JR, Stangel JJ, et al. Aspiration cytology of ovarian cysts in in-vitro fertilization patients. Acta Cytol 1992;36: 11.
23. Stanley MW, Horwitz CA, Frable WJ. Cellular follicular cyst of the ovary: fluid cytology mimicking malignancy. Diagn Cytopathol 1991;7:48.
24. Selvaggi SM. Fine-needle aspiration cytology of ovarian follicle cysts with cellular atypia from reproductive-age patients. Diagn Cytopathol 1991;7:189.

Gynecologic Cytopathology. Edited by
Thomas A. Bonfiglio and Yener S. Erozan.
Lippincott–Raven Publishers, Philadelphia, © 1997.

CHAPTER 10

Fine-Needle Biopsy in the Staging of Gynecologic Malignancy

Thomas A. Bonfiglio

Fine-needle aspiration biopsy (FNAB) has gained wide acceptance as a diagnostic modality. It is used extensively to evaluate both superficial and deep-seated lesions. Its role in gynecologic practice, and particularly in gynecologic oncology, has been primarily in the evaluation of intraabdominal and pelvic mass lesions, including ovarian tumors. This application of the technique is discussed in detail in Chapter 9. FNAB has perhaps seen most extensive utilization in association with the investigation of possible metastatic disease and the staging of gynecologic malignancy.[1-5] The technique, which can be employed with the aid of various imaging modalities, is a minimally invasive method of sampling pelvic and intraabdominal lymph nodes, pelvic and abdominal masses, and the retroperitoneal space. In addition, it is commonly used to evaluate possible metastases to other sites, including the lungs and liver.

FNAB of lymph nodes in gynecologic oncology patients has been the subject of several reports in the literature. Although lymphography was often employed as the imaging method of choice in earlier studies on the utility of this technique, computerized axial tomography scans and ultrasonography are the most common modalities employed today to direct lymph node sampling.

The cytologic preparation and subsequent interpretation of samples obtained by this technique are quite straightforward. In brief, direct smears are made of the aspirated sample. The specimens on slides are then fixed in 95% ethanol and stained by the Papanicolaou technique, or are air-dried and Giemsa-stained. The two stains are complementary, and both techniques are performed on each sample. If sufficient material is obtained,

cell block preparations can also be made. This facilitates the use of special stains and immunocytochemical techniques if necessary.

The cytologic characteristics of metastatic gynecologic malignancies in FNAB samples are similar to those of the tumors at their primary sites. Squamous cell carcinoma of the cervix or vagina typically metastasizes to pelvic and periaortic lymph nodes, whereas vulvar cancer usually first involves inguinal nodes. Aspirates of these involved nodes are characterized by minibiopsies of tumor and, usually, numerous single tumor cells (Figs. 10-1 and 10-2). The metastatic deposits may be centrally necrotic, and the aspiration of such a focus could result in a sample that contains only necrotic cellular debris with few, if any, identifiable tumor cells. In other cases,

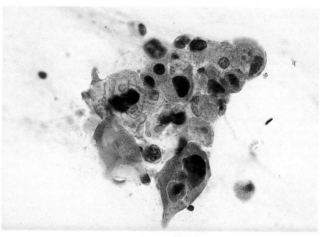

FIG. 10-1. Metastatic squamous cell carcinoma in fine-needle aspiration biopsy specimen of pelvic lymph node. The abundant, dense orangeophilic cytoplasm, sharp cell borders, and opaque nuclei are characteristic of a metastasis from a keratinizing squamous cell carcinoma of the cervix.

T. A. Bonfiglio: Department of Pathology and Laboratory Medicine, University of Rochester Medical Center, Rochester, New York 14642.

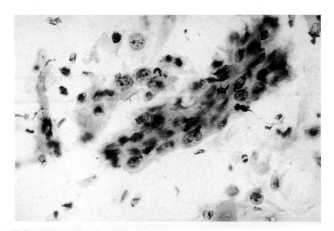

FIG. 10-2. The cells in this example of a metastatic squamous cervical carcinoma have a syncytial like arrangement in this small biopsy fragment seen in an fine-needle aspirate biopsy sample.

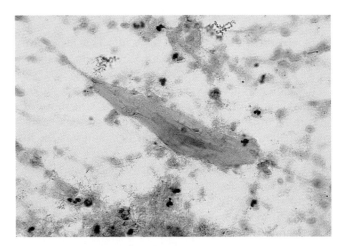

FIG. 10-3. Fine-needle aspirate biopsy specimen of a pelvic node involved by metastatic well-differentiated squamous cell carcinoma. There is only a suggestion of a degenerated nucleus in the center of this keratinized from. Aspirates from the center of a metastatic focus of keratinizing carcinomas may contain only keratin debri and anucleate cells.

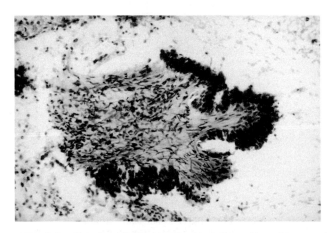

FIG. 10-4. This field is from an fine-needle aspirate biopsy of a pelvic node from a patient with metastatic papillary endocervical adenocarcinoma. The tumor cells here are seen in association with a dense fibrous stroma. The papillary nature of the neoplasm is obvious even in this small biopsy specimen.

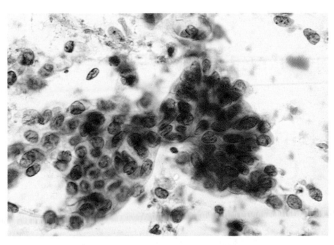

FIG. 10-5. Metastatic endocervical adenocarcinoma in periaortic node biopsy specimen. This is a moderately differentiated tumor. Note the suggestion of a pallisading arrangement.

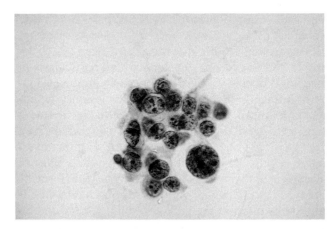

FIG. 10-6. Poorly differentiated endocervical adenocarcinoma in fine-needle aspirate biopsy specimen of a pelvic node.

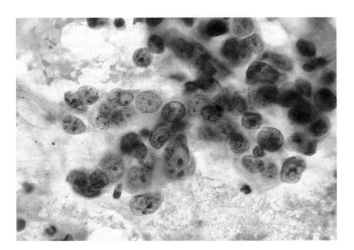

FIG. 10-7. This is an fine-needle aspirate biopsy specimen of medistinal nodes from a patient with metastases from a grade 3 endometrial adenocarcinoma. The cytologic findings are those of a high-grade adenocarcinoma. There is nothing specific that identifies this as endometrial. Comparison with the appearance of the primary neoplasm established a strong cytologic similarity.

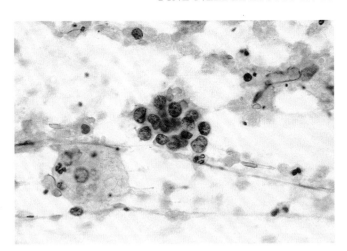

FIG. 10-8. Metastatic moderately differentiated endometrial adenocarcinoma in a lymph node aspirate. This tight cluster of smaller tumor cells is more typical of endometrial carcinoma than the cells seen figure 10-7.

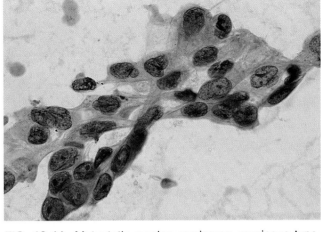

FIG. 10-11. Metastatic ovarian carcinoma, mucinous type. Notice the colunar configuration of some of the tumor cells in this group.

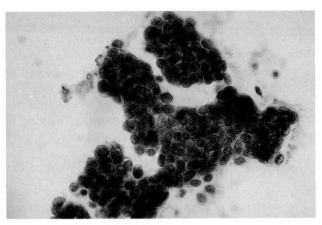

FIG. 10-9. Periaotic node fine-needle aspirate biopsy specimen, positive for metastatic papillary serous carcinoma of the ovary.

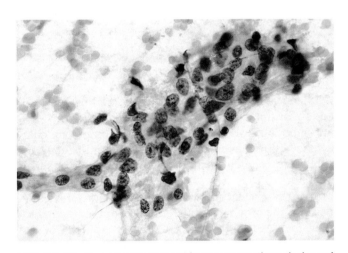

FIG. 10-12. Tumor cells derived from metastatic endodermal sinus tumor in fine-needle aspirate biopsy specimen of retroperitoneal mass. The granular eosinophilic cytoplasm is typical. Intracytoplasmic or extracellular eosinophilic droplets (not evident in this field) representing alpha-fetoprotein are often a cytologic feature of these tumors.

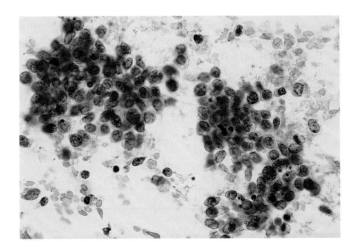

FIG. 10-10. These tumor cells from a metstatic endometrioid carcinoma of the ovary were present in a fine-needle aspirate biopsy specimen of an enlarged pelvic node. Although the cytologic features are certainly consistent with endometrioid differentiation in this case, definitive classifcation as endometrioid versus serous carcinoma is not always possible in this type of biopsy.

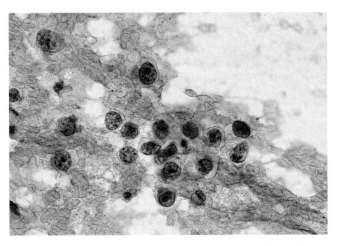

FIG. 10-13. Dysgerminoma cells in periaotic node aspirate. Note the large nuclei and prominent nucleoli. The cytoplasm, which is obscured by the blood in the background, is relatively scant with a pale, finely granular or clear appearance.

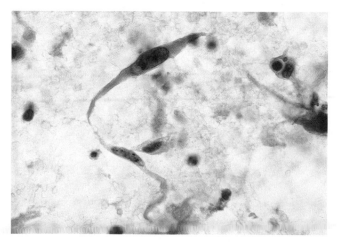

FIG. 10-14. Leiomyosarcoma in an fine-needle aspirate biopsy specimen of an abdominal mass from a patient with a uterine primary. The spindle appearance and the bluish staining cytoplasm represent characteristic cytologic features of this neoplasm.

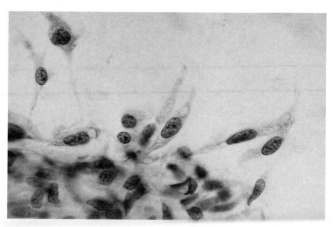

FIG. 10-15. Aggregate of cells from a leiomyosarcoma in a fine-needle aspirate biopsy specimen of a pelvic mass. Note the enlongate nature of the cells at the periphery and the variability of the nuclei.

there is extensive keratinization, and pleomorphic keratin debris dominates the sample (Fig. 10-3).

Adenocarcinomas arising from the uterine cervix or endometrium also metastasize to pelvic and, later, periaortic nodes. In FNAB samples, these tumors are characterized by the presence of three-dimensional clusters, acinar arrangements, papillary configurations, or sheets of abnormal cells. The cells reflect the appearance of the primary neoplasm, and their cytologic characteristics depend on the origin and differentiation of the original tumor. Figures 10-4 through 10-7 depict examples of several variants of metastatic endometrial and endocervical adenocarcinoma.

Ovarian neoplasia is characterized by a large morphologic spectrum of tumors. The most common epithelial malignancies include those tumors that arise from the germinal epithelium of the ovary, that is, serous, mucinous, clear-cell, and endometrioid adenocarcinomas. Some typical examples of FNAB samples of metastatic foci of these types of neoplasms are found in Figures 10-8 through 10-11. Germ-cell neoplasms make up another large group of ovarian tumors. Dysgerminomas, malignant teratomas, and endodermal sinus tumors may

be readily diagnosed at metastatic sites by FNAB (Figs. 10-12 through 10-14. Metastases from other, less common neoplasms of the ovary may also be encountered.

Sarcomas arising in the gynecologic organs less commonly metastasize to regional nodes, but may spread by direct extension into adjacent pelvic tissues and the abdomen. FNAB is an easy method of sampling in order to confirm involvement or provide an initial diagnosis.

ACCURACY OF THE METHOD

Fine-needle aspiration biopsy for the detection of metastatic disease has a high overall sensitivity and specificity. In a study of 109 cases from the laboratory at the University of Rochester, which was reported some years ago, no false-positive determinations were made and four false-negative interpretations were rendered. Therefore, the specificity was 100% and the sensitivity was 91%, with a diagnostic accuracy of 94%. The overall results are summarized in Table 10-1.[6] Similar results have been obtained in other studies. For example, in a study of fluoroscopically guided aspirates of pelvic lymph nodes in urologic malignancies, Piscioli and colleagues reported an accuracy rate of 93%.[7]

TABLE 10-1. *Calculated determinants of accuracy of pelvic and periaortic lymph node fine-needle aspiration biopsy for metastatic disease*

Site	Sensitivity	Specificity	Accuracy	PV+ result	PV− result
Periaortic	96%	100%	98%	100%	97%
Pelvic	84%	100%	94%	100%	90%
All sites	91%	100%	96%	100%	94%

PV+/−, predictive value of positive or negative result.

Bonfiglio TA, Fallon MA. Fine-needle aspiration biopsy of pelvic and periaortic lymph nodes in the evaluation of neoplastic disease. In Luciani L, Piscioli F (eds). Aspiration cytology in the staging of urological cancer. New York: Springer-Verlag, 1988:63.

REFERENCES

1. Zornoza J, Lukeman JM, Jing BS, et al. Percutaneous retroperitoneal lymph node biopsy in carcinoma of the cervix. Gynecol Oncol 1977;5:43.
2. Bonfiglio TA, MacIntosh PK, Patten SF, et al. Fine needle aspiration cytopathology of retroperitoneal lymph nodes in the evaluation of metastatic disease. Acta Cytol 1979;23:126.
3. Edeiken-Monroe BSE, Zornoza J. Carcinoma of the cervix: percutaneous lymph node aspiration biopsy. AJR Am J Roentgenol 1982; 138:655.
4. Dunnick NR, Fischer RI, Chu EW. Percutaneous aspiration of retroperitoneal lymph nodes in ovarian cancer. AJR Am J Roentgenol 1980;135:109.
5. Zornoza J. Abdomen. In Zornoza J (ed). Percutaneous needle biopsy. Baltimore: Williams & Wilkins, 1981:102.
6. Bonfiglio TA, Fallon MA. Fine needle aspiration biopsy of pelvic and periaortic lymph nodes in the evaluation of neoplastic disease. In Luciani L, Piscioli F (eds). Aspiration cytology in the staging of urological cancer. New York: Springer-Verlag, 1988:63.
7. Piscioli F, Scappini P, Luciani L. Aspiration cytology in the staging of urologic cancer. Cancer 1985;53:553.

Gynecologic Cytopathology. Edited by
Thomas A. Bonfiglio and Yener S. Erozan.
Lippincott–Raven Publishers, Philadelphia, © 1997.

CHAPTER 11

New Technology in Gynecologic Cytology: Automation in Cytology Screening and Thin-Layer Preparation Techniques

David C. Wilbur

The automation of the cytologic screening process has been a goal of analytical cytology research for many years.[1] Computerization of the screening process is highly desirable because of the repetitive nature of the process, the need to examine thoroughly each preparation, and the need to maintain reproducibility of interpretation utilizing known cytologic criteria. Computers are excellent tools for performing highly repetitive tasks, can be programmed to examine every cell over the entire surface of each slide, and are generally better than humans at maintaining consistency (or reproducibility) when making measurements, and thereupon applying set criteria for diagnosis. Theoretically, therefore, the computerized screening device should be able to perform the task of slide screening with few omission errors (failure to identify abnormal cells when present) or interpretation errors, based, of course, on the quality of the criteria that have been programmed into its differential algorithms. Much like the human screener, the computer can perform analyses of many features of each cell in a uniform fashion according to its programmed algorithms. This characteristic allows for the consistent use of objective morphometric criteria. In other words, the computer should label the same cell in the same way on every analysis. This cannot be said about human observation, where a cell labeled "atypical" on one examination may be labeled "normal" or "dysplastic" on subsequent examinations. The computerized system, therefore, allows for a potentially more uniform and less temporally biased assessment of a given cytologic sample. Last, the reliability of modern computer hardware allows for essentially continuous operation with minimal downtime of the screening instrumentation. Tireless operation is a potentially significant advantage of a computerized approach to screening over currently utilized human-based systems. Based on these distinct advantages of computerization in cytologic examination, one must ask the question: Why has it taken so long? Several important reasons can be put forth.

First, the tasks involved are complex. Human screeners must synthesize a vast amount of information when evaluating a case. In cytology slides, cells may present with a variety of artifacts and appearances, and with significant cellular overlap. Many diagnoses require a composite of many features or patterns present in a given case. The ability to define adequately the wide variety of abnormalities in a format that is adaptable to computerized analysis is difficult. Computers must be programmed in such a way that no positive case will be missed and that as few as possible false-positive cases will be "detected." Thus, the instrument will have high sensitivity and acceptable specificity rates for the detection of gynecologic lesions. Computerized instruments are generally programmed to examine the features of individual isolated cells or cell groupings. In addition to the single cells present, the complexity of the overall case must be taken into account in the programming in order to achieve results comparable or superior to current human screening.

Second, cytologists needed to develop and test cytologic criteria that could form the basis for the programming to differentiate all the entities that we now look for in the cytologic smear.

D. C. Wilbur: Department of Pathology and Laboratory Medicine, University of Rochester Medical Center, Rochester, New York 14642.

Third, computers have only recently entered a stage of sophistication where they are capable of analyzing all the above-noted features on many cells in a cost- and time-effective fashion.

Because the three reasons noted above are now essentially realities, instrumentation has been developed that can begin to address successfully the problem of gynecologic smear screening and interpretation. With a goal of providing more accurate and cost-effective cytologic services, a number of manufacturers of such instrumentation are currently testing the advantages of performing cervical cytologic screening procedures utilizing computerized scanning systems. Clinical trials ultimately will determine whether these advantages are realized, and whether the systems are practical to implement into common usage.

CURRENT STATUS OF AUTOMATION IN THE SCREENING OF GYNECOLOGIC CYTOLOGY SPECIMENS

The goal of computerization in gynecologic cytology is to develop instrumentation that will relieve human beings from the currently tedious and error-prone method of cervical smear evaluation; to provide equal or greater degrees of accuracy; and to do this in a timely and cost-effective manner. With the recent two decades of explosive growth in computing power and software development, many of the operational tasks required for computers to address the complex procedure of slide screening and evaluation can now be effectively addressed. Companies have been formed that are moving the process of computerized cytologic evaluation from the research laboratory into the setting of the clinical laboratory. Preliminary studies from several of the commercial ventures (see later) have shown promising results. Clinical trials designed to facilitate introduction of the technology into common usage have been recently completed, or are in the final planning stages at the time of this writing.

Initial attempts to introduce computerized scanning into practice will come with use of the instruments as quality control devices. Such instruments will be utilized to rescreen slides previously deemed to be within normal limits by cytotechnologists. Such devices would be expected to decrease overall laboratory false-negative rates, but will increase the cost of the test without concomitant direct economic savings. The more important task of automation will be to provide for primary screening of cervical cytology preparations. In such systems, the instrument would perform the initial evaluations on slides received in the laboratory. Several general approaches to automated prescreening have been identified and encompass the degree of "responsibility" that will be placed on the instrument in making the ultimate diagnosis on a given case. In addition, an important question in the process of automated screening revolves around the type of specimen preparation the screening instrumentation will utilize.

AUTOMATED VERSUS SEMIAUTOMATED APPROACHES TO INSTRUMENT SCREENING

The ultimate in computerization for cytology screening would be the scenario of slides being processed by an instrument, with a complete and final diagnosis being rendered in each case. Such a process would require that the instrument perform in a virtually flawless manner, with little room for error, given the current regulatory and liability environment. The availability of such instrumentation in the near future is unlikely at present. The next level of an "automated triage" instrument is more realistic. Under this scenario, slides would be classified automatically as "within normal limits," requiring no further review, or "potentially abnormal," requiring cytotechnologist screening. Because most cervical smears are indeed within normal limits, setting "sort rates" at progressively higher levels based on continued improvements and experience could effect significant gains in terms of cytotechnologist productivity and potential cost savings to the laboratory, hopefully with the advantage of decreased false-negative rates. In addition, such a system would provide for significantly more "interesting" material for the cytotechnologist to screen, relieving some of the tedium of the task and providing an impetus for improved accuracy in the routine screening process.

In contrast to these automated routines, in which the computer is allowed to make judgments on all or some cases without direct human input, the semiautomated approach represents an intermediate approach with decreased machine "responsibility." In this schema, the computer presents to the cytologist a series of images of cells that it has deemed the most abnormal. This is generally done via a reviewing station equipped with a video screen. The cytologist can then decide, upon reviewing the images, whether the slide requires screening or is within normal limits. This approach places the responsibility for each case on the human observer; however, the computer continues to be responsible for presenting relevant cells for human interpretation. Clinical trials of such instrumentation, in addition to showing that the computer is capable of finding and classifying abnormal cells, will have to prove that the human observer is capable of distinguishing abnormal from normal cases on the video display screen. Preliminary studies have shown that the task of reviewing video images is more rapid than screening slides. Therefore, in addition to diminished omission errors, cytologist screening productivity is improved as well. Semiautomated screening is the approach that several manufacturers of computerized

SPECIMEN TYPE AND THE IMPLICATIONS FOR AUTOMATED SCREENING

In the design of automated screening devices, decisions needed to be made regarding the types of specimens that would be utilized in the instruments. Some of the instruments have been designed to analyze conventionally prepared cervical smears. However, screening and interpretation of conventionally prepared cervical smears are very complex tasks for the computer. Routine smears may contain cells that are densely packed into groups, cells that lie atop one another, or cells that are covered by inflammation or blood, and that may have a variety of processing, staining, and other technique-related artifacts. All these features make conventional smears challenging for human observers, but they make the image recognition and interpretation necessary for computer analysis even more difficult.

One of the major problems for the computer is being able to separate visually one cell (or nucleus) from another. This is known as cell segmentation, and it allows the computer to measure discrete parameters of each individual cell. For instance, if one nucleus overlies another, as schematically shown in Figure 11-1A, the computer will have a complex task in determining the nuclear area and perimeter of each cell because it cannot easily tell where one nucleus ends and the other begins.

For the human, this is a relatively simple task. In order to address this difficulty for the computer, investigators must either develop sophisticated methods of analysis, which allow the computer to break down these overlapping cells into their component parts, or they must pre-process specimens into cell spreads that allow for better segmentation of individual cells, making cellular material more amenable to discrete individual cell analysis (see Fig. 11-1B). As the end result, a number of instrument manufacturers have chosen thin-layer processing techniques as the preferred preparation method for cellular samples analyzed by their devices.

MONOLAYER VERSUS THIN-LAYER PREPARATIONS

For many years, investigators in the field of computerized cell analysis have utilized monolayer preparations to achieve adequate cell segmentation for discrete cell measurement. Original techniques utilized harsh conditions with high shearing forces and digestive reagents to produce complete separation of all cells and form a uniform "monolayer," or single cell layer, on the two-dimensional slide plane.[2-4] Such techniques allowed for excellent visualization of individual cells, which greatly simplified computer analysis. However, such techniques have significant disadvantages for practical clinical cytology. Because of the disruptive forces utilized in the preparations, contextual features that have relevance to the overall interpretation of the slide usually are lost. Elements of the cytologic pattern, such as the presence and

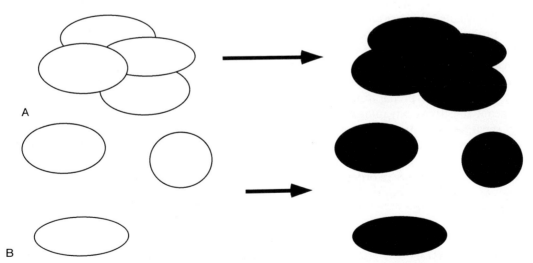

FIG. 11-1. **(A,B)** Adequate segmentation allows each cell or nucleus to be analyzed individually. On the left in **(A)**, a group of overlapping cells is schematically illustrated as it may be seen by a human observer. In distinction, the right-sided view is how a computer might visualize the same group. Individual cells are not easily separated in such groupings. Thin-layer processing allows for improved physical separation of cells, which improves optical segmentation during computer analysis. This principal is illustrated in **(B)**, again with the human and computer analyses on the left and right, respectively. Using this type of preparation, the computer is able to provide accurate individual cell morphometric measurements.

configuration of cellular groupings, are not available to add to the overall cytologic impression. In addition, the presence of background material, such as blood, inflammation, necrotic debris, and mucus, provides significant information in the overall assessment of each case. The loss of such features decreases the sensitivity and, therefore, the overall accuracy of the complete cytologic interpretation. In the circumstance of semiautomated screening and interpretation, where the human is in the position of making the final diagnosis, loss of these contextual features represents a major drawback of the monolayer method.

In an effort to maintain many of the contextual features of cell grouping, group configuration, and background material, investigators began to experiment with more gentle cell dispersion techniques that maintained some of the important visual cues for diagnosis.[5] These preparations were not true monolayers because they maintained many cell groupings and also contained many cells with some degrees of three-dimensional nuclear and cytoplasmic overlap. However, the task of cell segmentation was made significantly easier because most of the squamous cells were dispersed and remained free of obscuring background elements. Such smears have been found to be more amenable to computerized analysis while continuing to provide the additional contextual features necessary for utmost accuracy in final human diagnosis.

During initial investigations into the operating characteristics of thin-layer preparations as compared with routinely prepared conventional smears, it was noted that final readings of matched pairs of thin-layer and conventional cases derived from the same patient at the same sampling event showed a high degree of correlation.[6] In addition, it was noted that readings on the thin-layer preparations produced greater numbers of cases of squamous intraepithelial lesions than did the matched conventional smears. Because of these initial observations, it was suggested that the performance of gynecologic cytology by the thin-layer preparation technique might have significant sensitivity advantages when utilized, completely separate from its use as a method of preparation, for the computerized scanning instruments.

Because of these initial results, full-scale clinical trials have been initiated by two companies in order to explore thin-layer cytology as a new preparatory technique for use in routine screening situations.

THE THIN-LAYER METHOD

The two companies with products for the preparation of thin-layer cytology specimens are the Cytyc Corporation (Marlborough, MA) and Roche Image Analysis Systems (Elon College, NC). The Cytyc product is the ThinPrep Processor and the Roche instrumentation is the Cyto-Rich Processor. The two instruments work on different principles, but produce slides that are very similar in appearance and morphologic characteristics.

Specimen Procurement

Thin-layer processing differs from routine gynecologic cytology because specimen processing and slide preparation take place in the laboratory, rather than being performed by the clinician who takes the patient sample. Specimens are collected in a normal fashion with routine sampling devices. At this point, rather than smearing the collected cells onto the slide surface, the sampling device is immersed in a fluid fixative or transport medium and is agitated, thereby allowing the cellular and noncellular material obtained from the patient to be suspended in the fluid. No slide is made at this point, as in the conventional method. The suspension of cells then is transported to the cytology laboratory, where all specimen processing takes place. This manner of specimen procurement has obvious advantages in allowing specimen collection practices to remain uniform, while eliminating the inherently nonuniform process of office slide preparation. This change in slide preparation allows for significantly enhanced quality control of the slide-making process, leading to more uniform slide quality and fewer technique-related artifacts. Because the transport medium contains a fixative solution, cells are fixed immediately upon immersion. This eliminates any possibility of air-drying artifact in the final slides, and allows the material to remain stable during transport and subsequent storage.

Instrumentation

Cytyc ThinPrep Processor

The ThinPrep Processor (Fig. 11-2A) is a filter transfer device. Cell suspensions received in the cytology laboratory can be loaded directly into the instrument in the proprietary transport vials (PreservCyt) (see Fig. 11-2B). The device then lowers a plastic tube (TransCyt) (see Fig. 11-2B) with a polycarbonate filter on its end into the cell suspension. The filter tube is spun, acting as a vortex, allowing for the homogenization of the cell sample, which is crucial to the production of a well-distributed sample. After vortexing, negative pressure is created within the filter tube, drawing fluid through the filter and depositing cellular and noncellular material onto the surface of the filter. Pressure within the tube is monitored, thereby allowing a uniform amount of material to be deposited onto the filter in each case. When a pressure level is reached indicating appropriate cell density on the filter, the pressure is relieved and the process stops. The filter and tube are then removed from the cell suspen-

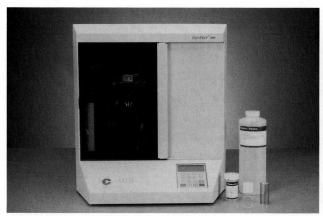
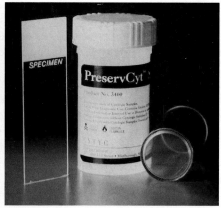

FIG. 11-2. (A) Cytyc ThinPrep 2000 Processor (courtesy of David Zahniser, PhD, Cytyc Corporation, Marlborough, MA). **(B)** Cytyc PreservCyt fixative/transport media and TransCyt vortexing filter for use in the ThinPrep Processor (courtesy of David Zahniser, PhD, Cytyc Corporation, Marlborough, MA).

sion, inverted, and blotted onto the surface of a glass slide. The filter places cells in a uniform 20-mm circle in a constant position in the central portion of the slide. During this blotting process, positive air pressure is applied to the filter, aiding in complete cell transfer to the glass slide surface. The glass slide is then immediately immersed in 95% ethanol to complete the fixation process.

The slide and cell suspension must be manually loaded and removed from the ThinPrep instrument. The slide may then be stained by whatever process is routinely utilized in each individual laboratory. No instrumentation is currently available for processing multiple specimens as a batch, although the company has reported plans to make such a device available in the future.

Roche Cyto-Rich Processor

The Cyto-Rich instrument (Fig. 11-3) is a density gradient sedimentation device. Because solution homogeni-

zation does not occur in the instrument phase of the process, as with the Cytyc device, preprocessing of the specimen received in fixative or transport media is required. Preprocessing is performed by a syringing process that forces the suspension through a series of baffle chambers, thereby applying shearing forces that break up mucus and cell aggregates, and effect the homogenization process achieved with the Cytyc instrument during its vortexing phase. The homogenized cell suspension is then processed through a series of centrifugation steps prior to transfer to the instrument, where it is automatically aliquoted into sedimentation vials that are placed over the surface of a glass slide. Cells are deposited directly onto the slide via the sedimentation process, in a uniform 13-mm circle located in the central portion of the slide.

The Cyto-Rich instrumentation has the advantage of preparing multiple slides (currently 48) at the same time,

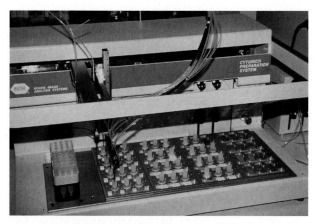

FIG. 11-3. Roche Image Analysis Systems Cyto-Rich Processor (courtesy of Ernest Kneisel, Roche Image Analysis Systems, Elon College, NC).

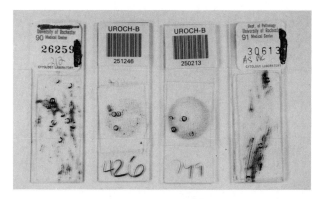

FIG. 11-4. Examples of thin-layer slides (inner two), as compared with their mated conventional smears from the same clinical sample (outer two), are shown. Note that the thin-layer preparations show cells only in a well-defined and uniform central area of each slide, as opposed to the conventional smears, which may show cellular material anywhere on the slide, including areas outside of the optimal viewing portions, such as under the label, or outside the coverslipped area.

offsetting somewhat the time spent in the syringing and centrifugation steps required in the preprocessing stages. After specimens have been preprocessed and loaded onto the instrument, the device proceeds with slide-making in a hands-off, unattended fashion. In addition, the Cyto-Rich device will fix and stain the slides prior to removal from the instrument, leaving coverslipping as the only task that needs to be performed on the slides after removal from the instrument. Trials are currently under way for automation of the preprocessing stages. Mechanization of these stages will greatly improve the efficiency of the Cyto-Rich method, because preprocessing is the most labor- and time-intense portion of preparation. Examples of thin-layer slides with their paired conventional smears derived from the same clinical samples are illustrated in Figure 11-4.

CLINICAL TRIALS OF THIN-LAYER INSTRUMENTATION FOR USE IN ROUTINE SCREENING

Study Design

Most studies performed and published to date regarding the use of thin-layer cytology preparations in gynecologic specimens have utilized very similar protocols. A basic schematic of most trial designs is illustrated in Figure 11-5. Specimens are obtained from participating women utilizing an endocervical broom device (Cervex-Brush, Rovers, Boonton, NJ) with standard collection techniques as recommended by the manufacturer. This type of device was chosen because of the high cell yields noted with the endocervical broom[7] and the ability to utilize the device to make single slide cases. A cervical smear is then made in a routine fashion, and the sampling device is suspended and agitated in the proprietary

transport media for suspension of the remainder of cells. The conventional smear and the cell suspension are then transported to the cytology laboratory. The conventional smear is routinely processed, screened, and reported. Thin-layer slides are made utilizing the respective instrumentation, the slides generated are screened, and diagnoses are rendered in a manner blinded to the results of the conventional smear. The results of each method are then compared, with final diagnoses on discrepant cases being resolved by a review process. A rigorous reconciliation of the two methods is designed to eliminate the possibility of false-negative errors related to screening or interpretation on both types of specimens. From this comparison, data are tabulated detailing the correlation of the two methods, as well as generating cases in which a discrepancy has favored one method over the other.

Results

Cytyc ThinPrep Processor

The initial study using the ThinPrep Processor was reported by Hutchinson and colleagues in a pilot group of 446 patients.[6] This study first identified the potential advantages of utilizing thin-layer cytology preparations for routine manual screening. In this study, thin-layer cytology cases produced lower rates of less than optimal specimens compared with paired conventional cases, and also showed slightly increased rates of detection of low-grade squamous intraepithelial lesions (LSIL; Table 11-1). Overall, the correlation rate for exact Bethesda System diagnosis between thin-layer and conventional specimens was 97%.

After the initial trial, the Cytyc Corporation sponsored a full-scale clinical trial utilizing five independent sites.[8] A total of 3218 patient specimens were examined, with

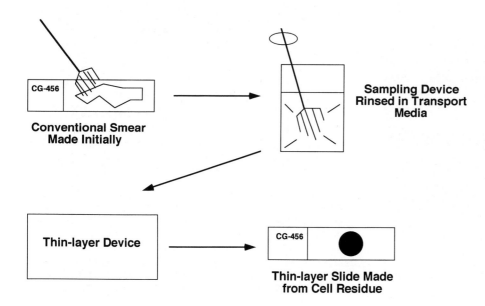

Conventional Smear Made Initially

Sampling Device Rinsed in Transport Media

Thin-layer Device

Thin-layer Slide Made from Cell Residue

FIG. 11-5. A schematic representation of the technical aspects of thin-layer clinical trials specimen processing is shown. Conventional smears are always generated first in an entirely routine fashion. The sampling device is then rinsed in the preservative transport media, removing the remaining cells and placing them in suspension. Thin-layer slides are generated from this cell suspension. This process allows no compromise of the conventional method, but may bias the study against the thin-layer procedure, because the intended use of the thin-layer technology is for all cells collected to be placed into the cell suspension.

TABLE 11-1. *Correlation between results of paired conventional and thin-layer slides in pilot study*

| | | Conventional Smear | | | | | |
		NG	AS	LG	HG	CA	TOT
Thin Layer	NG	349	0	2	0	0	351
	AS	1	3	0	0	0	4
	LG	5	0	57	0	0	62
	HG	0	0	1	23	0	24
	CA	0	0	0	0	2	2
	TOT	355	3	60	23	2	443

This study suggested that the thin layer method may be more sensitive for the detection of squamous abnormalities of the uterine cervix.

NG, negative; AS, atypical cells of undetermined significance; LG, low-grade squamous intraepithelial lesion; HG, high-grade squamous intraepithelial lesion; CA, carcinoma; TOT, total.

an exact correlation of diagnoses between the two techniques (by Bethesda System diagnosis) in 2840 cases (88.3%; Table 11-2). No discrepancies were identified in any of the carcinomas examined (7 cases). Comparison of the results between the categories of negative or atypical versus squamous intraepithelial lesion and carcinoma produced a correlation rate of 96% (3091 of 3218 cases; Table 11-3). There were 117 cases in which the thin-layer preparation was interpreted at a higher diagnostic level than the conventional smear, and 26 cases in which the opposite occurred. Among the 117 cases noted earlier, 18 cases of LSIL and 8 cases of high-grade squamous intraepithelial lesion (HSIL) were present on thin-layer slides, whereas the accompanying conventional slide was negative. In the other 26 cases, 3 cases of LSIL and 1 case of HSIL were present on the conventional slide, whereas the thin-layer slide was negative.

Follow-up studies at three of the clinical trial sites have shown that biopsy results obtained on patients with positive cytologic studies have correlated more closely with the thin-layer results than with the conventional smear re-

TABLE 11-2. *Correlation between results of paired conventional and thin-layer slides in the Cytyc clinical trials*

| | | Conventional Smear | | | | | |
		NG	AS	LG	HG	CA	TOT
Thin Layer	NG	1823	128	3	1	0	1955
	AS	97	497	19	3	0	616
	LG	18	72	366	10	0	466
	HG	3	8	16	147	0	174
	CA	0	0	0	0	7	7
	TOT	1941	705	404	161	7	3218

NG, negative; AS, atypical cells of undetermined significance; LG, low-grade squamous intraepithelial lesion; HG, high-grade squamous intraepithelial lesion; CA, carcinoma; TOT, total.

Modified from Wilbur DC, Cibas ES, Merritt S, et al. Thin Prep Processor. Clinical trials demonstrate an increased detection rate of abnormal cervical cytologic specimens. Am J Clin Pathol 1994;101:209.

TABLE 11-3. *Correlation between results of paired conventional and thin-layer slides in the Cytyc clinical trials: categories grouped by potential treatment schemes*

| | | Conventional Smear | | |
		NG/AS	LG/HG/CA	TOT
Thin Layer	NG/AS	2545	26	2571
	LG/HG/CA	101	546	647
	TOT	2646	572	3218

NG, negative; AS, atypical cells of undetermined significance; LG, low-grade squamous intraepithelial lesion; HG, high-grade squamous intraepithelial lesion; CA, carcinoma; TOT, total.

Modified from Wilbur DC, Cibas ES, Merritt S, et al. Thin Prep Processor. Clinical trials demonstrate an increased detection rate of abnormal cervical cytologic specimens. Am J Clin Pathol 1994; 101:209.

sults, further documenting the accuracy of the thin-layer approach.[9,10]

Additional studies have been performed after the clinical trials and also have shown that thin-layer processing with manual screening of slides produces equivalent or slightly better rates of abnormality detection.[11,12] Other studies have shown statistically significant improvements in specimen adequacy utilizing the thin-layer method.[13] A further study was designed to address specifically the question of thin-layer cytology in HSIL and cancer.[14] This study found good comparison between the methods (Table 11-4). The thin-layer method missed two endometrial cancers, but in one case, the thin-layer slide was unsatisfactory because of complete lack of cellularity. On the other hand, the thin-layer method detected one squamous cell carcinoma that was missed by the conventional smear. This study characterized key morphologic features of high-grade lesions and carcinomas on thin-layer preparations, which are detailed later. In one of the abovementioned studies, the sampling devices utilized were the endocervical brush and the spatula, which produced results similar to those derived from the endocervical broom–based studies noted earlier.[11] This finding suggests that specimens derived from other sampling devices will perform in a similar manner when applied to the thin-layer method.

Roche Cyto-Rich Processor

In a preliminary evaluation of the Cyto-Rich thin-layer processing device, Geyer and associates reported results similar to those obtained in the Cytyc ThinPrep Processor studies detailed earlier.[15] These authors studied 557 patients with paired thin-layer and conventional slides. They found that thin-layer slides were superior in satisfactory rates and in the detection of endocervical cells. Overall agreement between slides for Bethesda diagnosis was reported to be 99%. Agreement was 100% for HSIL and carcinoma (37 and 4 cases, respectively). As in

TABLE 11-4. *Results of a study comparing paired conventional and thin-layer (thin prep) slides in a high-risk gynecologic oncology practice**

		Conventional Smear							
		US	NG	AS	AG	LG	HG	CA	TOT
	US	0	1	0	0	1	0	1	3
	NG	3	187	0	0	0	1	1	192
	AS	1	6	9	0	4	0	0	20
Thin Layer	AG	0	3	0	1	0	0	0	4
	LG	0	0	3	0	8	0	0	11
	HG	1	0	1	0	0	9	1	12
	CA	0	0	0	0	0	0	17	17
	TOT	5	197	13	1	13	10	20	259

* In this population, the detection rates for lesions is virtually equivalent between the two methods. The increased rate of AGUS on thin-layer slides predicted, is noted in this study. *AG,* atypical glandular cells of undetermined significance; NG, negative; AS, atypical cells of undetermined significance; LG, low-grade squamous intraepithelial lesion; HG, high-grade squamous intraepithelial lesion; CA, carcinoma; TOT, total; US, unsatisfactory.

the Cytyc studies, a slight increase in the detection of LSIL was noted using the Cyto-Rich thin-layer method. The results of this study are shown in Table 11-5. In another preliminary study utilizing the Roche Cyto-Rich device, Azlin and colleagues reported a 14% reduction in limited and unsatisfactory results, and a 2% reduction in atypical squamous cells of undetermined significance (ASCUS) diagnoses.[16] Geyer and associates found improved false-negative rates for LSIL, HSIL, and carcinoma when more than 3000 paired thin-layer and conventional smears were rereviewed in a blinded fashion and the results of each review were compared.[17] This finding again points out the potential improvement in uniformity that may be realized using thin-layer technology.

Full-scale clinical trials of the Cyto-Rich instrument are under way at the time of this writing, and should be available for review in 1996.

THE PROBLEM OF "SUBSAMPLING"

An early criticism of the thin-layer systems has centered around the fact that thin-layer slides are produced

by taking aliquots of cell suspension in amounts necessary to produce cell spreads of uniform density on each slide. This process generally does not utilize all the cellular material available in the suspension. This phenomenon is referred to as "subsampling," and it was hypothesized that utilizing only a portion of the available material made false-negative results more likely because of a lack of diagnostic cells being transferred.

A study to test this hypothesis was reported by Hutchinson and colleagues, in which the authors made multiple thin-layer slides from many cell suspensions utilizing the ThinPrep Processor.[7] They found diagnostic cells on every preparation (up to 10) in all 27 cell suspensions tested. They postulated that randomization of the cell suspension during the vortexing step caused the cells to be distributed uniformly throughout the suspension and to have equal likelihood of being deposited on any given slide. They termed this process *random subsampling.*

During the course of the above-noted study, the possibility of subsampling in conventional smear preparation was also suggested and documented. The authors noted that an average of only 35% of the cellular material col-

TABLE 11-5. *Results of an initial comparison of paired conventional and Cyto-Rich thin-layer slides**

		Conventional Smear					
		NG	AS	LG	HG	CA	TOT
	NG	462	2	0	0	0	464
	AS	0	14	0	0	0	14
Thin Layer	LG	0	4	28	0	0	32
	HG	0	0	0	37	0	37
	CA	0	0	0	0	4	4
	TOT	462	20	28	37	4	551

* Excellent correlation and increased identification of squamous lesions also was noted in this study.
NG, negative; AS, atypical cells of undetermined significance; LG, low-grade squamous intraepithelial lesion; HG, high-grade squamous intraepithelial lesion; CA, carcinoma; TOT, total.
Modified from Geyer JW, Hancock F, Carrico C, et al. Preliminary evaluation of Cyto-Rich: an improved automated cytology preparation. Diagn Cytopathol 1993;9:417.

TABLE 11-6. *Important morphologic characteristics of thin-layer preparations*

Even distribution of cellular material
Lack of obscuring blood and inflammation
No air-drying artifact
Infectious agents (*Candida* and *Trichomonas*) easily identified
Cellular groupings are generally more three-dimensional
Individual cells may show rounding-up
Nuclei appear slightly smaller than in conventional smear
Diagnostic criteria for atypical squamous cells of undetermined significance and low-grade squamous intraepithelial lesion are virtually identical to conventional smear
High-grade squamous intraepithelial lesion often presents as small, isolated cells only
Because of three-dimensionality of groupings, glandular lesions are more difficult to evaluate than in conventional smear
Invasive carcinomas show a distinctive diathesis background pattern

lected in the taking of a cervical sample was deposited on the conventional slide (range 2.3% to 69.1%). The remainder of the cellular material left over after the conventional smear is made normally is discarded in the clinician's office. In addition, cells are collected on the sampling device in a nonrandom distribution (ie, cells are present only on those portions of the sampling device that come in contact with the lesion). Without further

processing, the cells are transferred to the glass slide in a nonrandom fashion. The difference between random and nonrandom subsampling forms the basis for one of the hypotheses as to why the thin-layer method may be more sensitive for the detection of squamous intraepithelial lesions, which has been shown in the clinical trials of the device. Without randomization of the specimen in the conventional smear, cells may be preferentially applied to the slide from some areas of the sampling device but not others. This difference in subsampling type may account for a source of false-negative results in the cervical smear method that is related to conventional slide preparation technique.

MORPHOLOGY OF THIN-LAYER PREPARATIONS

During the course of the studies performed on thin-layer and conventional preparations, numerous morphologic observations were made regarding the differences and similarities between the two techniques. A summary of these major morphologic characteristics of thin-layer preparations are shown in Table 11-6.

Thin-layer preparations provide a uniform distribution of cellular material across the surface of a 13- or 20-mm circle in a consistent position in the central portion of the slide. Because cell deposition on the filter or slide

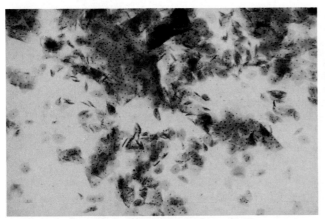

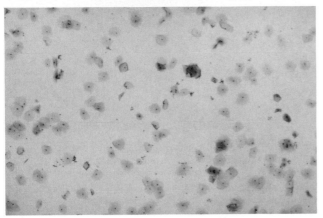

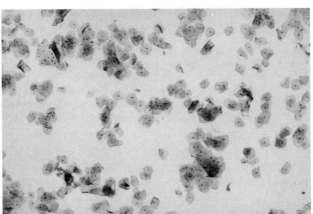

FIG. 11-6. Low-magnification images of conventional (**A**), ThinPrep (**B**) and Cyto-Rich (**C**) slides are shown. Note that compared with the conventional smear, cells in the two thin-layer preparations are more evenly distributed across the slide surface, and individual cells show significantly improved segmentation (**A,B,C**, 20×; Papanicolaou stain).

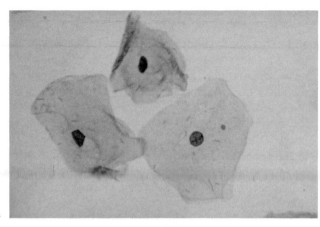
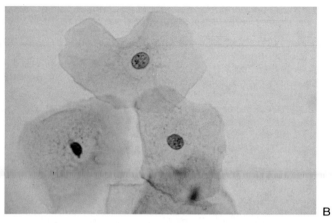

A   B

FIG. 11-7. High-magnification images of ThinPrep (**A**) and Cyto-Rich (**B**) slides are shown. Cellular conformation and nuclear chromatin detail is well-preserved in each specimen. General cellular preservation in each of these two processes is very similar (**A,B,** 200×; Papanicolaou stain).

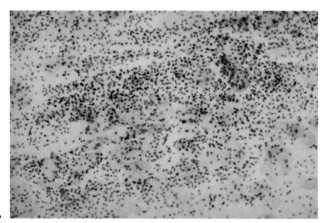
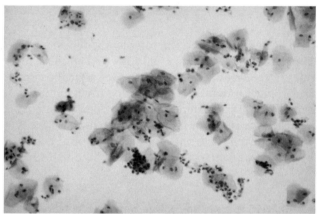

A   B

FIG. 11-8. Examples of inflammatory smears are shown. (**A**) shows a conventional smear, which was interpreted as having significant obscuring acute inflammation that impaired interpretation. (**B**) shows the same sample processed as a thin-layer slide (ThinPrep). An abnormal number of inflammatory cells can be seen in the slide, preserving this important contextual feature; however, thin-layer processing causes significant aggregation of these cells, thereby clearing the background and allowing adequate visualization of epithelial cells for a satisfactory examination (**A,B,** 50×; Papanicolaou stain).

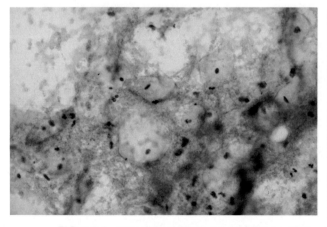
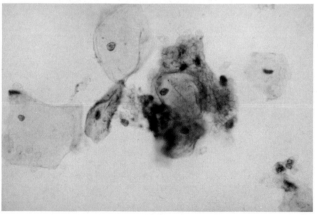

FIG. 11-9. Examples of bloody smears are shown. (**A**) shows a conventional smear that was interpreted as unsatisfactory due to excessive blood obscuring epithelial elements. (**B**) shows the same case prepared by the thin-layer (ThinPrep) process. Although the contextual feature of blood on the slide is preserved in the thin-layer specimen, the blood is coagulated and appears predominantly as erythrocyte ghosts, allowing for substantially improved epithelial cell visualization. This thin-layer specimen was interpreted as satisfactory for evaluation (**A,B,** 132×; Papanicolaou stain).

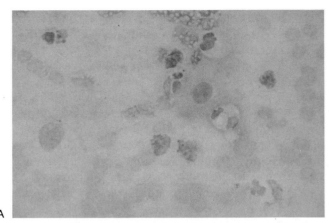

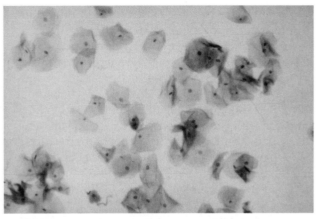

A ... **B**

FIG. 11-10. Thin-layer processing eliminates air-drying artifact. Because cells are immediately fixed in transport media during the making of the cell suspension, no air-drying artifact is seen in these specimens. (**A**) shows a conventional smear with marked air drying of cells, which inhibited an optimal interpretation. (**B**) shows the same specimen processed as a thin-layer slide. No air-drying artifact is present and the smear could be optimally evaluated (**A**, 132×; **B**, 50×; Papanicolaou stain).

is controlled, cell density is relatively uniform from one case to another. Cells are dispersed, allowing for generally good cell segmentation (Figs. 11-6 and 11-7). During the making of the cell suspension, red blood cells are lysed and remain only as a residue on the final slide. In addition, inflammatory cells such as neutrophils and lymphocytes are clumped and dispersed from epithelial cells, making obscuring of epithelial cells unusual. After

experience is gained with the technique, the amount of red blood cell residue and inflammatory component can be recognized and estimated, providing the key contextual feature of a bloody or inflamed specimen, similar to this evaluation process in conventional smears (Figs. 11-8 and 11-9). Because cells are transferred directly from the sampling device to the fixative transport media, the problem of air-drying artifact is virtually non-

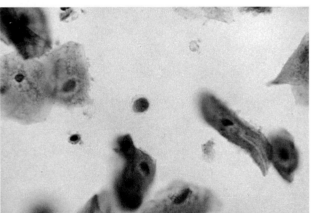

A ... **B**

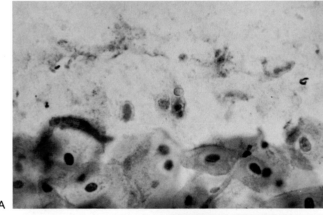

FIG. 11-11. Examples of Trichomonas vaginalis are illustrated in conventional (**A**), ThinPrep (**B**), and Cyto-Rich (**C**) slides. The organisms are easily visualized on thin-layer preparations with morphology identical to that noted on conventional smears (**A,B,C**, 200×; Papanicolaou stain).

C

existent in thin-layer studies, eliminating an important cause of technically inadequate smears (Fig. 11-10).

The identification of infectious organisms such as *Trichomonas* and *Candida* is easily accomplished in thin-layer smears. Trichomonads appear similar on conventional and thin-layer smears (Fig. 11-11). Candidal organisms are more easily identified in thin-layer slides as compared with conventional smears. Organisms generally are found on top of groups in these preparations, and stand out well from the epithelial cells (Fig. 11-12). Several studies have shown similar identification rates for these organisms in matched pairs of thin-layer and conventional slides.[15,18]

As mentioned previously, homogenization of the cellular material in thin-layer suspensions is gentle, allowing the maintenance of diagnostic groupings, such as endocervical and endometrial cells. These types of cells appear virtually identical to their morphology in conventional preparations. Patterns such as reparative changes in endocervical cells and the breakdown "exodus" balls of endometrial cells are maintained in each type of preparation (Figs. 11-13 and 11-14).

Because thin-layer specimens are collected in fluid medium, many of the changes seen in thin-layer preparations are similar to those that have been well recognized in other fluid-medium cytology studies.[19] Many of the changes are generic to fluid-based preparations and consist of cells and groups rounding up, with concomitant decreases in two-dimensional size. Because of this phenomenon, when compared with conventional smears, individual cells on thin-layer slides appear smaller, and groups are more three-dimensional with tighter, more cohesive architecture. In addition, because thin-layer preparations are blotted or sedimented onto the slide surface, cell groups retain a prominent three-dimensional architecture rather than undergoing the flattening that occurs when cells are sheared onto the glass surface in the making of a conventional smear. This accentuation of three-dimensionality causes cells at the edges of groups to be less visible on thin-layer slides in comparison with conventional smears, on which such cells may provide the best clues as to the origin of cells present within the group. This feature of thin-layer smears makes investigation of cell groupings more difficult. Hence, classification of lesions and normal cells presenting primarily as groups may be more difficult than in conventional smears.

Because thin layers are made from aliquots of the cell suspension, a uniform number of cells (about 50,000 versus as many as 300,000 on conventional smears) is deposited on each slide. A key feature generally noted in examples of all varieties of abnormalities presenting in

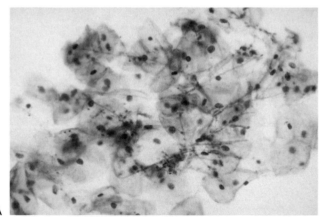

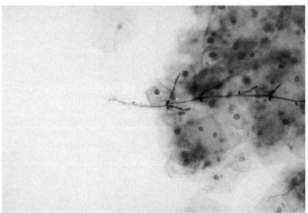

FIG. 11-12. *Candida* organisms are easily identified in thin-layer smears. Examples of *Candida* are shown in conventional (**A**), ThinPrep (**B**) and Cyto-Rich (**C**) slides. In thin-layer preparations, *Candida* organisms appear to stand out from, or "float" on the surface of epithelial groups (**B** & **C**), rather than being intermingled with the epithelial cells as routinely noted in conventional slides (**A**). This feature generally makes *Candida* more readily identified on thin-layer smears (**A,B,C,** 100×; Papanicolaou stain).

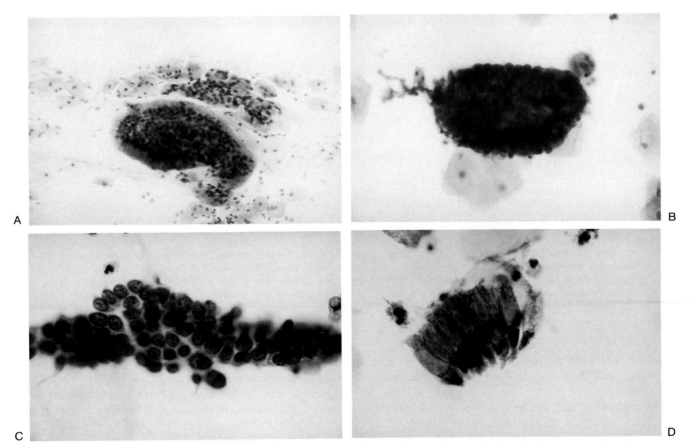

FIG. 11-13. Normal endocervical cells are shown in the conventional (**A**), ThinPrep (**B**), and Cyto-Rich (**C,D**) smears. Normal groupings of endocervical cells remain intact in the thin-layer slides. Note the typical honeycomb (**C**) and picket fence (**D**) arrangements which are well-preserved and illustrated in the thin-layer samples (**A**, 33×; **B**, 66×; **C**, 200×; **D**, 200×; Papanicolaou stain).

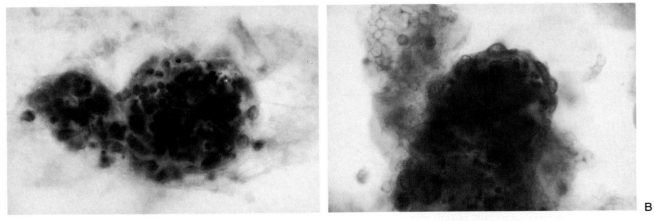

FIG. 11-14. Examples of normal endometrial cells in the typical "exodus" pattern seen on conventional (**A**) and thin-layer (ThinPrep) (**B**) slides from the same clinical sample (**A,B**, 132×; Papanicolaou stain).

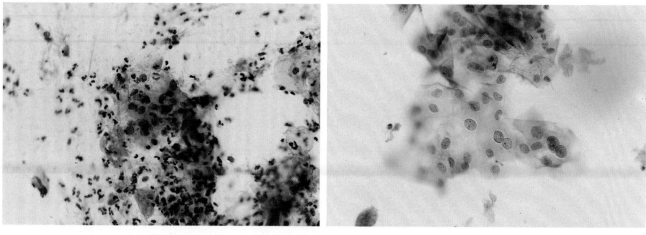

A   B

FIG. 11-15. The nuclear criteria for atypical squamous cells of undetermined significance (ASCUS) can be directly translated from conventional to thin-layer smears. Examples of ASCUS from conventional (**A**) and thin-layer (ThinPrep) (**B**) slides derived from the same clinical sample are shown. Thin-layer preparations often show improved visualization of ASCUS cells, allowing more definitive assessments of benign reactive changes as non-ASCUS cases (**A,B**, 66×; Papanicolaou stain).

thin-layer preparations has been the presence of fewer abnormal cells than may be found on paired conventional smears.

The squamous cell abnormalities of atypia (ASCUS) and LSIL present virtually identical morphologic appearances in thin-layer and conventional slides. The diagnosis of ASCUS (Fig. 11-15) often is more precise in thin-layer smears because of the improvement in nuclear visualization that occurs in thin layers unencumbered by cell overlap and obscuring background factors. In clinical studies, it has been well documented that despite increasing rates of LSIL detection, rates of ASCUS detection in thin layers have decreased.[14] This decrease almost certainly has resulted from improved cellular visualization, which allows for a more precise diagnosis of squamous intraepithelial lesions, benign cellular changes, or

normal findings. A great advantage of thin-layer preparations, therefore, has been diminution of the "wastebasket" portion of ASCUS diagnoses, which includes many cases that show either technical artifact or poorly presented squamous cells that are therefore of unknown significance. Cases of LSIL, including pure cytopathic effect of the human papillomavirus (koilocytotic atypia) and classic mild dysplasia (cervical intraepithelial neoplasia grade I), show entirely similar morphologies using the two techniques (Figs. 11-16 and 11-17).

Cells of HSIL may show similar appearances in thin-layer and conventional slides in many cases (Fig. 11-18). However, significant differences that may be of diagnostic importance have been noted in other cases. Lesions of HSIL tend to show fewer numbers of cells in thin-layer preparations when compared with paired conventional

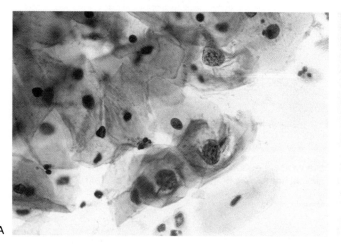
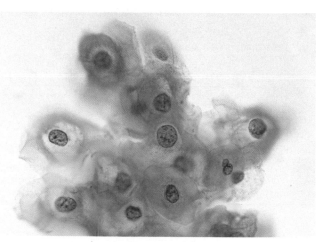

A   B

FIG. 11-16. Koilocytotic atypia, or the cytopathic effect of the human papillomavirus, appears virtually identical in conventional (**A**) and thin-layer (ThinPrep) (**B**) slides (**A,B**, 132×; Papanicolaou stain).

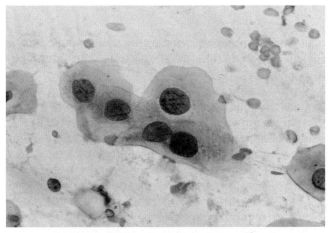

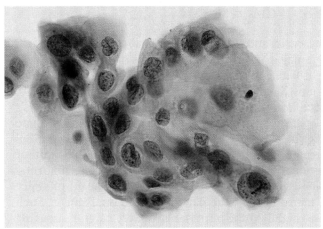

A

B

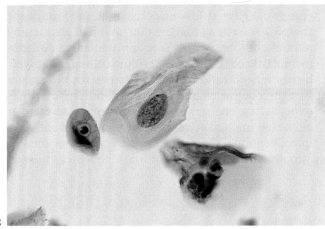

C

FIG. 11-17. Examples of low-grade squamous intraepithelial lesion (LSIL) are shown in conventional (**A**), ThinPrep (**B**), and Cyto-Rich (**C**) slides. (**A & B**) are from the same clinical sample. Criteria for the diagnosis of LSIL are directly transformable between conventional and thin-layer preparations (**A,B,C**, 200×; Papanicolaou stain).

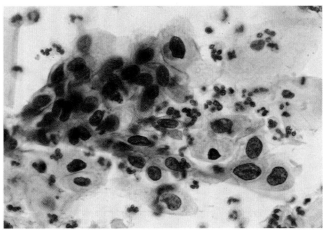

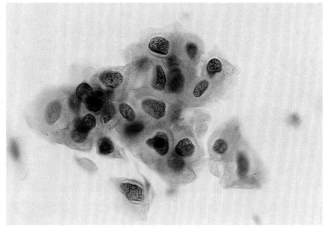

A

B

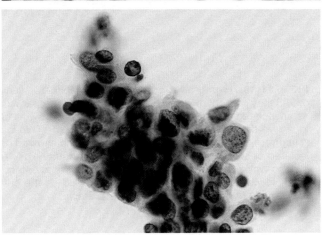

C

FIG. 11-18. Examples of high-grade squamous intraepithelial lesion (HSIL) are shown in conventional (**A**), ThinPrep (**B**), and Cyto-Rich (**C**) slides. (**A & B**) are from the same clinical sample. In these examples, HSIL appears identical in conventional and thin-layer specimens (**A,B**, 200×; Papanicolaou stain).

smears. In addition, fluid suspension and homogenization may cause increasing numbers of abnormal cells to be isolated or to present in small, rather than large, groups. Such cells may have the appearance of immature metaplastic cells,[20,21] which may be mistaken for reserve cells, histiocytes, or small glandular cells. As such, these types of cells need to be searched for carefully on initial screening of thin-layer slides (Fig. 11-19). This author has identified cases of HSIL in which only one abnormal cell was present on a thin-layer slide, despite the presence of many cells on the paired conventional smear. Such cases highlight the importance of very careful screening of thin-layer slides in order to achieve sensitivities of detection similar to those reported earlier in the clinical trials of the instruments. Further discussion of training issues regarding thin-layer cytology is presented later.

The most challenging area of thin-layer cytology is the identification and classification of malignant lesions. Many types of invasive carcinoma that present in the lower female genital tract have appearances that are identical on both types of preparations. Pleomorphic keratinized cells from keratinizing squamous cell carcinoma are illustrated in Figure 11-20, showing main-

tenance of irregular cytoplasmic shapes and conformations in the thin layers despite the liquid-phase suspension.

Nonkeratinizing squamous cell carcinomas and adenocarcinomas of the endocervix and endometrium are types of tumors that present more difficulty for the cytologic observer of thin-layer slides. These tumors are more likely to present with cell groupings that may appear different from conventional preparations because of fluid suspension and lack of shearing force in the making of the final thin-layer slide. Figure 11-21 illustrates examples of nonkeratinizing squamous cell carcinomas that presented on thin-layer slides predominantly as groups of cells. At low magnification, the groups show sharply demarcated borders that, at initial glance, might remind the observer of a group of benign squamous metaplastic cells. It is not until the cells are observed at higher magnification that it becomes readily apparent that the nuclear characteristics are indicative of malignancy. These changes are in distinction to the easily recognizable malignant cells at the margins of the groups in conventional smears. Squamous cells associated with atrophy also may present initial differential diagnostic

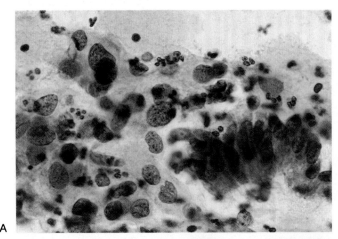

A

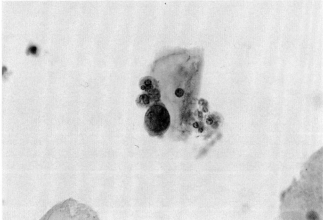

B

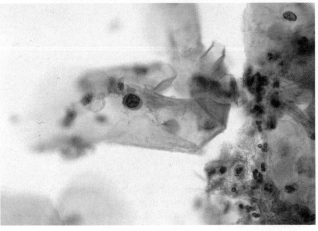

C

FIG. 11-19. High-grade squamous intraepithelial lesion (HSIL) may present more commonly in thin-layer preparations as an isolated cell pattern. (**A**) Conventional smear with HSIL in a two-dimensional sheet-like arrangment. (**B**) Thin-layer (ThinPrep) from the same clinical sample, which showed only isolated or small groups of HSIL cells. (**C**) Another ThinPrep slide in which the single isolated cell present in the center of the field was the only dysplastic cell identified on the entire preparation (**A,B,C**, 132×; Papanicolaou stain).

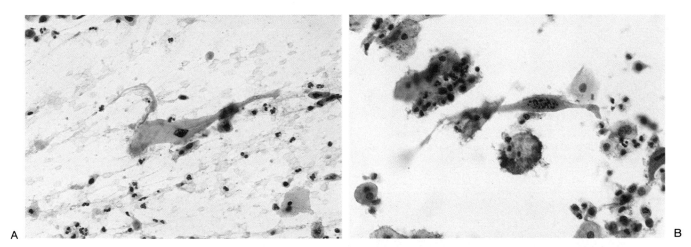

FIG. 11-20. Isolated pleomorphic cells from keratinizing squamous cell carcinoma from the same clinical sample are shown from the conventional (**A**) and thin-layer (ThinPrep) (**B**) slides. These cells have similar morphologic features in the two types of preparations (**A,B**, 132×; Papanicolaou stain).

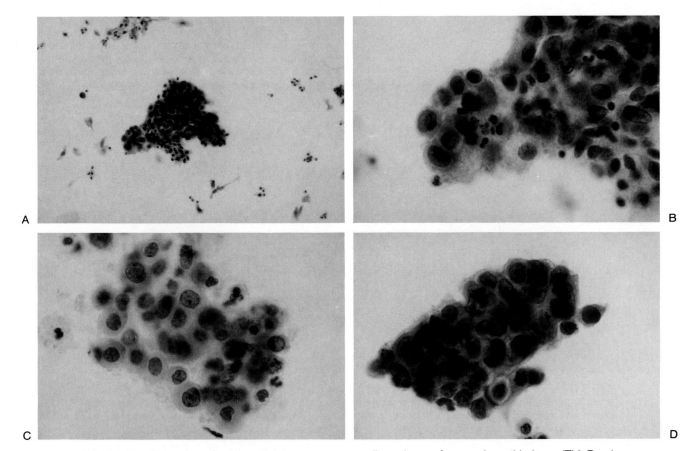

FIG. 11-21. Examples of nonkeratinizing squamous cell carcinoma from various thin-layer (ThinPrep) slides (**A-D**), are shown. At low magnification, groups of nonkeratinizing squamous cell carcinoma may resemble the sharp-bordered groups of benign squamous metaplasia (**A**), which may cause false-negative screenings. When viewed at higher magnification, typical nuclear features of malignancy become obvious, allowing the correct diagnosis to be rendered (**B-D**) (**A**, 50×; **B-D**, 200×; Papanicolaou stain).

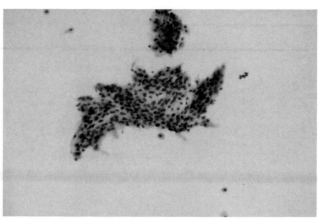

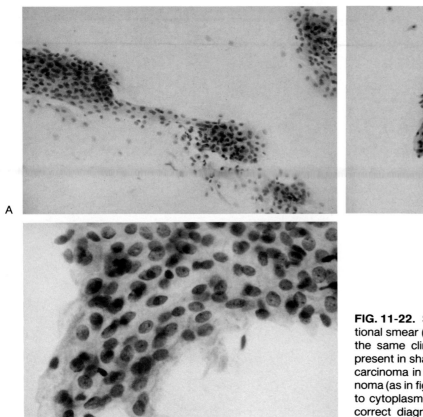

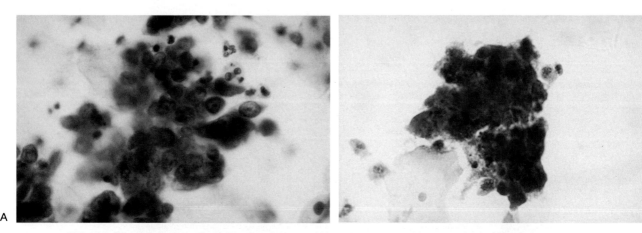

FIG. 11-22. Squamous cells in atrophy are shown in conventional smear (**A**) and in thin-layer (ThinPrep) slides (**B,C**) from the same clinical sample. In thin-layer slides, atrophy can present in sharp boardered groups reminiscent of squamous carcinoma in situ or as nonkeratinizing squamous cell carcinoma (as in figure 21**B**). Close attention to uniformity, nucleus to cytoplasmic ratio, and lack of nuclear atypia will allow a correct diagnosis when evaluated carefully (**A-B**, 50×, **C**, 200×; Papanicolaou stain).

FIG. 11-23. Examples of conventional smear (**A**) and thin-layer (ThinPrep) (**B**) slides from a case of adenosquamous carcinoma of the uterine cervix. Malignancies of glandular type which present predominantly as three-dimensional epithelial clusters may be very difficult to classify due to density and nuclear overlapping in such groups. Cases such as these could potentially increase the number of diagnoses of atypical glandular cells of uncertain significance (AGUS) in the thin-layer systems (**A**, 132×; **B**, 66×; Papanicolaou stain).

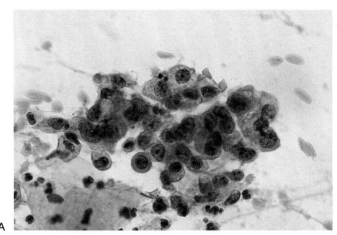
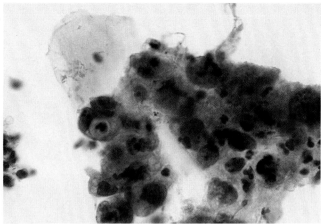

A

B

FIG. 11-24. In this case of endocervical adenocarcinoma, conventional (**A**) and thin-layer (ThinPrep) (**B**) slides were made from the same clinical sample (**A,B**, 198×; Papanicolaou stain).

difficulties. In thin-layer preparations, atrophic cells form sharply marginated groups (Fig. 11-22) that, at low magnification, may mimic the groups of nonkeratinizing squamous cell carcinoma described earlier, or the syncytial groups of squamous carcinoma in situ. Again, high-magnification reviews of such cases aid in correct diagnosis because of the uniformity of the nuclei, lack of atypical nuclear characteristics, and low nucleus-to-cytoplasm ratio.

In cases of adenocarcinoma, malignant cells are routinely present in conventional smears as two- and three-dimensional groups. When suspended and fixed in fluid transport media, these groups become more spherical or clustered. This phenomenon makes normally two-dimensional groups of endocervical adenocarcinoma cells appear more three-dimensional, making it more difficult to differentiate this lesion from endometrial tumors. In addition, nuclei present in such groups show less "visual accessibility" because of overlap and increased cytoplasmic thickness resulting in less cytoplasmic transparency. Therefore, when dealing with cases involved by carcinomas presenting primarily as groups of cells, the thin-layer preparation may show degrees of sensitivity to an abnormality similar to those of the conventional smear; however, there may be a drop in specificity for the correct categorization, which is related to inferior visualization of characteristic differential diagnostic features, as discussed elsewhere in this monograph. Examples of this phenomenon are illustrated in Figures 11-23 through 11-26, which represent examples of groups of glandular neoplasia cells from the two preparation types.

This problem with cellular groupings also may relate to benign cells presenting in three-dimensional configurations. Groups of endocervical and endometrial cells commonly are difficult to evaluate, particularly when re-

active. This circumstance may translate to increased diagnoses of atypical glandular cells of undetermined significance (AGUS) on thin-layer slides (Fig. 11-27).

The background patterns, or contextual features, that often are utilized as important adjuncts to diagnosis can be evaluated on thin-layer preparations. As mentioned previously, inflammatory and bloody smear patterns can be appreciated, as well as the presence and conformation of cell groups. In addition, it is possible to identify tumor diathesis in thin-layer slides. In conventional smears, tumor diathesis appears as necrotic and inflammatory debris spread evenly throughout the smear background. In thin-layer slides, the cellular debris making up the diathesis is coagulated and aggregated in the fluid transport medium, and may appear as coagulated groups of debris

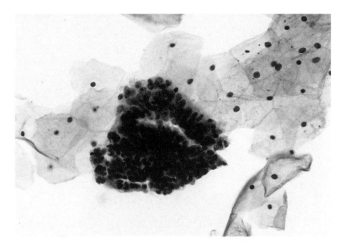

FIG. 11-25. Endometrial hyperplasia is illustrated in a thin-layer (ThinPrep) slide. Uniformity and small size of nuclei differentiate this case from adenocarcinoma (132×; Papanicolaou stain).

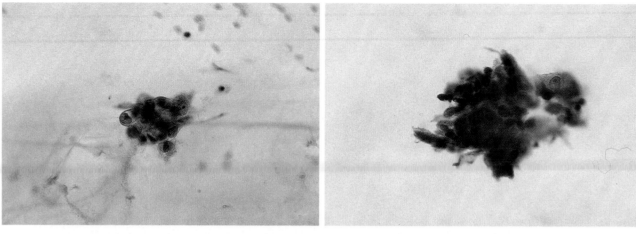

FIG. 11-26. Endometrial adenocarcinoma in conventional (**A**) and thin-layer (Cyto-Rich) (**B**) slides is shown. Note the tight packing and nuclear overlapping in the thin-layer slides. This feature can make definition classification of glandular lesions difficult (**A & B**, 132×; Papanicolaou stain).

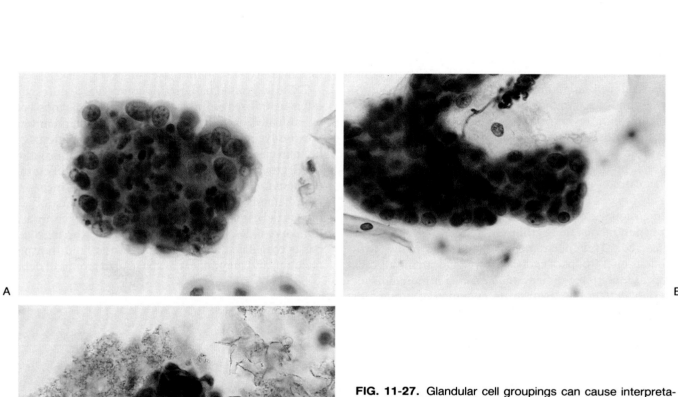

FIG. 11-27. Glandular cell groupings can cause interpretation difficulties in thin-layer preparations. Their three-dimensionality is enhanced in fluid cellular suspensions and as such, groupings may be dense and thick. This may lead to poor visualization of individual cells or nuclei, which may limit optimal specificity of interpretation. Shown are examples of difficult three-dimensional groupings, which were all diagnosed as AGUS. (**A**) Benign reactive endocervical cells, (**B**) papillary serous endometrial carcinoma, and (**C**) endometrial adenocarcinoma, typical form (**A**, ThinPrep, 200×; **B**, ThinPrep, 200×; **C**, Cyto-Rich, 200×; Papanicolaou stain).

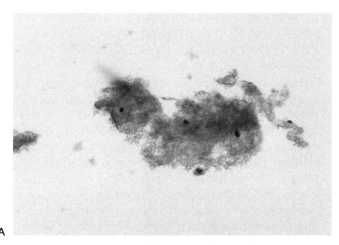
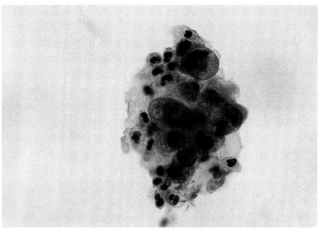

A   B

FIG. 11-28. The typical "clinging" diathesis pattern that is noted in invasive lesions on thin-layer preparations. Glandular debris and inflammatory cells cling to groups of both normal (**A**) and abnormal cells from endocervical adenocarcinoma (**B**), across the smear in a very distinctive and recognizable pattern. Compare with tumor diathesis in conventional smears shown in Figure 6-84 from section on squamous lesions of the cervix (**A,B**, 132×; Papanicolaou stain).

in a clear background. In cases where diathesis debris is less pronounced, it may be found in close association with normal and abnormal cells in the smear. Therefore, the author's group has termed this pattern *clinging diathesis.* This type of diathesis is observed commonly in cases of invasive carcinoma presented in thin-layer slides (Fig. 11-28). A prominent granular diathesis pattern also has been seen in cases of endometrial adenocarcinoma, akin to the "watery" diathesis pattern that is seen on conventional smears in such cases (Fig. 11-29). Such diathesis patterns can be detected easily on initial low-power scanning of the slide, and when present, should immediately raise suspicion of an abnormality.

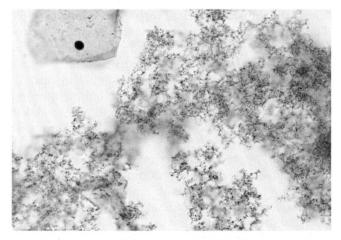

FIG. 11-29. Granular debris in the background of this Cyto-Rich slide having endometrial adenocarcinoma is a correlate of the "watery" diathesis pattern that can be seen in conventional smears with this entity. (See Figure 7-5 from glandular lesions section) (Papanicolaou stain).

OTHER FEATURES OF THIN-LAYER CYTOLOGY

Archival Storage of Cell Suspensions

Because only an aliquot of each cell suspension is utilized in making a standard thin-layer slide for analysis, additional cells are available in storage for further processing. As mentioned above, studies have shown the relative equivalency of multiple slides made from the same suspension, on the basis of randomization of the sample during the homogenization process.[7] This aspect of thin-layer processing allows for the unique advantage of being able to store archival material (analogous to paraffin blocks in histopathology) for future use. Therefore, additional slides can be made for replacement sets, special studies, teaching material, or further diagnostic slides to confirm or enhance an impression. In our laboratory, thin-layer slides have been found to be an entirely appropriate medium on which to perform special histochemical, immunocytochemical, and in situ nucleic acid hybridization assays. In addition, we have found long-term storage to be stable, with specimens prepared after up to 2 years of storage showing morphology identical to that of newly processed material.

Effect of Thin-Layer Technology on Screening Time and Workload

Hypothetically, a cytologist might be able to screen a thin-layer preparation, on average, more rapidly than a corresponding conventional smear. There are several reasons for this conjecture. In the thin-layer preparation, cellular material is located in a consistent 13- or 20-mm circle in a constant central region of the slide. Therefore, cells should be located more rapidly and the number of microscopic fields to be examined should be reduced based on decreased screening area. In addition, clean backgrounds, lack of obscuring elements, and excellent segmentation of epithelial cells should provide for faster analysis. A number of preliminary studies have supported the concept of faster screening of these preparations. Reports have found screening throughput of thin-layer preparations to be as much as 3.39 times higher,[15] but most studies reporting timing data show ratios with an approximately twofold gain using thin-layer preparations.[11,12]

In our own laboratory, we have not done formal time studies to test this hypothetical advantage of thin-layer preparations for cervical cytology. Several points need to be made in overall assessment of the time it takes to examine a thin-layer slide. As noted earlier, many of the morphologic features of abnormalities appearing on thin-layer preparations may require closer scrutiny than on conventional smears. The search for the rare, small, isolated cells of HSIL and close evaluation of normal and atypical groups of cells may require increased vigilance on the part of the screening cytologist. Such morphologic pitfalls may not have been fully appreciated in the initial studies reporting timing data; therefore, this author recommends that additional formalized time studies be conducted by experienced observers before final conclusions are presented regarding workload advantages of thin-layer technology in gynecologic cytology.

Educational Requirements for Initiation of Thin-Layer Technology for Gynecologic Specimens

After final Food and Drug Administration (FDA) approval is obtained for the use of thin-layer technology in cervical cytology, educational programs will need to be developed for laboratory personnel planning to implement this system. Cytotechnologists and pathologists should be familiar with the operating characteristics of the thin-layer systems and with the differences in the morphologic appearances of the normal and abnormal cells present on these slides. Programs must be designed that acquaint cytologists with the full variety of unusual lesions and ensure an initial level of screening competence. One strong recommendation in the ongoing educational process is parallel processing of cervical specimens in a manner analogous to the clinical trials noted earlier, with correlation of paired results and a reconciliation process to point out potential false-negative screening and interpretation results on thin-layer preparations. The length of time this process should be continued is variable and depends on laboratory volume, case mix, and individual experience.

SUMMARY OF THIN-LAYER PREPARATION TECHNIQUES FOR GYNECOLOGIC CYTOLOGY

Thin-layer preparation techniques have been shown to provide some advantages over conventionally prepared cervical cytology specimens. The thin-layer method provides significant opportunities for improvement of quality control in the processing of gynecologic cytology specimens. Cell fixation and slide making are taken out of the hands of clinicians and brought into the laboratory, where uniform processing techniques and quality control of the processing method can produce improved and far more reproducible cytologic slides.

Because cell fixation occurs immediately after collection and slides are made directly from cell suspensions, air-drying artifact is virtually eliminated and factors such as inflammation and blood, which commonly obscure epithelial elements in conventional smears, can be controlled. Slide backgrounds are clean and cells are deposited in uniform areas on each slide produced, promoting ease of screening and interpretation.

It appears that the sensitivity of thin-layer preparations for the detection of squamous intraepithelial lesions may be higher than that of paired conventional smears. This observation has been made in multiple studies, despite the fact that each experimental protocol has favored the conventional slide, with thin-layer cell suspensions being made from the cells that remain after the conventional smear has been produced. Clinical trials also have noted a decrease in squamous atypia (AS-CUS) rates when thin-layer cytology is utilized. This finding indicates greater specificity of the diagnosis, presumably based on improved preservation and visualization of cells. Morphologically, the major disadvantage of thin-layer cytology relates to increased difficulty in visualizing the individual cells of three-dimensional groups. This feature may lead to decreased specificity in discriminating between choices in the differential diagnoses of such groups. In addition, decreased numbers of abnormal cells and the presence of isolated cells in cases of HSIL are features that require additional attention to screening detail in the evaluation of thin-layer slides. Fortunately, these deficiencies have not led to decreased sensitivity of the overall process for positive diagnoses, as exemplified by the presented clinical trial data.

The thin-layer process has additional advantages relating to the ability to maintain archival cell suspension material for future use and the ability to make additional slides for special studies.

One important factor that must be considered in evaluating the usefulness of thin-layer processing is the ratio of additional cost to additional benefit. Because of the need for new processing equipment and disposable items for transport and instrument processing, the cost of uti-

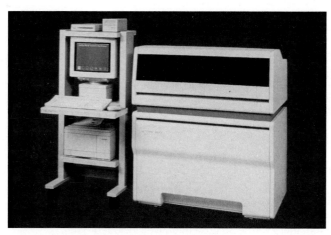

FIG. 11-30. NeoPath AutoPap 300 instrument (courtesy of Stanley F. Patten, Jr., MD, PhD, NeoPath Corp).

lizing thin-layer preparation technology will be greater than that of conventional smears. The additional cost of using this technology ultimately will be determined by the marketplace, but initial estimates are in the range of $2 to $3 per case. Whether or not this increase in cost creates a favorable cost-benefit ratio in an individual laboratory will be determined by potential cost savings in terms of lower unsatisfactory rates, improved screening volumes, and increased overall accuracy.

AUTOMATED SCREENING DEVICES

Three companies have been actively developing computerized screening devices for potential marketing in the United States. They are the NeoPath Corporation (AutoPap 300 and 300QC), Neuromedical Systems (PAPNET), and Roche Image Analysis Systems (AUTO-cyte). All the systems consist of an automated microscope into which slides are automatically loaded via a robotic device. Slides are scanned, with the output of the device being either an overall assessment of the case (NeoPath) or a storing of images of abnormal cells for later presentation to cytologists (Neuromedical, Roche).

NeoPath and Neuromedical instruments utilize conventionally prepared slides, whereas the Roche instrument utilizes thin-layer preparations made via the Cyto-Rich method. Several of the companies have reported preliminary data utilizing their instrumentation, as detailed later.

NeoPath AutoPap 300 and 300 QC (Seattle, WA; Fig. 11-30)

The NeoPath instrumentation has been designed at two levels. The first is a quality control screening device (AutoPap 300 QC) that will review slides previously reported as "within normal limits" and satisfactory after manual screening by a cytotechnologist (Fig. 11-31). The device will identify the cases that are at highest risk for representing false-negative abnormalities, which then can be rescreened by cytotechnologists as replacement for the 10% quality control rescreening mandated by Clinical Laboratory Improvements Act of 1988 (CLIA). Therefore, utilizing this type of device will not increase the laboratory's overall screening workload. In this mode, the instrument can decrease a laboratory's overall false-negative rate. The theoretical advantages of the use of this system are illustrated in Figure 11-32. Clinical trials to document this utility have recently been completed and show that use of the AutoPap 300 QC device increases the number of false-negative cases in the pool of slides entered into quality control screening by a factor of threefold to fivefold (FDA Scientific Advisory Panel Meeting, August 8, 1995; Table 11-7). Human screening of this enhanced quality control pool presumably will result in decreased false-negative rates for the cytology laboratory. The FDA granted approval to this device on September 29, 1995, making the AutoPap 300 QC the first FDA-approved device for automated cytology.

In its second application mode, the instrumentation (AutoPap 300) will operate as a prescreener in order to identify cases that have the highest probability of representing abnormalities. In doing so, the operation of the instrument will be set at such a level that cases falling

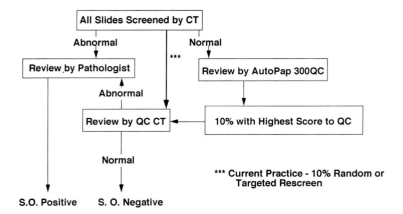

FIG. 11-31. Use of the AutoPap 300QC to select cases for the CLIA '88-mandated quality control rescreening process has been shown to significantly increase the ability to detect false-negative cases (abbreviations: CT, cytotechnologist; QC, quality control; S.O., signout; CLIA '88, Clinical Laboratory Improvement Act of 1988).

Assumptions:

| 5% FN Rate | 50% Sensitivity of AP for FN Cases |

Routine 10% Random Rescreen	AutoPap Rescreening
1000 Cases	1000 Cases
50 FN Cases	50 FN Cases
Random Review of 100 Cases	All Slides Reviewed by AP - 10% Selected
100 Cases with 5 FN Included	100 Cases with 25 FN Included
Cases Rescreened by QC CT	Cases Rescreened by QC CT
4.75 FN Identified	23.75 FN Identified

Theoretical Improvement of FN Identification of 5 fold

FIG. 11-32. This illustration depicts the theoretical advantage in the use of the NeoPath AutoPap 300QC device for selection of the 10% quality control rescreening pool. Assumptions made in the hypothesis are a 5% false negative screening rate, and a 50% sensitivity to false negative case inclusion, within the top 10% of cases. For every 1000 positive cases reviewed, there will be 50 false negatives included. The highest possible number of false negative cases included within the QC screening pool for a random process will be 5. With a 50% sensitivity, 25 false negative cases will be present in the AutoPap-selected quality control pool. After rescreening the selected cases, the AutoPap pool will have identified false negative cases at 5 times the rate as will the random selection process. Data from the clinical trials, testing the device sensitivity assumption, and hence the overall utility of the process, are presented in table 7 (abbreviations: FN, false negative; QC, quality control; CT, cytotechnologist; AP, AutoPap).

below a certain point or "score" can be reliably designated as being "within normal limits" without requiring further human review. Slides whose review triggers an instrument score above this setpoint will be referred on for human screening. An initial sort rate of approximately 50% is the goal for the clinical trials, which are set to begin in 1996. Further refinements and testing are anticipated to achieve an ongoing reduction in the percentage of slides requiring manual screening. Preliminary studies to date have reported comparable rates of sensitivity for abnormal cases between computerized and human screeners, when the instrument is used in the prescreener mode.[22]

Neuromedical Systems: PAPNET (Suffern, NY; Fig. 11-33)

The PAPNET system is designed to identify and present cells and cell groupings to the cytologic observer that

TABLE 11-7. *AutoPap 300QC sensitivity for false-negative cases at the 10% threshold level**

All false-negative	33% (67/203)
All false-negative ≥ low-grade squamous intraepithelial lesion	56.3% (18/32)

* This table shows the sensitivity of the Neopath AutoPap 300 QC device for the detection of false-negative cases within the top 10% of instrument "scores." When compared with the assumed sensitivity of the device shown in Figure 11-32, these figures translate to an approximately 3-fold increase in false-negative case detection (all categories of abnormality), and to a 5-fold increase in false-negative case detection at the level of low-grade squamous intraepithelial lesion and above. These data from the clinical trials clearly show the potential advantage of this process when utilized for quality control in the cytology laboratory.

have the highest probability of being abnormal, according to the neural network computer. Conventionally prepared slides are screened by the device, and a recording of the findings is transmitted to a cytologist reviewing station, where the images are displayed. The cytologist observer may decide that none of the cells or cell groupings presented represents an abnormality and, therefore, immediately diagnose the case as "within normal limits." The observer also may decide that a case has a high likelihood of having an abnormality and that it must be screened by a human cytotechnologist. The intended use of this device is as an adjunctive test to be performed on cases previously diagnosed as "within normal limits" that already have cleared the routine quality control process of the laboratory. As such, additional screening resources need to be allocated in a user's laboratory in order to view the images of cells identified, and rereview slides that are deemed to have a potential abnormality.

Studies performed to date have shown that cellular abnormalities can be discerned on the video screen presentation in virtually all abnormal cases. Koss and colleagues showed that abnormal cells were identified and displayed by the instrument in 97% of cases tested. In this study, the PAPNET system identified additional cases of squamous intraepithelial lesions when it was utilized in a quality control screening mode.[23] In another study, Boon and Kok studied 10 cases of known false-negative cervical smears that were detected in women with invasive carcinoma.[24] In all 10 cases, the PAPNET instrument detected and presented cells or cell groupings that were identified as at least "suspicious." Known carcinoma smears also were detectable using the PAPNET system, and known benign cases were reported to be easily discernible as such in this study. In a separate study, Boon and associates reported on 62 false-negative smears

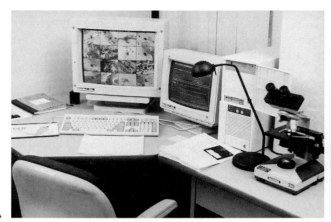
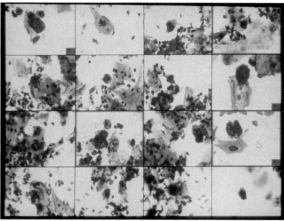

A   B

FIG. 11-33. Neuromedical PAPNET instrument (**A**), review station, which presents abnormal cells and groups to the cytologic observer; (**B**), illustration of video "tiles," which show cells or cell groupings identified as potentially abnormal by the PAPNET instrument. (Courtesy of Laurie Mango, MD, Neuromedical Corp.)

that were rereviewed utilizing the PAPNET method.[25] They found high rates of detection and greater consistency of diagnosis when the PAPNET system of review was employed in the evaluation of each case. Elgart and colleagues also utilized the PAPNET System as a quality control device to rescreen presumably negative smears.[26] The use of PAPNET to select cases for manual rescreening was reported to detect false-negative cases of squamous intraepithelial lesions at a higher rate than does routine human rescreening of cervical smears.

Roche AUTOcyte (Elon College, NC; Fig. 11-34)

The Roche AUTOcyte is reported to operate with an approach similar to that utilized by the PAPNET system. The major difference between the two systems is that the Roche instrument is designed to utilize thin-layer preparations produced with the Cyto-Rich preparation device, as opposed to conventional smears. Theoretically, the use of thin-layer preparations with automated analysis

may produce improved results compared with the same analyses performed with conventional smears. This hypothesis is based on the potential improvement of sensitivity that already has been reported with manual screening of thin-layer preparations. The Roche system, like PAPNET, is designed to screen smears and present video images of abnormal cells to the cytologic observer. The human observer then may diagnose the case immediately as "within normal limits," with no need for further review, or pass the slide along for human review if an abnormality is suspected. In addition, the instrument makes its own in depth assessment of the slide, much like the NeoPath device.

At the time of this writing, promising preliminary studies have been published regarding the operating characteristics of this device. In a study of 1272 cases (728 normal and 544 abnormal), the AUTOcyte instrument showed false-negative rates of 0%, 0.5%, and 2.3% for carcinoma, HSIL, and LSIL, respectively. Interestingly, the false-positive rate for the normal cases was 44.3%. Such data indicate good sensitivity but relatively poor specificity for abnormal cases at present.[27]

THE ROLE OF THE FOOD AND DRUG ADMINISTRATION IN THE IMPLEMENTATION OF AUTOMATED TECHNOLOGY

New devices for medical use must be reviewed by the FDA prior to introduction into general use. The FDA's charge is to determine the safety of the device and the efficacy for the device's intended use, and to perform a risk-benefit analysis of the product. Based on the complexity of the proposed test, the FDA assigns a classification to each new device or test proposed for the market. Automated cervical cytology instrumentation has been placed in the highest class of devices (class III),

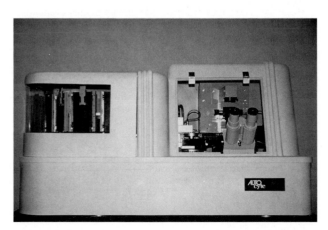

FIG. 11-34. Roche AutoCytc instrument (courtesy of Ernest Kneisel, Roche Image Analysis Systems).

which requires extensive laboratory testing and clinical studies prior to marketing approval. This comprehensive assessment, or premarket approval, is required for all the automated preparation and screening devices mentioned in this chapter. The premarket approval process is lengthy, requiring clinical trials to demonstrate the three aspects of the FDA charge noted earlier. At this writing, no manufacturer of thin-layer technology has received FDA approval for its device. As previously stated, Neo-Path has received FDA approval to market its device for selection of the 10% quality control population and for adjunctive testing of negative smears, and the PAPNET device has received approval only for use as an adjunctive test.

Thin-layer preparation may be utilized for nongynecologic cytology because the FDA has deemed that there is no current standard for nongynecologic specimen preparation. Therefore, thin layers do not represent a new methodology that must be compared with a standard of practice. Hence, FDA approval is not required for their use in these types of specimens.[28]

SUMMARY

Automated thin-layer preparation in gynecologic cytology has been shown to be an effective and potentially improved method of making cervical smears. The major advantages include the potential for standardization of cervical smear preparation, with quality control monitors being applicable. A change to this method will yield improvements in slide quality and consistency, and in accuracy of interpretation. In addition, the process itself appears to be more sensitive for the detection of squamous lesions of the cervix, presumably because of the randomization process during preparation, improved visualization of the lesions that are present, and fewer unsatisfactory or less than optimal slides. Findings supporting these improvements have been demonstrated in multiple cited studies.

In the arena of automated screening of cervical cytology specimens, preliminary studies also have shown promising results, which, if ultimately proven to be accurate, will enhance the productivity and reliability of cytologic evaluations. The ability to add quality control instrument screening to current quality control procedures in the laboratory should improve overall false-negative rates. The addition of instrument-based prescreening of cervical smears will alleviate a significant amount of work in the laboratory, allowing the cytotechnologist to concentrate on more challenging and rewarding specimens while increasing overall productivity. It is the burden of the corporations bringing the described products to market, to convince the regulatory agencies and the consuming public, through the conduct of scientific trials, that these devices will enhance the overall quality of care in a cost-efficient manner. With increasing demand for cervical screening programs and decreasing resources available in the cytology laboratory, such devices will be welcome upon their ultimate approval for clinical use.

REFERENCES

1. Husain OAN. The history of automated cell scanners. In Grohs HK, Husain OAN (eds). Automated cervical cancer screening. New York: Igaku-Shoin, 1994:3.
2. Wheeless LL. Onderdonk MA. Preparation of gynecologic cytology specimens for automated analysis: an overview. J Histochem Cytochem 1974;22:522.
3. Mead JS, Horan PK, Wheeless LL. Syringing as a method of cell dispersal: I. effect on intermediate and superficial squamous cells. Acta Cytol 1978;22:86.
4. Rosenthal DL, Stern E, McLatchie C, et al. A simple method of producing a monolayer of cervical cells for digital image processing. Anal Quant Cytol 1979;1:84.
5. Oud PS, Zahniser DJ, Harbers-Hendriks R, et al. The development of a cervical smear preparation procedure for the BioPERP image analysis system. Anal Quant Cytol 1981;3:74.
6. Hutchinson ML, Cassim CM, Ball HG. The efficacy of an automated preparation device for cervical cytology. Am J Clin Pathol 1991;96:300.
7. Hutchinson ML, Isenstein LM, Goodman A, et al. Homogeneous sampling accounts for the increased diagnostic accuracy using the ThinPrep processor. Am J Clin Pathol 1994;101:215.
8. Wilbur DC, Cibas ES, Merritt S, et al. ThinPrep processor. Clinical trials demonstrate an increased detection rate of abnormal cervical cytologic specimens. Am J Clin Pathol 1994;101:209.
9. Cibas ES, Constantine NM, Dinisco S, et al. The accuracy of a new cervical cytology preparation device compares favorably to conventional smears as correlated with colposcopically directed biopsy results. Acta Cytol 1992;36:579.
10. James LP, Knapp D. New cervical cytology preparation device shows improved sensitivity to abnormal findings over the conventional Papanicolaou smear. Acta Cytol 1992;36:579.
11. Awen C, Hathway S, Eddy W, et al. Efficacy of ThinPrep preparation of cervical smears: a 1,000 case, investigator-sponsored study. Diagn Cytopathol 1994;11:33.
12. Knowles K, Bur M, Otis C, et al. Comparison between conventional Papanicolaou smears and ThinPrep preparations for evaluation of cervicovaginal cytology. Acta Cytol 1992;36:582.
13. Kish J, Vallera D, Ruby S, et al. ThinPrep gynecologic study: a review of 488 cases. Acta Cytol 1994;38:806.
14. Wilbur DC, Dubeshter B, Angel C, et al. Use of thin-layer preparation for gynecologic smears with emphasis on the cytomorphology of high-grade intraepithelial lesions and carcinomas. Diagn Cytopathol (In Press)
15. Geyer JW, Hancock F, Carrico C, et al. Preliminary evaluation of Cyto-Rich: an improved automated cytology preparation. Diagn Cytopathol 1993;9:417.
16. Azlin T, Smith S, Lambird PA. A comparison study of gynecologic specimens using the Roche Cyto-Rich monolayer Papanicolaou smear and the conventional Papanicolaou smear methods. Acta Cytol 1994;38:805.
17. Geyer JW, Heinzerling R, Kirkpatrick M, et al. An analysis of the false-negative rates in the various diagnostic categories for matched Cyto-Rich cervical and conventional Papanicolaou smear preparations. Acta Cytol 1994;38:806.
18. Evans SK, Wilbur DC. Identification of endocervical cells and microorganisms on cervical thin-layer cytology specimens: comparison to paired conventional smears. Acta Cytol 1993;37:776.
19. Reagan JW, Lin F. An evaluation of the vaginal irrigation technique in the detection of uterine cancer. Acta Cytol 1967;11:374.
20. Sheils L, Wilbur DC. The significance of atypical cells of squamous type (AS) on Papanicolaou smears: a 5 year follow-up study. Acta Cytol 1992;36:580.
21. Dressel DM, Wilbur DC. Atypical immature squamous metaplastic cells in cervical smears: association with high grade squamous

intraepithelial lesions (HGSIL) and carcinomas of the cervix. Acta Cytol 1992;36:630.

22. Richart RM, Nelson AC, Wood T. Clinical test results for automated quality control and primary screening of cervical smears using the NeoPath AutoPap 300 system. Acta Cytol 1994;38:805.

23. Koss LG, Lin E, Schreiber K, et al. Evaluation of the PAPNET cytologic screening system for quality control of cervical smears. Am J Clin Pathol 1994;101:220.

24. Boon ME, Kok LP. Neural network processing can provide means to catch errors that slip through human screening of Pap smears. Diagn Cytopathol 1993;9:411.

25. Boon ME, Kok LP, Nygaard-Neilsen M, et al. Neural network processing of cervical smears can lead to a decrease in diagnostic vari-

ability and an increase in screening efficacy: a study of 63 false-negative smears. Mod Pathol 1994;7:957.

26. Elgart PA, Suhrland MJ, Re E, et al. Prospective quality control of cervical smears using the PAPNET system. Acta Cytol 1994;38:804.

27. Knesel E. Roche Image Analysis Systems. In Weid GL, Bartels PH, Rosenthal DL, et al (eds). Compendium on the computerized cytology and histology laboratory. Chicago: Tutorials of Cytology, 1994:353.

28. Brindza LJ. Governmental approval of technology and equipment and related issues. In Grohs HK, Husain OAN (eds). Automated cervical cancer screening. New York: Igaku-Shoin, 1994:249.

Gynecologic Cytopathology. Edited by
Thomas A. Bonfiglio and Yener S. Erozan.
Lippincott–Raven Publishers, Philadelphia, © 1997.

CHAPTER 12

Quality Assurance in the Cytopathology Laboratory

Karen M. Atkison

The primary function of the cytopathology laboratory is to evaluate and report cytologic findings on gynecologic and nongynecologic specimens. The goal of the laboratory is to ensure that the reported results are accurate, reliable, and meaningful to the physician or health care provider. Accuracy in reporting is key because the clinician relies on the laboratory results as one of the parameters used in treating and managing the patient.

To achieve accurate and reliable test results, the laboratory must monitor and assess the quality of all phases of the testing process, including specimen collection, accessioning, microscopic evaluation, reporting, and record retention. In order to accomplish this, the laboratory should establish quality assessment parameters to evaluate the effectiveness of its processes as well as the competency of the individuals performing the tests. Quality assessment parameters include quality control data, laboratory statistics, and personnel performance indicators. The documentation and subsequent analysis of these parameters can be used to identify and correct deviations (errors) from established standards of laboratory practice in any phase of the testing process. This permits continuous quality improvement and maximizes the effectiveness and quality of the health care delivery system in cytology.

The specific components of a comprehensive quality assurance program for the cytology laboratory are determined by the laboratory director. It should be noted, however, that federal and, in many instances, state regulations define mandatory standards for cytology laboratory practice. These regulations detail the quality control

and quality assurance activities and the personnel standards that must be in place.

MANDATORY REGULATION OF LABORATORY PRACTICE

The federal government is the primary player in the regulatory arena. The Clinical Laboratory Improvement Amendment of 1988 (CLIA 88) established principles that resulted in regulations for clinical practice in any laboratory that performs tests and receives financial reimbursement for Medicare patients. The Health Care Financing Administration established the federal regulations to comply with the law established by CLIA 88 and is responsible for monitoring and enforcing compliance.

The Health Care Financing Administration may monitor regulatory compliance through certifying or licensing agencies, such as state departments of health, the College of American Pathologists, and the Joint Commission on the Accreditation of Hospitals. These agencies perform clinical laboratory inspections and certify that the laboratory meets the minimum requirements to provide clinical laboratory service in each specialty. In 1995, the Health Care Financing Administration granted deemed status to the College of American Pathologists, the Joint Commission on the Accreditation of Hospitals, and New York state. Therefore, the clinical laboratory inspection programs of these agencies meet the requirements of the federal government. These certifying agencies evaluate compliance of clinical laboratory practice with the requirements detailed in the CLIA 88 regulations.

Each certifying agency may establish its own guidelines or regulations that meet the standards found in the

K. M. Atkison: Department of Pathology and Laboratory Medicine, University of Rochester Medical Center, Rochester, New York 14642.

CLIA 88 regulations. However, each agency may set more stringent standards for any area of laboratory practice. For example, in cytology, some states have set the workload limit of slides screened per 24-hour period at 80 compared with the limit of 100 established in CLIA 88. If the regulation of a certifying agency is more stringent than that of CLIA 88, it supersedes the federal regulation.

The cytology laboratory may be inspected by more than one agency. For example, in New York state, a hospital cytology laboratory may be inspected by both the state department of health and the Joint Commission on the Accreditation of Hospitals. The laboratory must comply with the regulations of all the certifying agencies that directly approve that laboratory to practice cytology. Therefore, because regulations may vary between agencies, it is important to become familiar with each set of regulations or guidelines. These regulations can provide a framework that can be used as an outline for an effective quality assurance program. Overall, the cytology laboratory quality assurance program must be designed to meet mandatory regulatory requirements.

A copy of the interpretive guidelines that detail the CLIA 88 regulations and accompanying examples of how the regulations should be interpreted can be obtained by contacting National Technical Information Services, App C. PB92146174 (800-553-6847 or 703-487-4650).

QUALITY ASSURANCE PROGRAM

Meeting the requirements of established regulations is an important aspect of a quality assurance program. However, the real purpose and objective of a good quality assurance program is to provide the means for the laboratory to ensure that it is providing the best possible service to the patient.

Quality assurance is a comprehensive process. Its systems evaluate and monitor all aspects of specimen testing and laboratory operations. In cytology, the evaluation includes specimen collection by the health care provider; the testing process (accession, cytologic evaluation, and reporting of test results); the competence of the individuals performing the tests; the maintenance of quality control and statistical data; the use of appropriate facilities and equipment for testing; and established methods for correcting identified problems.

STANDARD OPERATING PROCEDURE MANUAL

The laboratory is required by law to have available a standard operating procedure manual (SOPM). The SOPM should contain a description of all laboratory policies, procedures, and methods pertaining to testing, laboratory operations, and personnel. Any activity performed by the laboratory should be detailed in the SOPM. All policies, procedures, and methods appearing in the SOPM should be followed and adhered to by all laboratory personnel. In effect, the SOPM functions as a handbook of operations and should be detailed enough to guide any new employee with little or no supervision.

The laboratory's medical director is responsible for approving all policies and procedures in the SOPM. The director must sign and date each procedure; however, a coversheet may be used to approve the manual in its entirety. If the directorship changes, the procedures must be reapproved by the new director. Each change in a procedure must be approved, signed, and dated by the director. If a procedure changes, the date of its initial use and discontinuance must be maintained for a minimum of 2 years.

CYTOTECHNOLOGIST QUALIFICATIONS AND CONTINUING EDUCATION

The laboratory director is responsible for hiring adequately trained individuals to perform the laboratory tests. On hiring, a cytotechnologist should be able to evaluate accurately gynecologic and nongynecologic cytologic specimens. Qualifications include successful completion of specialized training in cytology at an approved and accredited school of cytotechnology, a baccalaureate degree, and registration as a cytotechnologist after successful completion of the Board of Registry examination in cytotechnology.

To maintain competence, the cytotechnologist should participate in some form of continuing education. Federal law does not directly mandate a specified number of continuing education hours for cytotechnologists. However, CLIA 88 regulations state that the laboratory director is responsible for ensuring that the individuals performing the tests are competent and that they remain competent. The director must identify the needs of individuals for remedial training or continuing education to improve detection and interpretation skills. Other certifying agencies require a minimum number of documented continuing education hours in cytology in order to remain qualified to practice. New York, Florida, and California are examples of states that require cytotechnologists to provide formal documentation of participation in continuing education.

FACILITIES AND EQUIPMENT

It is the responsibility of the laboratory director to provide a safe and efficient working environment for the performance of all testing events. Adequate space and ventilation must be available for all laboratory personnel to carry out the functions required in the testing process.

Appropriate equipment must be provided that contributes to accurate and reliable testing.

The laboratory should be arranged to provide adequate space for cytologic preparation, data processing, interpretation of glass slide material, and storage of glass slides and records. The contaminated preparation area should not be contiguous with the noncontaminated screening or data processing area. Clearly delineated and separate spaces should be provided.

Adequate ventilation (fume hoods) to accommodate the elimination of fumes from alcohol, xylene, or any other chemicals used in the testing process must be available. Frequent monitoring of air quality with the use of button- or badge-like detectors or more elaborate systems should be routinely performed and documented.

The laboratory must establish a policy for monitoring and documenting the maintenance of all equipment used in the cytology laboratory. This policy must be available in the SOPM. Microscopes should be cleaned and serviced semiannually. All fume and biologic hoods, centrifuges, and ovens must be serviced, calibrated, or checked for safety, efficiency, and accuracy annually. A policy stating the course of action to be taken in the event of equipment malfunction or failure should be established and available in the SOPM.

A safe environment must be provided that protects employees from physical, chemical, and biologic harm. A separate safety manual should be available detailing the safety precautions observed by the laboratory as well as the appropriate course of action for an emergency such as a chemical spill. Posting of safety precautions is recommended. Maps detailing exit routes in the event of fire or other large-scale disaster (evacuation plan) should be posted and plainly visible to all employees. Emergency telephone numbers for fire and hazardous waste removal should be readily available. Protective clothing and equipment should be available for any personnel handling biologically hazardous material.

SPECIMEN COLLECTION

Because the procurement of an adequate specimen for gynecologic testing begins with specimen collection by the health care provider, the laboratory must provide detailed instructions on how to obtain an adequate Papanicolaou smear. A client service manual detailing how to collect and submit cytologic specimens should be made available by the laboratory and distributed to all clients.

The information in the manual can be distributed in any format. A brochure, newsletter, test requisition, or manufacturer's instruction booklet can be used. A separate client service manual can be created for cytology, or it can be included in the general manual covering all laboratory services provided by the clinical laboratory. The manual should contain information on laboratory service hours and the telephone numbers of key individuals to contact with questions or concerns.

Specifically, Papanicolaou smear collection instructions provided to the clinician should include detailed specimen identification procedures; a list of materials required to obtain a Papanicolaou smear (ie, sampling devices, glass slides, fixative); the appropriate method of collection, cell spread, and fixation; and the best means of packaging and sending the specimen to the laboratory.

The clinician should be instructed on how to properly label the glass slide with the patient's name or other unique identifier that matches the information on the accompanying test requisition or test request form. Some laboratories require that the glass slide be labeled with the patient's last name and first initial. Others supply multiple matching, preassigned labels to be affixed to the glass slide and test requisition. The exact method of specimen identification required by each laboratory should be specified to the health care provider.

Instructions detailing significant clinical and demographic information required by the laboratory should also be included in the client service manual and communicated to the health care provider. Clinical information such as last menstrual period; age (date of birth); hysterectomy status; previous abnormal cytology, histology, or colposcopy; and any clinical history placing the patient at high risk for the development of cervical disease are examples of the information that should be requested and provided. The use of check boxes on the test request form facilitates the submission of this information.

SPECIMEN RECEIPT AND ACCESSION

Once the specimen is received by the laboratory, it is good laboratory practice to assess its integrity prior to accession. However, the laboratory should first establish specimen rejection criteria in the form of a written policy, which should be communicated to the clinician. If a specimen fails to meet acceptable standards, the event and the course of action taken should be documented. Acceptance standards usually include correlation of the identifying information on the glass slide and the accompanying requisition, submission of the name and address of the referring physician, and receipt of an intact glass slide. The actions the laboratory may take when acceptance standards are not met include returning the specimen to the referring physician and telephoning the physician to obtain information necessary to correct the discrepancy.

The laboratory is responsible for tracking the dates related to the course of events specimens undergo once they have been received in the laboratory. At a minimum, these should include the date of receipt of the specimen in the laboratory, the date of slide review, and the date of the final report. These dates can then be compared with the date of specimen collection and can be used to monitor any significant delays in transportation as well as the time frame associated with routine processing, evaluation, and reporting.

QUALITY CONTROL: STAINING

Once the specimen has been deemed acceptable and is subsequently accessioned, it must be stained using a standard Papanicolaou stain. The quality of stained slides must be assessed and documented by laboratory personnel on a daily basis. Acceptable standards for staining intensity and color, as well as what constitutes a deviation from acceptable standards (ie, too dark or light, water contamination, air bubbles) should be established in the form of a written policy. If a staining problem is identified, the type of problem and the action taken to correct it should be documented on the daily record. The dates of all events and identities of all personnel involved should be recorded (see Appendices 1 and 2).

Nongynecologic specimens must be stained separately from gynecologic specimens. If space permits, a separate staining set-up with dishes dedicated to nongynecologic samples should be used. If space does not permit, all solutions must be either discarded or filtered between gynecologic and nongynecologic staining.

A copy of the staining protocol for both gynecologic and nongynecologic specimens, with associated flow charts, should be posted in the staining area. The dishes should be labeled as to their contents. The lids should not be labeled because they may be mismatched on the dishes. Any commercial stain or alcohol should be dated on receipt in the laboratory and the expiration date monitored. A record documenting when the stains are changed or filtered and by whom should be kept by the cytopreparatory personnel. All containers of any solution found in the laboratory must be labeled as to their contents and dated.

EVALUATION OF THE CELLULAR SAMPLE

Prior to evaluation and interpretation of the cellular findings, the cytotechnologist should be aware of laboratory policy and procedure related to cytologic evaluation. The following policies or procedures should be detailed in a step-by-step fashion in the SOPM and made available to all laboratory personnel:

1. The recommended method of screening (ie, horizontal or vertical screening motion, manual or mechanical stage)
2. A list of the diagnostic terminology used by the laboratory, with a brief description of the criteria used to assess all diagnostic categories (ie, within normal lim-

its, satisfactory but limited by specific factors, unsatisfactory, premalignant, malignant)
3. A list of the categories of diagnoses that require a pathologist's review
4. The protocol for routine evaluation and signout of any Papanicolaou smear that does not require review by a pathologist, including selection and documentation of cases to be screened, recording of diagnoses, report generation, and slide storage
5. The method for identifying and marking cells to be referred to a pathologist for review
6. The protocol for submitting a case that qualifies for 10% routine quality control rescreening as well as the protocol for rescreening a 10% quality control case
7. Workload standards (ie, limits for individual cytotechnologists)

It is important to note that records documenting the date the case was screened, the identity of the individual screening the case, the identity of the pathologist reviewing the case, and the date of final signout must be maintained by the laboratory. This information can be recorded on the test requisition, worksheet, or laboratory information system. According to CLIA 88 regulations, any records established by the laboratory should be kept on file and available for review for a minimum of 2 years. If a worksheet is used to record dates or cytologic interpretations, the worksheet is considered to be a record that must be maintained by the laboratory. This documentation allows the laboratory to evaluate the timeliness of the testing system, to identify the personnel involved, and to track a specimen throughout the testing process.

It is also important for the laboratory to keep a record of the cytotechnologist's interpretation, especially if the case has been referred to a pathologist for review. Care should be taken when using a laboratory information system for reporting to avoid deleting from the electronic record evidence of all interpretations by signout personnel.

DOCUMENTATION OF CYTOTECHNOLOGIST WORKLOAD AND COMPETENCE

State and federal laws mandate the maximum number of slides that any individual (cytotechnologist or pathologist) performing primary evaluation (screening) can evaluate in a 24-hour period. However, this maximum allowable limit should not be used by the laboratory director as a minimum standard output for all cytotechnologists. Each individual cytotechnologist must be evaluated by the laboratory director for accuracy and competence, and assigned a daily average volume in keeping with his or her ability.

The law requires that this performance assessment be conducted and documented by the laboratory director semiannually. Various performance indicators established by the laboratory director and documented in writing in the SOPM can be used to evaluate competence. Examples of suitable performance indicators include false-negative rate, individual positive rate compared with overall laboratory positive rate, ratio of cases referred to the pathologist for review that were signed out positive versus negative, total daily volume, interpretation skills, and type and amount of continuing education.

To monitor the daily volume, each cytotechnologist is responsible for documenting the actual number of slides screened and the number of hours spent screening per 24-hour period. The recording of other related activities, such as assisting on fine-needle aspiration procedures, preparing nongynecologic specimens, and accessioning specimens received in the laboratory, aids the supervisor and laboratory director in assessing fluctuations in daily output (see Appendix 3).

A cytotechnologist who is employed by more than one laboratory must sign a qualifying statement indicating this fact. The cytotechnologist is responsible for supplying workload information to all employers so that each laboratory can determine whether the individual is remaining within maximum workload limits for any given period. Workload limits prevent excessive volume screening, which can result in fatigue and a potential subsequent increase in undetected abnormalities.

ACCURATE REPORTING OF RESULTS

It is the goal of the cytology laboratory to report accurate and reliable test results in a timely fashion. To ensure accuracy, the laboratory's quality assurance program should include a system for verifying a final report before it is released to the referring physician. The patient's demographic and clinical information as it appears on the final report should match that on the test request form. The final diagnosis, dates of testing events, and identity of personnel involved should match internal laboratory records. Verification of a final report can be performed by manual review or by use of a mandatory review step on a laboratory information system.

FINAL REPORTS: VERIFICATION OF REVIEW BY A PATHOLOGIST

Federal law requires that all gynecologic cases interpreted as reactive, premalignant, or malignant, and all nongynecologic specimens be reviewed by a pathologist. The date and outcome of the review must be documented in the record system. If the laboratory is computerized and does not utilize an electronic signature, or if the laboratory is not computerized, the pathologist must manually verify and sign each final report before releasing it to the health care provider. This review serves a quality control function to ensure the accuracy of all abnormal and nongynecologic cytology reports generated.

For clarification, a signature or name generated by a computer does not constitute an electronic signature. To qualify as an electronic signature, the system must be secure. The release of any final report must be initiated by the pathologist using a secure code accessible only to that pathologist. If data entry personnel or a cytotechnologist can edit a final report, the laboratory is not utilizing an electronic signature.

A written policy and procedure for the signout of any case requiring review by a pathologist must be available in the SOPM. Step-by-step instructions detailing report generation and verification must also be provided in the SOPM.

QUALITY CONTROL: DETECTION OF ERRORS IN EVALUATION

The primary goal of quality assurance is to detect errors or deviations from acceptable laboratory standards. False-negative cases and discrepancies between cytologic interpretation and histologic confirmation provide a means of detecting errors through quality control review. Quality control systems that previously were utilized voluntarily in most high-quality laboratories are now mandated by federal regulations. These include 10% rescreening of cases previously diagnosed as negative or within normal limits, retrospective review of the last 5 years of slides previously diagnosed as negative on any case currently diagnosed as a high-grade squamous intraepithelial lesion or above, and cytology-histology correlation studies.

Ten Percent Quality Control

Although not regarded as the most effective method of detecting false-negative cytology cases, one of the most commonly utilized systems in the cytology laboratory is the random rescreening of a minimum of 10% of cases deemed to be within normal limits on initial screening. Cases should be randomly selected for rescreening and should include patients who are considered to be at high risk for the development of cervical neoplasia. A written policy detailing how a case qualifies for routine 10% rescreening should be available in the SOPM. The rescreening can be performed by either a cytotechnologist with a minimum of 3 years of full-time experience or a pathologist. The rescreening of cases must be performed prior to the release of the final report.

Documentation of the cases selected, the date of the rescreening, and the identity of rescreening personnel should be maintained in the record system. Although rescreening of 10% of the total eligible population is sufficient, it is recommended that 10% of each individual's workload be rescreened. In the event a false-negative case is detected, documentation must be maintained. The primary screening cytotechnologist who did not detect the abnormality should be given the case for review, and this review should be documented. These quality control results can be used as performance indicators to monitor the competence of individual cytotechnologists (see Appendix 4).

Retrospective Review of Cases Previously Diagnosed as Negative

One of the more effective quality control methods used for the detection of false-negative gynecologic cytology is the review of slides previously diagnosed as negative on any case that currently is diagnosed as a high-grade squamous intraepithelial lesion, invasive cancer, or atypical glandular cells of undetermined significance (AGUS). By regulation, the review should encompass the previous 5 years of available cytology. A written policy detailing which abnormalities warrant initiation of a retrospective review and the documentation procedures associated with the review should be available in the SOPM.

The record system for the 5-year retrospective review should include documentation of the following: the date of the search for cases previously deemed to be negative, the identity of the individual performing the search, the results of the search (ie, cases found or not found), the accession numbers of the cases found, and the interpretation(s) on rescreening. Documentation of review of a false-negative case by a pathologist and the original primary screening cytologist should also be maintained in the record system. This review ensures that continuing education for remediation is used to minimize future errors by the cytotechnologist (see Appendix 5).

The laboratory should establish a written policy for the issuance of revised or corrected reports on false-negative cases detected on retrospective rescreening. Federal law requires that revised reports be issued if the revised interpretation is clinically significant and would alter the current management protocol for the patient.

Cytology-Histology Correlation

Cytology-histology correlation incorporates the review of all positive gynecologic cases with the available corresponding biopsy specimens and all positive biopsy specimens with the available corresponding cytology specimens. This quality control review assesses diagnostic accuracy and may detect false-negative or false-positive cytology results. The cytology laboratory should assess and document the total number of gynecologic cases with available and unavailable histologic correlation, the number of correlates and noncorrelates, and the

reasons for any discrepancies. The findings generated from the cytology-histology review can be used as indicators for evaluating the performance of individual cytotechnologists and pathologists (see Appendix 6).

REVISED OR CORRECTED REPORTS

A revised report is generated when an original diagnosis that has been reported to a health care provider requires revision due to a significant change that might have an impact on clinical management. Most frequently, the change in diagnosis occurs when a false-negative or false-positive case is detected during the quality control process.

In the event it is necessary to issue a revised interpretation, the laboratory must ensure that a copy of all the original information, including the preliminary and final interpretations, is maintained in the laboratory record system. Any revised or corrected report that is generated must clearly delineate the original diagnosis from the revised diagnosis and include an explanation of why the report was revised. If the laboratory is computerized and utilizes a laboratory information system for operations, a program must be established that allows the user to maintain the original information and not replace it with the revised diagnosis. This requirement extends to all clinical information, including dates of testing events and identities of personnel.

The laboratory director must establish a written policy detailing the circumstances that warrant the issuance of a revised report. This policy should be available in the SOPM. As stated previously, federal law requires that a revised report be issued if the revised diagnosis will have an impact on the current course of clinical management.

RECORDS

The laboratory is required to maintain numerous quality control records for 2 years per federal regulations. A record is the documentation of an activity, event, or data collected in the testing process. These records provide useful information that, when analyzed, monitors laboratory operations and may detect deviations from standards. The following records should be incorporated into the cytology quality assurance program:

Daily Papanicolaou stain assessment
Change and filter stain log
Specimen rejection and course of action log
Temperature control charts for refrigerator and oven
Telephone call log to document calls received and made, especially those that involve problem resolution or reporting of diagnoses

Test requisition or test request form; this record contains all the original patient demographic and clinical information

Any worksheet used to document preliminary interpretations, dates, or personnel; if a "sticky" note is used for this purpose, it is considered to be a record and must be maintained

Any record used to track specimens (ie, accession log, referenced material log, slides loaned to other laboratories, list of nongynecologic specimens received, list of gynecologic cases taken to be screened by cytotechnologist)

List of cases that qualified for 10% quality control rescreening

Workload recording and semiannual assessment of workload and competence

Retrospective review of previous 5 years of negative cytology reports on cases currently diagnosed as high-grade squamous intraepithelial lesions

Revised reports (keep copy of original and revised reports)

Continuing education activity, including conferences, journals, and reviews of cases with pathologists

False-negative case log

RETENTION REQUIREMENTS

Federal regulations state that all laboratory records must be retained by the laboratory for 2 years. The original hard copies of all records do not need to be maintained. Electronic files, microfilm, and microfiche are acceptable alternatives. Regardless of the type of storage selected, the records must be filed in a fashion that allows accessibility and timely retrieval. The laboratory must determine how records are filed and must establish a written policy in the SOPM. For example, records may be filed by accession number, patient name, collection date, or referring physician. Records are not required to be stored on site.

Test reports must be retained by the laboratory for 10 years. An exact duplicate of the original report is not required, but all the clinical, demographic, and diagnostic information that was submitted on the original report must be retained. This information includes the dates of collection, signout, and report.

All gynecologic glass slides interpreted as being within normal limits must be stored for a minimum of 5 years. All gynecologic glass slides interpreted as not being within normal limits or as abnormal must be stored for a minimum of 10 years. Glass slides must be accessible and able to be retrieved in a timely fashion. Glass slides are not required to be stored on site.

ANNUAL STATISTICS

Annual statistics on laboratory volume and general diagnostic categories provide the laboratory with feedback on the case mix of the population and the work flow, and average values against which to compare an individual's performance. CLIA 88 regulations require that certain statistics be maintained; however, the laboratory can collect additional data at its discretion to monitor specific trends in the laboratory.

The laboratory must collect the following on an annual basis: the total number of cytology cases examined, the number of specimens processed by specimen type, the volume of patient cases reported by diagnosis, the number reported as unsatisfactory, the number in which the cytology and available histology were discrepant, the number of gynecologic cases in which any rescreening of a normal or negative specimen resulted in reclassification as malignant or premalignant, and the number of gynecologic cases for which histology results were unavailable to compare with malignant or premalignant cytology.

If an excessive number of unsatisfactory cases are reported, this information can be used to determine whether the trend involves one or more physicians. If a consistent problem is identified, the laboratory can use the statistical data to compare the physician's unsatisfactory rate to the overall client population. Feedback comparing the specific data from the providers in question with that of the overall group is more meaningful to those who receive the information.

SUMMARY

In summary, a good quality assurance program can help ensure the provision of excellent services to patients and their health care providers. The laboratory must design a system that monitors all aspects of laboratory operations, including laboratory personnel. With the capture and analysis of quality control data, statistics, and performance indicators, any deviation from acceptable laboratory standards can be detected and corrected, resulting in improved quality of care.

ADDITIONAL READING

1. Health Care Financing Administration interpretive guidelines. National Technical Information Services. Appendix C, PB92146174. 1-800-553-6847 or 703-487-4650.
2. Keebler C, Somrak T. The manual of cytotechology. Chicago: American Society of Clinical Pathologists Press, 1993.
3. Triol J. ASCT cytopathology quality assurance guide, vol I. 1992.

Gynecologic Cytopathology. Edited by
Thomas A. Bonfiglio and Yener S. Erozan.
Lippincott–Raven Publishers, Philadelphia, © 1997.

APPENDIX

Sample Forms for Use in a Cytopathology Laboratory Quality Assurance Program

FORM 1

Daily Stain Evaluation Log

Date	Reviewed by	LGT	DK	MS	W	B	Other	COA	COA Documented by	

LGT, light stain; *DK,* dark or overstained; *MS,* meets standards as defined in standard operating procedure manual; *W,* water contamination; *B,* brown artifact; *COA,* course of action.

FORM 2

Sample Quality Control: Papanicolaou Staining Set-up

Date								
Filter nongyn stain								
Change nongyn stain								
Change gyn staining set-up								
Change Diff-Quik solution								
Change xylene								
Daily change 95%, 99%, base								
Hydrometer check - ETOH								

Any activity associated with the routine staining of gynecologic and nongynecologic specimens should be documented (ie, changing or filtering stains). *Nongyn,* nongynecologic; *gyn,* gynecologic; *ETOH,* ethyl alcohol.

FORM 3

Workload Recording Records

XYZ Cytology Laboratory
444 East Main St.
Java, New York 11111

Cytotechnologist   License/Registration #

Date								
# Gyn slides								
# Gyn cases								
# Gyn 1 slide cases								
# Gyn 2 slide cases								
# Nongyn slides								
# Nongyn cases								
# 10% Q.C. slides reviewed								
# Cases RTP (gyn)								
# Cases S/O pos. (gyn)								
# Procedures-FNAs								
# Stats/rushes								
Hrs. cont. education								
Sick/vac./holiday								
Hours worked								
Hours screened								

Capture of related activities will provide additional information in assessing each individual's work output and overall performance in the laboratory. The comparison of number of cases referred to a pathologist (RTP) versus those signed out (S/O) positive will indicate whether the cytotechnologist is able to adequately differentiate between negative and positive cases. The individual's positive rate can be compared with the overall laboratory's positive rate to determine whether the cytotechnologist is detecting the expected number of abnormal cases when compared with daily screening volumes.

A disclaimer on the workload recording form indicating whether the ctyotechnologist has or has not interpreted cytologic samples at other sites is recommended. If the cytotechnologist has screened at another site, the workload volume and location should be noted on the form for the laboratory director to assess.

The workload data can be collated with the use of any commercially available software program.

FORM 4

False-Negative Documentation

False-Negative Cases Found on 10% or 5-Year Retrospective Rescreening Log

Cytotechnologist _____

Accession # of Negative QC Case Missed	Revised Interpretation	FN Case Reviewed by		Date of Final Signout
		QC CT	MD	

QC, quality control; CT, cytotechnologist; MD, medical doctor.

FORM 5

Five-Year Retrospective Rescreening Search Log

Cytotechnologist _____

Date of Review	Accession # of Current HGSIL, AGUS, Cancer	Previous Negative	
		Not Found	Found (Refer to RRS Log)

HGSIL, high-grade squamous intraepithelial lesion; *AGUS*, atypical glandular cells of undetermined significance; *RRS*, retrospective rescreening.

FORM 6

Five-Year Retrospective Rescreen (RRS) of Previous Negative Cytology Log

Cytotechnologist _____

Accession # Current HGSIL, AGUS, Cancer	Accession #(s) Previous Negative Cytology	CT/MD ID on Previous Negative	Confirmed Negative Dx on Rescreen	Final DX if not Negative	Date and MD on Final S/O

HGSIL, high-grade squamous intraepithelial lesion; *AGUS*, atypical glandular cells of undetermined significance; *CT*, cytotechnologist; *MD*, medical doctor; *ID*, identification; *Dx*, diagnosis; *S/O*, signout.

FORM 7

Cytology–Histology Correlation

Cytology Accession #	Cytology Diagnosis	CT/MD	Surgical #, Diagnosis	Correlation Yes, No, NA	Reason for Discrepancy	Date of Review and ID of Reviewer

Cytology–histology correlation is a quality control method used to detect false-negative and false-positive cases. It can be used to determine whether a cytologic false-negative case is the result of sampling, screening, or interpretation error. A sampling error indicates that a lesion is present on the cervix as verified by the surgical specimen but the corresponding cells were not represented on the Papanicolaou smear. A screening error indicates the abnormality is present on the Papanicolaou smear but was not detected by the cytotechnologist. An interpretation error on a false-negative case indicates the abnormal cells were detected on the Papanicolaou smear but were interpreted as "within normal limits" by the cytotechnologist (CT) or cytopathologist (MD).

Cytology–histology correlation can be used as a continuing education tool. Review of discrepancies related to false-positive cytology or grading of a lesion that resulted in incorrectly interpreting the cytologic changes can be used to develop cytomorphologic criteria that can be applied more consistently. It also can be used to identify and recognize cytologic patterns that result in more frequent false-negative or false-positive cases (ie, excessive inflammatory exudate obscuring small, isolated, high-grade squamous intraepithelial lesion cells, tissue fragments resembling reactive endocervical cells, and tubal metaplasia).

Miscellaneous Forms for Quality Control

FORM 8

Follow-up Correlation Log

Date	Patient Name	Accession #	Diagnosis	Follow-up/Comments

This log can be used by cytotechnologists to track interesting cases. It should not be used for cytology–histology correlation.

FORM 9

Case Review Log

Accession #	Reason for Review	Comments	Date Reviewed

This log documents the review of discrepant or interesting cases. It can be used to verify review of false-negative cases and discrepant cytology–histology correlations, and for continuing education purposes.

FORM 10

Telephone Call Log

Date	Accession #	Patient Name	Location, Name of Person Taking Call	Reason for Call

Documentation of telephone calls can be beneficial, especially if it concerns problem resolution or relaying a diagnosis that initiates significant or immediate clinical follow-up. It is important to note the name of the individual taking the call in case the office staff claims they were never alerted to the results or problem.

SUBJECT INDEX

Page numbers followed by *f* indicate figures; page numbers followed by *t* indicate tabular material.

A

Actinomyces, 39f, 39–40
   invasive, 39, 39f
   in IUD user, 39, 39f
Adenocarcinoma
   Arias-Stella reaction *vs.,* 49
   endocervical. *See* Endocervical adenocarcinoma.
   endometrial. *See* Endometrial adenocarcinoma.
   HPV prevalence in, 58, 59f
   in situ
      HPV cytopathic effect in, 65
      squamous carcinoma in situ *vs.,* 96–97
Adenoid basal cell carcinoma, 147–148, 148f
Adenoid cystic carcinoma, 147–148, 148f
Adenosis, vaginal, in diethylstilbestrol exposure in utero, 149–150, 150f
Adenosquamous cervical carcinoma, thin-layer cytology specimen in, 188f, 189
Adenosquamous endometrial adenocarcinoma, 136
Adenovirus, 41
AGCUS. *See* Atypical glandular cells of undetermined significance (AGCUS).
Air-drying artifact(s), 12, 12f–13f
   thin-layer cytology and, 181f, 181–182
Alternaria, as smear contaminant, 29–31, 30f
Anisonucleosis, in tubal (ciliated cell) metaplasia *vs.,* 123, 123f
Antioncogene(s), HPV and, 61–62
Arias-Stella reaction, 48f–49f, 48–49

Artifact(s)
   air-drying, 12, 12f–13f
      thin-layer cytology and, 181f, 181–182
   blue blobs, 29, 30f
   brown (corn flaking), 14, 14f
   brush, 122
ASCUS. *See* Atypical squamous cells of undetermined significance (ASCUS).
Atrophic cell(s)
   endometrial adenocarcinoma *vs.,* 141
   high-grade intraepithelial lesions *vs.,* 26f
   in postmenopausal smear, 26, 26f
      severe intraepithelial lesions *vs.,* 93–94, 94f
   in postpartum smear, 26, 26f
   in thin-layer cytology specimen, 188f, 189
Atrophic vaginitis, "blue blobs" in, 29, 30f
Atypical cells of immature squamous metaplastic type, 77f–78f, 77–78
   high-grade squamous intraepithelial neoplasia *vs.,* 95, 96f
   histologic counterpart of, 78, 78f
Atypical cells of squamous metaplastic type, 76, 76f
Atypical endocervical cells of undetermined significance, 117–120, 119t, 120f–121f
   endometrial cells and, 119
   endometriosis and, 119
   follow-up for, 128t, 128–129
   goblet colonic cells and, 119, 121f
   IUD use and, 119, 121f
   management of, 129t, 129–130
   normal cells *vs.,* 117, 120f
   reactive cells, 117, 119, 120f
   squamous neoplasia *vs.,* 126–128, 127f–128f
Atypical glandular cells of undetermined significance (AGCUS), 107

Atypical squamous cells of undetermined significance (ASCUS), 73–81
   atypical repair in, 78t, 78–79, 79f
   benign reactive changes *vs.,* 74
   binucleation in, 76, 76f
   biologic potential of, 73, 74f
   diagnostic criteria for, 74f–76f, 74–76
   differential diagnostic features of, 74t
   follow-up studies in, 79–80
   management of, 80–81
      in atypical repair, 80
      immature squamous metaplasia and, 80
      mature squamous cells and, 80
      in postmenopausal patient, 80
   nuclear enlargement in, 74f–76f, 76
   other classifications compared to, 67t
   squamous intraepithelial lesion and decreasing maturity levels and, 80
      rate of association of, 79–80
   squamous intraepithelial lesions *vs.,* 93, 94t
   thin-layer cytology specimens in, 184, 184f
AUTOcyte (Roche), 195, 195f
Automated cytology screening, 171–197
   "automated triage" method in, 172
   complications in development of, 171–172
   current status of, 172
   devices for, 193–195
   Food and Drug Administration and, 195–196
   monolayer preparations for, 173–174
   NeoPath AutoPap 300 and 300 QC for, 193f–194f, 193–194, 194t
   Neuromedical Systems: PAPNET for, 194–195, 195f
   Roche AUTOcyte for, 195, 195f
   semiautomated approach *vs.,* 172–173
   specimen type for, 173, 173f

211